AF572384

Contemporary Pharmacotherapy of Overactive Bladder

Lindsey Cox • Eric S. Rovner
Editors

Contemporary Pharmacotherapy of Overactive Bladder

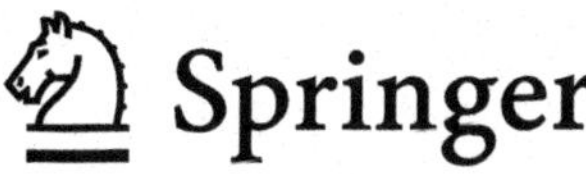

Editors
Lindsey Cox
Department of Urology
Medical University of South Carolina
Charleston, SC
USA

Eric S. Rovner
Department of Urology
Medical University of South Carolina
Charleston, SC
USA

ISBN 978-3-319-97264-0 ISBN 978-3-319-97265-7 (eBook)
https://doi.org/10.1007/978-3-319-97265-7

Library of Congress Control Number: 2018957309

This Springer imprint is published by the registered company Springer Nature Switzerland AG
The registered company address is: Gewerbestrasse 11, 6330 Cham, Switzerland

Foreword

The significant prevalence and adverse impact on the quality of life of overactive bladder (OAB) is fairly well-defined. Clinicians—not just urologists or urogynecologists—of diverse backgrounds are often challenged by these patients. For decades, treatment relied on behavioral techniques and antimuscarinc monotherapy. However, there have been promising advancements in treatment, with expanding pharmacotherapeutic options along with onobotulinumtoxinA and neuromodulation. These advancements are promising, yet it is challenging to remain well-versed and to correlate these developments with the care of our patients. In addition, our patients are becoming more proactive and are demanding optimal therapies.

Clinical guidelines are available for reference; however, a contemporary background on the pathophysiology, diagnosis, and pharmacology is lacking. For anyone involved in the care of these patients, *Contemporary Pharmacology for Overactive Bladder* will be an extremely valuable resource. Lindsey Cox and Eric S. Rovner, widely recognized authorities in this field, have put together a very thoughtful, concise, and comprehensive overview. This text, with contributions from many of the internationally recognized thought leaders in the diagnosis and management of OAB, starts with a timely review of the pathophysiology and diagnosis of OAB. This is followed by unique insights into patient expectations, outcome measures, as well as OAB nuances in select patient populations. It has been quite some time since I have read such an extensive review of pharmacotherapy for OAB. These chapters are highly valuable for anyone involved in OAB treatment. Great effort is taken to describe each drug class and associated pathophysiology. Combination therapy as well as future therapies are presented in a manner that illustrates the potential roles in the treatment of these often complex patients. This book will undoubtedly advance the knowledge of all medical professionals caring for OAB.

The editors of this book are to be congratulated for providing us with a highly relevant text that will serve as a frequently read reference in the pharmacotherapy of OAB. This text is without question "one for the bookcase."

New Orleans, LA, USA — J. Christian Winters
June 3, 2018

Preface

For decades, oral pharmacotherapy for urinary urgency, frequency and urgency urinary incontinence (overactive bladder, or OAB) consisted primarily of antimuscarinic compounds such as oxybutynin. However, since the mid 1990s, the understanding of the basic science, physiology, and pharmacology of OAB has greatly evolved. Improved drug delivery systems, as well as better characterized receptors, neurotransmitters, and neural pathways have led to a vast array of novel options for treatment of this highly prevalent and bothersome condition. Indeed, the number of pharmacological agents has rapidly expanded. Most notably, this includes a number of unique antimuscarinic agents as well as an entirely new class of therapeutic agents for OAB termed β3-agonists. Furthermore, several other oral and intravesical compounds are in development with additional novel mechanisms of delivery and action.

Not surprisingly, given these rapid changes, several national and international organizations have recently published guidelines and/or clinical pathways for the management of OAB, including the American Urological Association; the Society of Urodynamics, Female Pelvic Medicine & Urogenital Reconstruction; the European Association of Urology; and the National Institute for Health and Care Excellence (UK). Furthermore, the 6th International Consultation on Incontinence has recently updated the evidence basis for many of the currently available treatments. Nevertheless, a thorough review of the contemporary options and specific application of these agents for the clinician is lacking.

Contemporary Pharmacotherapy for Overactive Bladder is a comprehensive, state-of-the art review of the field of drug therapy for OAB. All of the chapters are written by acknowledged experts in OAB and include the most up-to-date scientific and clinical information. The goal of this work is to serve as a valuable resource for clinicians, surgeons, and researchers with an interest in OAB.

Charleston, SC, USA Lindsey Cox
Charleston, SC, USA Eric S. Rovner

Acknowledgements

The Editors would like to make several important acknowledgements. Firstly, we are grateful to each of the chapter authors for their outstanding contributions. It is their individual and collective expertise, and clear, concise writing that truly comprise the essence of this work. We would also like to thank Springer for giving us the platform and opportunity to produce this book, but especially Katherine Kreilkamp who kept us on task, on time and shepherded this project to completion. Finally, and most importantly, the Editors would like to express our everlasting gratitude to our respective spouses and families who graciously and lovingly provided the time and opportunity as well as the inspiration allowing us to pursue and complete this project.

Contents

Contributors

Karl-Erik Andersson Institute for Regenerative Medicine, Wake Forest University School of Medicine, Winston Salem, NC, USA

Institute of Laboratory Medicine, Lund University, Lund, Sweden

Márcio Augusto Averbeck, MD, MSc, PhD Neuro-Urology Coordinator, Videourodynamics Unit, Department of Urology, Moinhos de Vento Hospital, Porto Alegre, Brazil

Ari M. Bergman, MD Department of Urology, Donald and Barbara Zucker School of Medicine at Hofstra/Northwell, Hempstead, NY, USA

Smith Institute for Urology, Greenlawn, NY, USA

Rebecca Budish, MS LSU Health – Shreveport, Louisiana State University, Shreveport, LA, USA

Christopher R. Chapple, MD, FRCS (Urol), FEBU Department of Urology, Royal Hallamshire Hospital, Sheffield Teaching Hospitals NHS Foundation Trust, Sheffield, UK

Lindsey Cox, MD Department of Urology, Medical University of South Carolina, Charleston, SC, USA

Roger R. Dmochowski, MD, MMHC Urologic Surgery, Department of Urology, Vanderbilt University, Nashville, TN, USA

David A. Ginsberg, MD Department of Urology, University of Southern California, Los Angeles, CA, USA

Howard B. Goldman, MD Glickman Urologic and Kidney Institute, Cleveland Clinic, Cleveland, OH, USA

Alex Gomelsky, MD Department of Urology, LSU Health – Shreveport, Louisiana State University, Shreveport, LA, USA

Cristiano Mendes Gomes, MD Division of Urology, Hospital of the University of Sao Paulo School of Medicine, Sao Paulo, Brazil

Sophia Delpe Goodridge, MD Female Reconstructive Medicine and Reconstructive Surgery, Department of Urology, Vanderbilt University, Nashville, TN, USA

Alyssa Greiman, MD Department of Urology, Medical University of South Carolina, Charleston, SC, USA

Marcelo Hisano, MD Division of Urology, Hospital of the University of Sao Paulo School of Medicine, Sao Paulo, Brazil

Emily F. Kelly, MS, MD Department of Urology, LSU Health – Shreveport, Louisiana State University, Shreveport, LA, USA

Gary E. Lemack, MD Department of Urology, UT Southwestern Medical Center, Dallas, TX, USA

Alison C. Levy, MD Department of Urology, Lahey Hospital & Medical Center, Burlington, MA, USA

Svjetlana Lozo, MD, MPH Division of Urogynecology, Department of Obstetrics & Gynecology, University Health System, University of Chicago Pritzker School of Medicine, Skokie, IL, USA

Lara S. MacLachlan, MD Department of Urology, Lahey Hospital & Medical Center, Burlington, MA, USA

Rena D. Malik, MD Department of Urology, UT Southwestern Medical Center, Dallas, TX, USA

Victor Nitti, MD NYU Female Pelvic Medicine and Reconstructive Surgery Program, Departments of Urology and Obstetrics and Gynecology, NYU Langone, New York University, New York, NY, USA

Ricardo Palmerola, MD, MS NYU Female Pelvic Medicine and Reconstructive Surgery Program, Department of Urology, NYU Langone, New York University, New York, NY, USA

Joon Jae Park, MBBS, MRCS, FRCS(Urol)(Glasgow) Department of Urology, Changi General Hospital, Singapore, Singapore

Jennifer Rolef, MD Department of Urology, Medical University of South Carolina, Charleston, SC, USA

Eric S. Rovner, MD Department of Urology, Medical University of South Carolina, Charleston, SC, USA

Peter K. Sand, MD Department of Obstetrics & Gynecology, North Shore University Health System, University of Chicago Pritzker School of Medicine, Winnetka, IL, USA

Melissa T. Sanford, MD Department of Urology, University of Southern California, Los Angeles, CA, USA

Ariana L. Smith, MD Division of Urology, Penn Medicine University of Pennsylvania Health System, Philadelphia, PA, USA

Andrew A. Stec, MD Department of Urology, Medical University of South Carolina, Charleston, SC, USA

Adrian Wagg, FRCP (Lond), FRCP (Edin), FHEA Department of Medicine, University of Alberta, Edmonton, AB, Canada

Alan J. Wein, MD, PhD (Hon) Division of Urology, Penn Medicine University of Pennsylvania Health System, Philadelphia, PA, USA

Jeffrey P. Weiss, MD Department of Urology, SUNY Downstate Medical Center, Brooklyn, NY, USA

Chapter 1
Pathophysiology of Overactive Bladder

Márcio Augusto Averbeck and Howard B. Goldman

Introduction

Overactive bladder (OAB) syndrome is defined by the International Continence Society as urinary urgency, usually accompanied by frequency and nocturia, with or without urgency urinary incontinence (UUI), in the absence of urinary tract infection or other obvious pathologies [1]. OAB affects individuals of both genders and of all ages, imposing a detrimental impact on quality of life [2]. Despite the negative burden and the relevance of OAB in clinical practice, its underlying pathophysiology is not yet fully understood, which complicates the development of targeted therapeutic interventions.

OAB symptoms are commonly attributed to involuntary bladder muscle contractions known as detrusor overactivity (DO). However, DO is only observed in approximately 58% of women with reported UUI [3]. Thus, the link between OAB symptoms and DO represents a simplistic way to understand the pathophysiological mechanisms, which are usually multifactorial.

Various theories have been proposed to elucidate the pathophysiology of OAB. However, since the origin of OAB is often multifactorial, there is not a unique and widely accepted pathophysiological mechanism to explain this syndrome.

M. A. Averbeck (✉)
Neuro-Urology Coordinator, Videourodynamics Unit, Department of Urology, Moinhos de Vento Hospital, Porto Alegre, Brazil

H. B. Goldman
Glickman Urologic and Kidney Institute, Cleveland Clinic, Cleveland, OH, USA

L. Cox, E. S. Rovner (eds.), *Contemporary Pharmacotherapy of Overactive Bladder*, https://doi.org/10.1007/978-3-319-97265-7_1

Pathophysiological Mechanisms Related to OAB Symptoms

Table 1.1 lists a number of distinct theories to explain the pathophysiology of OAB [4–10].

Dysfunction of Afferent Signaling in OAB

OAB may be a result of increased, abnormal afferent sensory activity, resulting in increased efferent signaling. Consequently, voluntary control of micturition is compromised [4]. Small myelinated (Aδ) and unmyelinated (C-fiber) axons (responsive to chemical and mechanical stimuli) represent the primary afferent innervation of the urinary bladder [11]. Pathological conditions may alter the chemical and electrical properties of bladder afferent pathways, leading to urgency, increased voiding frequency, nocturia, UUI, and pain.

The urothelium plays a role as an active source of neurotransmitters and modulators such as acetylcholine (ACh), adenosine 5′-triphosphate (ATP), nitric oxide, prostaglandins, and neuropeptides. They exert both excitatory and inhibitory effects toward modulating urinary tract motility [12]. Stenqvist et al. demonstrated that ATP induces a release of urothelial ACh that contributes to the purinergic contractile response in the rat urinary bladder [13]. This observation may also help in the understanding of OAB pathophysiology.

In the setting of bladder outlet obstruction, plasticity of bladder afferent fibers likely plays a critical role in the subsequent manifestation of OAB symptoms [11]. Evidence obtained from ice water cystometry, which elicits a C-fiber-dependent spinal micturition reflex, suggests considerable C-fiber upregulation in symptomatic subjects with bladder outlet obstruction. Chai et al. [14] prospectively studied 111 consecutive patients who underwent videourodynamics. Symptoms of urgency, UUI, nocturia and daytime frequency, as well as the presence of neurological disease were obtained from history and physical examination. When patients with neurological disease were excluded, a positive ice water test was found in 71% of subjects with bladder outlet obstruction (12 of 17), which was significantly higher ($p < 0.0005$, Yates corrected chi-square test) than the 7% positive ice water test rate

Table 1.1 Hypothesized etiologies of overactive bladder

Hypothesized etiologies
Afferent signaling dysfunction
Altered brain responses
Myogenic dysfunction
Neurogenic-myogenic dysfunction
Urothelial dysfunction
Classic neurogenic – loss of inhibition
Microbiome alterations
Psychologic or environmental etiologies

in nonobstructed subjects (3 of 44) [14]. These results support the hypothesis of an enhanced spinal micturition reflex possibly due to plasticity of bladder afferents after bladder outlet obstruction.

Altered Brain Responses

It has been demonstrated that OAB patients may demonstrate abnormal brain responses in areas processing urge and social propriety [5, 6]. Diminished responses in areas responsible for voluntary voiding have also been previously described. According to functional magnetic resonance imaging (f-MRI) studies, poor bladder control is specifically associated with inadequate activation of the orbitofrontal cortex. More recently, Gill et al. [15] performed f-MRI to identify changes in brain activity during sacral neuromodulation (SNM) in women with OAB who were responsive to therapy. Sensory stimulation activated the insula but deactivated the medial and superior parietal lobes. Suprasensory stimulation activated multiple structures and the expected S3 somatosensory region. f-MRI confirmed that SNM influences brain activity in women with OAB who responded to therapy [15].

Myogenic Theory

The myogenic theory proposed that detrusor smooth muscle itself becomes more spontaneously active and generates abnormal excitatory rhythms, which reflects fundamental changes to detrusor muscle excitation-contraction coupling [16].

Localized movements of the urinary bladder, known as "micromotions," were described initially in animal models [17]. In the normal bladder, they are low-amplitude contractions with minimal effect on intravesical pressure and are undetected by standard urodynamic techniques. The origin of micromotions and their association with urinary tract sensations remain unanswered. However, some postulate that specific areas of the bladder which may be damaged generate aberrant activity, ultimately causing abnormal sensations or contractions [16]. Although different patterns of micromotions have already been previously described, their initiation and propagation are still not fully understood. Sadananda et al. developed a decerebrate arterially perfused rat model and demonstrated that bladder micromotions are more evident when the neuraxis becomes nonfunctional. Thus, neural modulation is possible [18].

Fry et al. proposed that bladder smooth muscle should not be regarded solely as a collection of independent cellular contractile units that are each activated by separate neural inputs, but also as a syncytium of cells; individual detrusor cells possess membrane properties that may lead to spontaneous activity fluctuations, which can affect adjacent cells and, thus, produce multicellular aberrant responses [19].

A better understanding of bladder wall micromotions in humans and its relationship to OAB relies on improvements of pressure and motion measurement techniques to allow routine recording of such subclinical events during urodynamics. Future research may also include changes to ionic channel activity in cells or tissue from OAB patients [16].

Neurogenic-Myogenic Theory

Partial denervation alters smooth muscle properties, which may result in increased excitability, coordinated myogenic contractions, and increased bladder pressure [7].

Conversely, "leakage" of ACh from parasympathetic nerves during bladder filling may be related to activation of detrusor bundles and afferent signaling [8, 9]. Kanai et al. examined the origin of spontaneous activity in neonatal and adult rat bladders and hypothesized that ACh that is released from the urothelium during bladder filling could enhance spontaneous activity [20].

Drake et al. carried out an observational study to establish whether localized activity arose in the normal human bladder, and whether it would correspond to changes in reported sensation [9]. Fourteen women presenting with increased bladder sensation during filling-phase cystometry were compared with six asymptomatic women volunteers. Localized bladder activity was assessed by the micromotion detection (MMD) method, using eight electrodes mounted on a Silastic balloon; local displacements of the electrodes were recorded as changes in electrical resistance, which were used to compute changes in the distance between each pair of electrodes. Women with increased sensation on filling cystometry had a significantly higher prevalence of localized activity than did the control group during MMD recording. The localized activity was more sustained and at a higher frequency than in asymptomatic women. All nine women reporting urinary urgency during MMD recording had localized contractile activity. The authors concluded that localized distortion of the bladder wall stimulates afferent activity and that the human detrusor may be functionally modular [9].

Urothelial Theory

The urothelium is no longer regarded as a silent barrier protecting the body from the toxic effects of urine, but instead produces a number of compounds that are related to cell signaling events, acting in an autocrine and paracrine manner [10, 21, 22].

Distension of the bladder wall stretches the urothelium, releasing adenosine 5′-triphosphate (ATP) and other substances such as ACh and nitric oxide [23–25]. ATP is linked to the activation of afferent signaling, whereas the role of ACh and nitric oxide is not fully understood [26]. Additionally, several subgroups of interstitial cells are located within the bladder wall and make structural interactions with nerves and smooth muscle, indicating integration with intercellular communication and key physiological functions [27, 28].

The main implication of the urothelial autocrine and paracrine function is related to lower urinary tract dysfunction. Sun et al. studied patients with painful bladder syndrome (PBS), demonstrating the link between urothelial ATP and increased sensitivity of the afferent nerve terminals [29]. Another example is the Ach effect on afferent muscarinic receptors, which is an important target for the treatment of OAB [30].

Classic Neurogenic: Lack of Central Inhibition

Small-vessel disease of the brain affecting the deep white matter has been classically associated with neurological syndromes, such as vascular dementia and vascular parkinsonism [31]. Nevertheless, there is increasing evidence to suggest that deep white matter disease (WMD), mostly in the prefrontal area of the brain, could also result in UUI and other OAB symptoms. Sakakibara et al. investigated 63 patients (mean age 73 years) with varying degrees of cerebral WMD. All patients underwent MRI, which allowed WMD grading on a scale of 0–4. The prevalence of nocturia in cases of grade 1 WMD was 60%; grade 2 was 58%; grade 3 was 93%; and grade 4 was 91%, respectively. The overall prevalence of nocturia was 75%, which was an earlier OAB feature than UUI (40%). The authors highlighted the fact that OAB was not always accompanied by a gait disorder or dementia, suggesting that OAB symptoms might be the first clinical manifestation of the observed WMD [32].

Once the pattern of LUT dysfunction following neurological disease is determined by the site and nature of the lesion, the occurrence of DO following cerebrovascular accident (CVA), multiple sclerosis, and suprasacral spinal cord injuries provides further evidence to support the classic neurogenic theory related to loss of inhibition due to damage to inhibitory centers or the nerves that transmit the inhibitory messages [33].

Microbiome Theory

Recent evidence suggests that the urinary tract harbors a variety of bacterial species, known collectively as the urinary microbiome, even when clinical cultures are negative [34]. Changes in the microbiome of the bladder may induce changes in sensitivity and/or responsiveness of urothelium and smooth muscle in the bladder.

Karstens et al. [34] prospectively studied the characteristics of the urinary microbiome in women with and without UUI. In order to characterize the resident microbial community, the bacterial 16S rRNA genes were amplified by polymerase chain reaction (PCR). The authors found that the relative abundance of 14 bacteria significantly differed between control and UUI samples. Additionally, an increase in UUI symptom severity was associated with a decrease in microbial diversity in women with UUI. According to this study, the urinary microbiome may play an important role in the pathophysiology of UUI, and the loss of microbial diversity may be associated with clinical severity of symptoms.

Psychological and Environmental Factors

OAB symptoms have long been associated with comorbid conditions such as anxiety and depression [35]. Melotti et al. [36] performed a systematic review and meta-analysis to assess the relationship between symptoms of depression, anxiety, and OAB using validated instruments. Eleven articles, containing 11,784 participants with depression and 10,436 with anxiety, were included in this review. Depression and anxiety were positively correlated with OAB. Men with OAB were considerably more likely than women to have anxiety (odds ratio [37], 1.56; 95% confidence interval [CI], 1.40–1.73), but there was no sex-related difference in depression (OR, 0.96; 95% CI, 0.77–1.21).

Dietary factors have long being associated with the development or worsening of OAB symptoms. Robinson et al. performed a literature review to investigate the association between OAB and specific dietary factors, such as consumption of caffeine, alcohol, and carbonated drinks [38]. The authors concluded that there is some evidence within the literature to support a role of these factors in the pathogenesis of OAB and UUI. Caffeine is reported to activate nonselective cation channels in rat primary sensory neurons indicated to be TRPV1 [39]. There have been many reported studies investigating the effect of caffeine on OAB symptoms although, overall, the results are conflicting [38, 40–42]. Evidence from the Leicester Medical Research Council (MRC) study has shown an association between consumption of carbonated soft drinks with OAB symptoms (OR, 1.62; 95%CI, 1.18–2.22) [43]. Concerning alcohol consumption, the Boston Area Community Health Survey of 3201 women suggested a link with UUI (OR, 3.51; 95% CI, 1.11–11.1) [37]. Conversely, there was no association found in the Norwegian EPINCONT study [40].

While some of the findings tend to be contradictory, others clearly show an association between the ingestion of caffeine, carbonated drinks, and alcohol with symptom severity. However, in view of the controversial evidence, more research is needed to determine the precise role of these factors in the pathogenesis and management of OAB [38].

How Does Neuromodulation Help Us to Understand the Origin of OAB?

The goal of SNM is to modulate abnormal sensations and involuntary reflexes of the lower urinary tract and restore voluntary control. The therapeutic benefits of SNM in patients with refractory OAB may arise from the effects of electrical stimulation on afferent and efferent nerve fibers connecting the pelvic viscera and the spinal interneurons to the central nerve system (CNS). SNM influences sacral afferents and modulates spinal cord reflexes and brain centers involved in lower urinary tract function [44]. From this perspective, it may be that patients whose neural system is not intact may not be ideal candidates for this therapy [45].

The neurostimulator provides an electrical charge to an area near the sacral nerve, resulting in altered neural activity. This stimulation depolarizes the nerve, causing an action potential. The signal propagates impulses along the axon as if the neuron had naturally fired an action potential. SNM electrically stimulates somatic afferent nerves in a sacral spinal root and sends signals to the CNS that may restore normal bladder function. Activation of somatic afferent nerves inhibits bladder sensory pathways and reflex bladder hyperactivity [4]. Unlike other therapies that target the bladder, bladder regulation occurs without physically influencing the bladder or sphincter muscles [46, 47]. The carry-over effect could be caused by negative modulation of excitatory synapses in the central micturition reflex pathway [46]. The fact that nerve stimulation modulates bladder function supports many of the hypotheses noted above that involve aberrant neural function as an etiology of OAB.

Evidence in the cat model suggests the inhibition of bladder activity occurs primarily in the CNS by inhibition of the ascending or descending pathways of the spinobulbospinal micturition reflex [48]. Still, according to experimental models, SNM delivers stimulation that is parameter dependent [49–51]. The inhibitory effects on bladder contraction may be mediated by both afferent and efferent mechanisms. Lower intensities of stimulation may activate large, fast-conducting fibers and actions through the afferent limb of the micturition reflex arc in SNM. Higher intensities may additionally act through the efferent limb [49].

Snellings et al. [50] studied the effects of acute electrical stimulation frequency and amplitude at the dorsal nerve of the penis (DNP), pudendal nerve (PN), and S1 sacral nerve (S1) on isovolumetric reflex bladder contractions and maximum cystometric capacity in anesthetized male cats. There was no significant difference in the maximum degree to which the respective optimum parameters inhibited bladder contractions or increased cystometric capacity by location. However, the range of amplitudes and frequencies that caused maximum inhibition was larger for DNP stimulation than for PN or S1 stimulation [50].

Peters et al. [51] studied three rate-setting sequences in OAB female patients undergoing SNM: 5.2, 14, and 25 Hz. Rate significantly affected the number of incontinence episodes and pad changes per day. Rate had a statistically significant effect on the number of incontinent episodes ($P < 0.001$) and number of pad changes ($P = 0.039$) with more incontinent episodes in the 5.2-Hz setting compared to the 14- and 25-Hz settings ($P < 0.04$) for both measurements. The number of adverse events was similar across the three rate settings with programming-related adverse events lowest in the 14-Hz group [51].

How Does Botulinum Toxin Help Us to Understand the Origin of OAB?

Botulinum toxin (BT) is potent neurotoxin produced from a gram-positive anaerobic bacterium [52]. Seven serotypes of BT have been identified, but only types A and B are used for medical purposes [53].

Intradetrusor BT injections for the treatment of neurogenic detrusor overactivity (NDO) were first described by Schurch et al., who reported the promising results in spinal cord-injured patients [54]. Since then a large number of clinical studies have been published, attesting to the efficacy and safety of BT injections in the bladder of patients with both neurogenic and idiopathic DO [55, 56]. BT injections into the bladder wall have been shown to be an effective alternative to antimuscarinics and more invasive surgery in those patients with multiple sclerosis and spinal cord injury with NDO and UUI. In August 2011, Botox® (onabotulinumtoxinA) received Food and Drug Administration (FDA) approval for this use [57].

Efferent System

Once depolarization of the presynaptic neuron occurs, the ACh vesicles fuse with the plasma membrane causing calcium influx and membrane depolarization, resulting in the release (exocytosis) of the ACh transmitter molecules into the synaptic cleft. The ACh then diffuses across the synaptic cleft and binds to and stimulates the postsynaptic ACh receptors. This phenomenon is essential for normal contraction of the detrusor, which is modulated by the autonomic parasympathetic nervous system [58].

BT disrupts the proteins that form the "soluble N-ethylmaleimide-sensitive factor attachment protein receptor" complex (SNARE) located at the presynaptic nerve terminal. This prevents the synaptic vesicles from attaching to the SNARE complex so that there is no membrane depolarization or exocytosis of the ACh from the presynaptic nerve terminal. Thus, BT inhibits detrusor overactivity by reducing the bioavailability of ACh in the neuromuscular junctions of the bladder [59].

Afferent System

The rationale for the success of intradetrusor BT injections in patients with OAB was initially thought to be solely related to blockage of presynaptic release of ACh from the parasympathetic efferent nerve. However, once refractory idiopathic OAB patients without detrusor overactivity on urodynamics were shown to also benefit from intradetrusor BT [60], it was postulated that the efficacy of intradetrusor BT might result not only from an inhibitory effect on detrusor muscle but also from inhibition of the afferent nerve input.

Khera et al. showed that BT inhibited the bladder sensory mechanisms in chronic spinal cord-injured rats [61]. Further studies evaluated the urothelial release of nerve growth factor (NGF) in rats [62]. Higher concentrations of NGF were demonstrated in those with DO compared to those without DO. However, following the administration of BT, NGF was found to significantly decrease [63].

Apostolidis et al. investigated potential effects of BT on human bladder afferent mechanisms by studying the sensory receptors P2X3 and TRPV1 in biopsies from patients with neurogenic or idiopathic DO [64]. Thirty-eight patients (22 with NDO, 16 with idiopathic DO) with refractory DO were treated with intradetrusor BT, and bladder biopsies were taken at 4 and 16 weeks. Specimens were studied immunohistochemically for P2X3 and TRPV1. P2X3-immunoreactive and TRPV1-immunoreactive (IR) fibers were decreased at 4 weeks after BT, and more significantly at 16 weeks (paired t test $P = 0.0004$ and $P = 0.0008$, respectively), when significant improvements were observed in clinical and urodynamic parameters. P2X3-IR fiber decrease was significantly correlated with reduction of urgency episodes at 4 and 16 weeks ($P = 0.0013$ at 4 weeks and $P = 0.02$ at 16 weeks), but not maximum cystometric capacity or detrusor pressures. TRPV1-IR fiber decrease showed a similar trend. The authors concluded that decreased levels of sensory receptors P2X3 and/or TRPV1 may contribute to the clinical effect of BoNT/A in detrusor overactivity.

While the exact mechanisms whereby BT affects the afferent system are not completely understood, there is increasing evidence both in animal and human studies that this occurs [57]. These actions of BT give us further insights into the overall pathophysiology of OAB.

Conclusions

OAB pathophysiological mechanisms are complex and multifactorial. A number of theories that explain the origin of OAB symptoms have been discussed above. In all likelihood there is not one single mechanism by which OAB occurs, but it is likely the ultimate symptomatic expression of one of any number of specific pathologies involving aberrant brain function, damaged nerves, alterations in the urothelium or detrusor muscle, or various bacteriologic, psychologic, or environmental factors. Ongoing research should provide further answers as to the underlying causes of OAB. Furthermore, examination of the mechanism of action of therapies that have helped treat the symptoms of OAB may allow for a better understanding and ultimately more opportunity for effective treatment of OAB.

References

1. Abrams P, Cardozo L, Fall M, Griffiths D, Rosier P, Ulmsten U, et al. The standardisation of terminology of lower urinary tract function: report from the Standardisation Sub-committee of the International Continence Society. Neurourol Urodyn. 2002;21(2):167–78.
2. Ouslander JG. Management of overactive bladder. N Engl J Med. 2004;350(8):786–99.
3. Hashim H, Abrams P. Is the bladder a reliable witness for predicting detrusor overactivity? J Urol. 2006;175(1):191–4. discussion 4–5

4. Leng WW, Morrisroe SN. Sacral nerve stimulation for the overactive bladder. Urol Clin North Am. 2006;33(4):491–501. ix
5. Griffiths D, Tadic SD. Bladder control, urgency, and urge incontinence: evidence from functional brain imaging. Neurourol Urodyn. 2008;27(6):466–74.
6. Griffiths D, Derbyshire S, Stenger A, Resnick N. Brain control of normal and overactive bladder. J Urol. 2005;174(5):1862–7.
7. Turner WH, Brading AF. Smooth muscle of the bladder in the normal and the diseased state: pathophysiology, diagnosis and treatment. Pharmacol Ther. 1997;75(2):77–110.
8. Andersson KE. Treatment-resistant detrusor overactivity – underlying pharmacology and potential mechanisms. Int J Clin Pract Suppl. 2006;60(151):8–16.
9. Drake MJ, Harvey IJ, Gillespie JI, Van Duyl WA. Localized contractions in the normal human bladder and in urinary urgency. BJU Int. 2005;95(7):1002–5.
10. Keay SK, Birder LA, Chai TC. Evidence for bladder urothelial pathophysiology in functional bladder disorders. Biomed Res Int. 2014;2014:865463.
11. de Groat WC, Yoshimura N. Afferent nerve regulation of bladder function in health and disease. Handb Exp Pharmacol. 2009;194:91–138.
12. Guan NN, Gustafsson LE, Svennersten K. Inhibitory effects of urothelium-related factors. Basic Clin Pharmacol Toxicol. 2017;121(4):220–4.
13. Stenqvist J, Winder M, Carlsson T, Aronsson P, Tobin G. Urothelial acetylcholine involvement in ATP-induced contractile responses of the rat urinary bladder. Eur J Pharmacol. 2017;809:253–60.
14. Chai TC, Gray ML, Steers WD. The incidence of a positive ice water test in bladder outlet obstructed patients: evidence for bladder neural plasticity. J Urol. 1998;160(1):34–8.
15. Gill BC, Pizarro-Berdichevsky J, Bhattacharyya PK, Brink TS, Marks BK, Quirouet A, et al. Real-time changes in brain activity during sacral neuromodulation for overactive bladder. J Urol. 2017;198(6):1379–85.
16. Chacko S, Cortes E, Drake MJ, Fry CH. Does altered myogenic activity contribute to OAB symptoms from detrusor overactivity? ICI-RS 2013. Neurourol Urodyn. 2014;33(5):577–80.
17. Drake MJ, Hedlund P, Harvey IJ, Pandita RK, Andersson KE, Gillespie JI. Partial outlet obstruction enhances modular autonomous activity in the isolated rat bladder. J Urol. 2003;170(1):276–9.
18. Sadananda P, Drake MJ, Paton JF, Pickering AE. An exploration of the control of micturition using a novel in situ arterially perfused rat preparation. Front Neurosci. 2011;5:62.
19. Fry CH, Sui GP, Severs NJ, Wu C. Spontaneous activity and electrical coupling in human detrusor smooth muscle: implications for detrusor overactivity? Urology. 2004;63(3 Suppl 1):3–10.
20. Kanai A, Roppolo J, Ikeda Y, Zabbarova I, Tai C, Birder L, et al. Origin of spontaneous activity in neonatal and adult rat bladders and its enhancement by stretch and muscarinic agonists. Am J Physiol Renal Physiol. 2007;292(3):F1065–72.
21. Birder L, Andersson KE. Urothelial signaling. Physiol Rev. 2013;93(2):653–80.
22. Fry CH, Vahabi B. The role of the mucosa in normal and abnormal bladder function. Basic Clin Pharmacol Toxicol. 2016;119 Suppl 3:57–62.
23. Olsen SM, Stover JD, Nagatomi J. Examining the role of mechanosensitive ion channels in pressure mechanotransduction in rat bladder urothelial cells. Ann Biomed Eng. 2011;39(2):688–97.
24. Yoshida M, Inadome A, Maeda Y, Satoji Y, Masunaga K, Sugiyama Y, et al. Non-neuronal cholinergic system in human bladder urothelium. Urology. 2006;67(2):425–30.
25. Andersson KE, Persson K. Nitric oxide synthase and nitric oxide-mediated effects in lower urinary tract smooth muscles. World J Urol. 1994;12(5):274–80.
26. Winder M, Tobin G, Zupančič D, Romih R. Signalling molecules in the urothelium. Biomed Res Int. 2014;2014:297295.
27. McCloskey KD. Bladder interstitial cells: an updated review of current knowledge. Acta Physiol (Oxf). 2013;207(1):7–15.

28. Andersson KE, McCloskey KD. Lamina propria: the functional center of the bladder? Neurourol Urodyn. 2014;33(1):9–16.
29. Sun Y, Keay S, De Deyne PG, Chai TC. Augmented stretch activated adenosine triphosphate release from bladder uroepithelial cells in patients with interstitial cystitis. J Urol. 2001;166(5):1951–6.
30. Yokoyama O, Yusup A, Miwa Y, Oyama N, Aoki Y, Akino H. Effects of tolterodine on an overactive bladder depend on suppression of C-fiber bladder afferent activity in rats. J Urol. 2005;174(5):2032–6.
31. Sakakibara R, Panicker J, Fowler CJ, Tateno F, Kishi M, Tsuyusaki Y, et al. Is overactive bladder a brain disease? The pathophysiological role of cerebral white matter in the elderly. Int J Urol. 2014;21(1):33–8.
32. Sakakibara R, Hattori T, Uchiyama T, Yamanishi T. Urinary function in elderly people with and without leukoaraiosis: relation to cognitive and gait function. J Neurol Neurosurg Psychiatry. 1999;67(5):658–60.
33. Groen J, Pannek J, Castro Diaz D, Del Popolo G, Gross T, Hamid R, et al. Summary of European Association of Urology (EAU) Guidelines on Neuro-Urology. Eur Urol. 2016;69(2):324–33.
34. Karstens L, Asquith M, Davin S, Stauffer P, Fair D, Gregory WT, et al. Does the urinary microbiome play a role in urgency urinary incontinence and its severity? Front Cell Infect Microbiol. 2016;6:78.
35. Sanford MT, Rodriguez LV. The role of environmental stress on lower urinary tract symptoms. Curr Opin Urol. 2017;27(3):268–73.
36. Melotti IGR, Juliato CRT, Coelho SCA, Lima M, Riccetto CLZ. Is there any difference between depression and anxiety in overactive bladder according to sex? A systematic review and meta-analysis. Int Neurourol J. 2017;21(3):204–11.
37. Maserejian NN, Kupelian V, Miyasato G, McVary KT, McKinlay JB. Are physical activity, smoking and alcohol consumption associated with lower urinary tract symptoms in men or women? Results from a population based observational study. J Urol. 2012;188(2):490–5.
38. Robinson D, Hanna-Mitchell A, Rantell A, Thiagamoorthy G, Cardozo L. Are we justified in suggesting change to caffeine, alcohol, and carbonated drink intake in lower urinary tract disease? Report from the ICI-RS 2015. Neurourol Urodyn. 2017;36(4):876–81.
39. Daher JP, Gover TD, Moreira TH, Lopes VG, Weinreich D. The identification of a caffeine-induced Ca2+ influx pathway in rat primary sensory neurons. Mol Cell Biochem. 2009;327(1–2):15–9.
40. Hannestad YS, Rortveit G, Daltveit AK, Hunskaar S. Are smoking and other lifestyle factors associated with female urinary incontinence? The Norwegian EPINCONT Study. BJOG. 2003;110(3):247–54.
41. Jura YH, Townsend MK, Curhan GC, Resnick NM, Grodstein F. Caffeine intake, and the risk of stress, urgency and mixed urinary incontinence. J Urol. 2011;185(5):1775–80.
42. Bryant CM, Dowell CJ, Fairbrother G. Caffeine reduction education to improve urinary symptoms. Br J Nurs. 2002;11(8):560–5.
43. Echeverri D, Montes FR, Cabrera M, Galán A, Prieto A. Caffeine's vascular mechanisms of action. Int J Vasc Med. 2010;2010:834060.
44. Bernstein AJ, Peters KM. Expanding indications for neuromodulation. Urol Clin North Am. 2005;32(1):59–63.
45. Kessler TM, Wöllner J, Kozomara M, Mordasini L, Mehnert U. Sacral neuromodulation for neurogenic bladder dysfunction. Urologe A. 2012;51(2):179–83.
46. van der Pal F, Heesakkers JP, Bemelmans BL. Current opinion on the working mechanisms of neuromodulation in the treatment of lower urinary tract dysfunction. Curr Opin Urol. 2006;16(4):261–7.
47. Chancellor MB, Chartier-Kastler EJ. Principles of sacral nerve stimulation (SNS) for the treatment of bladder and urethral sphincter dysfunctions. Neuromodulation. 2000;3(1):16–26.

48. Zhang F, Zhao S, Shen B, Wang J, Nelson DE, Roppolo JR, et al. Neural pathways involved in sacral neuromodulation of reflex bladder activity in cats. Am J Physiol Renal Physiol. 2013;304(6):F710–7.
49. Su X, Nickles A, Nelson DE. Optimization of neuromodulation for bladder control in a rat cystitis model. Neuromodulation. 2016;19(1):101–7.
50. Snellings AE, Grill WM. Effects of stimulation site and stimulation parameters on bladder inhibition by electrical nerve stimulation. BJU Int. 2012;110(1):136–43.
51. Peters KM, Shen L, McGuire M. Effect of sacral neuromodulation rate on overactive bladder symptoms: a randomized crossover feasibility study. Low Urin Tract Symptoms. 2013;5(3):129–33.
52. van Ermengem E. Classics in infectious diseases. A new anaerobic bacillus and its relation to botulism. E. van Ermengem. Originally published as "Ueber einen neuen anaëroben Bacillus und seine Beziehungen zum Botulismus" in Z Hyg Infekt. 1897;26:1–56. Rev Infect Dis. 1979;1(4):701–19.
53. Kuo YC, Kuo HC. Botulinum toxin injection for lower urinary tract dysfunction. Int J Urol. 2013;20(1):40–55.
54. Schurch B, Stöhrer M, Kramer G, Schmid DM, Gaul G, Hauri D. Botulinum-A toxin for treating detrusor hyperreflexia in spinal cord injured patients: a new alternative to anticholinergic drugs? Preliminary results. J Urol. 2000;164(3 Pt 1):692–7.
55. Soljanik I. Efficacy and safety of botulinum toxin A intradetrusor injections in adults with neurogenic detrusor overactivity/neurogenic overactive bladder: a systematic review. Drugs. 2013;73(10):1055–66.
56. Jo JK, Kim KN, Kim DW, Kim YT, Kim JY. The effect of onabotulinumtoxinA according to site of injection in patients with overactive bladder: a systematic review and meta-analysis. World J Urol. 2018;36(2):305–17. https://doi.org/10.1007/s00345-017-2121-6. Epub 2017 Nov 9.
57. Linsenmeyer TA. Use of botulinum toxin in individuals with neurogenic detrusor overactivity: state of the art review. J Spinal Cord Med. 2013;36(5):402–19.
58. Meier T, Wallace BG. Formation of the neuromuscular junction: molecules and mechanisms. BioEssays. 1998;20(10):819–29.
59. Chancellor MB, Fowler CJ, Apostolidis A, de Groat WC, Smith CP, Somogyi GT, et al. Drug insight: biological effects of botulinum toxin A in the lower urinary tract. Nat Clin Pract Urol. 2008;5(6):319–28.
60. Kanagarajah P, Ayyathurai R, Caruso DJ, Gomez C, Gousse AE. Role of botulinum toxin-A in refractory idiopathic overactive bladder patients without detrusor overactivity. Int Urol Nephrol. 2012;44(1):91–7.
61. Khera M, Somogyi GT, Salas NA, Kiss S, Boone TB, Smith CP. In vivo effects of botulinum toxin A on visceral sensory function in chronic spinal cord-injured rats. Urology. 2005;66(1):208–12.
62. Yokokawa R, Akino H, Ito H, Zha X, Yokoyama O. Nerve growth factor release from the urothelium increases via activation of bladder C-fiber in rats with cerebral infarction. Neurourol Urodyn. 2017;36(6):1448–55.
63. Yokoyama T, Chancellor MB, Oguma K, Yamamoto Y, Suzuki T, Kumon H, et al. Botulinum toxin type A for the treatment of lower urinary tract disorders. Int J Urol. 2012;19(3):202–15.
64. Apostolidis A, Popat R, Yiangou Y, Cockayne D, Ford AP, Davis JB, et al. Decreased sensory receptors P2X3 and TRPV1 in suburothelial nerve fibers following intradetrusor injections of botulinum toxin for human detrusor overactivity. J Urol. 2005;174(3):977–82; discussion 82–3.

Chapter 2
Diagnosis of Overactive Bladder

Eric S. Rovner and Jennifer Rolef

Overactive bladder (OAB) is a highly prevalent disorder impacting millions of people's lives throughout the world [1]. Despite prevalence estimates in men and women of 17% in the United States (National Overactive Bladder Evaluation Study) and 12–17% in six European nations, overactive bladder syndrome remains underdiagnosed and undertreated [2]. Over the last few decades, several changes in terminology and advances in therapy for this condition have occurred. Because of these developments, considerable confusion exists within, and outside, the medical community with respect to the diagnosis of this burdensome condition. In order to optimize the identification and subsequent diagnosis of individuals who may suffer from OAB, it is important to fully understand the current definition of the term.

The exact origin of the term "overactive bladder" is unknown, but nevertheless, it became widely utilized and popularized in the medical lexicon in the latter half of the 1990s. It is interesting that although much controversy was engendered by the use of the phrase "overactive bladder," this exact term was never actually defined or described by the International Continence Society (ICS) in prior terminology reports until 2001. The term overactive detrusor function (generally shortened to overactive detrusor) does appear [3] in the lexicon as a finding on urodynamic testing. This term is defined by the occurrence of involuntary detrusor contractions during the filling phase of cystometry, which may be spontaneous or provoked.

Thus, overactive detrusor function and the terms which correctly or incorrectly have been used as substitutes (overactive detrusor, detrusor overactivity, and, eventually, overactive bladder) were all urodynamic terms and were utilized to describe abnormalities of detrusor function during filling cystometry. Thus, a urodynamic study was required to describe the finding of detrusor overactivity, which, in turn then, provided the patient with a de facto diagnosis of overactive bladder despite the

E. S. Rovner (✉) · J. Rolef
Department of Urology, Medical University of South Carolina, Charleston, SC, USA
e-mail: rovnere@musc.edu

L. Cox, E. S. Rovner (eds.), *Contemporary Pharmacotherapy of Overactive Bladder*, https://doi.org/10.1007/978-3-319-97265-7_2

fact that the term did not yet exist in the urologic literature. The limitations of this model have been recognized by several authors [4]. It was apparent that the requirement of urodynamics in making the diagnosis placed an undue burden on the practicing physician, the patient, and the healthcare system in general. In addition, the term overactive bladder would need to be formally defined.

Several important ICS reports were subsequently published including a report on the Standardization of Terminology of Lower Urinary Tract Symptoms in 2002 [3].The definitions and descriptions were meant to restate or update those presented in previous ICS Standardization of Terminology reports [5]. Among other important changes and updates, this report addressed the definition and use of the term "overactive bladder" and classified it as a type of syndrome. According to this document, syndromes "describe constellations or varying combinations of symptoms but cannot be used for precise diagnosis…[syndromes] are functional abnormalities for which a precise cause has not been defined" [3]. Overactive bladder syndrome, or urgency-frequency syndrome, is thus defined as "urgency with or without urge incontinence, usually with frequency and nocturia." In 2010, the ICS together with the International Urogynecological Association (IUGA) restated this definition in their most recent joint report on the terminology for pelvic floor dysfunction [6]. The goal of this report was to better update terminology of the lower urinary tract by a "female-specific approach." Nevertheless, for the overactive bladder syndrome, the definition remained unchanged. It is important to recognize that while these symptoms are suggestive of detrusor overactivity, a urodynamic demonstration of detrusor overactivity is not necessary to make the diagnosis. Furthermore, the definition allows that a variety of other conditions of urethro-vesical dysfunction may result in a similar symptom complex.

Within the framework of this definition of OAB, it is important to emphasize that the use of the term overactive bladder is necessarily restricted to those situations in which local pathology, such as infection, and malignancy have been excluded. A large number of clinical conditions, both commonly encountered and rarely seen, can present with symptoms suggestive of OAB (Table 2.1). The goal of the practitioner in the evaluation of OAB should be to assess the individual for the presence of symptoms suggestive of OAB and then be able to comfortably, confidently, and accurately exclude the coexistence of most of these conditions. Fortunately, a well-done and complete medical history consistent with OAB, a normal physical examination, and an unremarkable urine analysis will usually be adequate to exclude many of these conditions and arrive at the proper diagnosis. The diagnosis of OAB is usually not difficult; however, in appropriate cases, the use of additional selected, adjunctive studies may be helpful as described below.

In this chapter, we will discuss the usual diagnostic evaluation of the patient with suspected OAB and briefly review some of the adjunctive studies that may be indicated in selected cases. The evaluation of an individual with suspected OAB should be simple, rapid, and accurate, in order to initiate effective therapy and alleviate the symptoms associated with the condition.

Table 2.1 Differential diagnosis of OAB

Differential diagnosis of OAB
Excessive fluid intake
Urinary retention (overflow)
Bacterial cystitis
Prostatitis
Radiation cystitis
Sexually transmitted disease (GC, chlamydia, etc.)
Interstitial cystitis, sensory urgency syndromes
Bladder cancer
Bladder stones
Pelvic mass (GI, GU, GYN, vascular aneurysm, etc.)
Gynecological problem
Vaginitis, endometriosis, malignancy, etc.
Postmenopausal atrophic vaginitis
Vaginal prolapse: cystocele, rectocele, etc.
Severe stress urinary incontinence
Medical illnesses producing fluid shifts: CHF, cirrhosis, etc.
Drugs (e.g., diuretics)
Other

OAB overactive bladder, *GC* gonococcus, *GI* gastrointestinal, *GU* genitourinary, *Gyn* gynecological

History

Symptom Assessment

As noted in the definition discussed above, OAB is a symptomatic diagnosis. Therefore, a proper symptom assessment, both qualitatively and quantitatively, is of paramount importance. Urgency is the primary symptom of OAB, and as such it is important to define [7]. The ICS defines urgency as a "sudden compelling desire to void that is difficult to defer," differentiated from the term urge, which is a normal feeling during bladder filling [6]. Urgency is the primary driver of OAB and leads to the typical symptoms including urinary frequency, nocturia, and, if the urgency cannot be suppressed, urinary urge incontinence [8]. According to the ICS, urinary frequency is a complaint of micturition occurring more frequently during the daytime hours. Nocturia is simply waking to urinate during sleep hours, and only one interruption of sleep is needed to qualify. Urinary incontinence occurring shortly after, or in concert with the sensation of impending leakage, is called urgency incontinence. Urinary incontinence is present in approximately one-third of patient with OAB and is termed "OAB wet" [7].

Frequency and nocturia can be assessed by patient report or voiding diaries (discussed below). Patient self-report of voiding frequency is quite variable, subject to considerable recall bias, and thus not generally considered highly reliable [9]. Normative values for 24-h urinary frequency are not universally agreed upon. Urinary frequency is obviously dependent on a number of variables including, but not limited to, volume intake (total fluid intake, etc.), insensible losses due to sweating and respiration, climate factors (ambient humidity, etc.), as well as the functional bladder capacity. Generally, urinary frequency of >8 episodes/24 h is considered consistent with a diagnosis of OAB and represents the threshold for inclusion into many OAB pharmacotherapy studies. The complaint of urgency is inherently subjective in nature and, therefore, particularly difficult to capture when evaluating patients. It is unclear whether the severity or magnitude of each episode of urgency is important or whether the total number of episodes of urgency is important. Urgency episodes can be quantified by patient report or by voiding diaries and are thus subject to the same limitations as quantifying frequency. Various urgency severity scales have been developed and validated [10–12]. Their role in assisting with the diagnosis of OAB is unknown.

In addition to assessing symptoms, a detailed past medical, gynecological, and surgical history should be obtained, specifically looking for possible causes of the patient's symptoms. The patient should be asked if he/she has a history of sexually transmitted diseases and vaginal or urethral discharge. The patient's menstrual history and bowel habits should be reviewed as it has been well established that bowel and bladder dysfunctions are intimately related. In men with constipation reporting three or fewer bowel movements weekly, for example, there is a significantly increased prevalence of LUTS [13]. The patient's medications, both prescription and over the counter, should be assessed as potential causes for his/her symptoms as many classes of medications can have wide-ranging and well-documented collateral effects on lower urinary tract function. The review of systems should concentrate on factors potentially related to etiology (e.g., neurologic, metabolic, medication(s)) or related diagnoses. A history of diabetes, neurologic disease, excess fluid intake, and prior pelvic/abdominal surgery are just some of the factors that should be specifically queried.

As noted previously, a number of conditions may contribute to or simulate the overactive bladder, and a careful history will allow the practitioner to begin to differentiate among the possibilities. For example, patients with stress incontinence may present with many of the symptoms of OAB in that they may void frequently in an attempt to avoid leakage, a behavior that is termed "defensive voiding." A careful history with special emphasis on onset, progression/regression, and response/non-response to treatments is valuable. The use of a diagnostic aid is sometimes helpful, in order to distinguish between the symptoms of OAB and stress incontinence (Table 2.2) [14]. However, it is important to realize that these two conditions often coexist.

Questionnaires

When assessing patient symptoms, it is important to remember that individuals experience different symptoms to varying degrees, which poses difficulties in accurately characterizing the condition and measuring the effect of treatment. There exist a wide variety of validated questionnaires for the study of voiding dysfunction, and there is some low-level evidence that the use of these questionnaires may help in the screening for or categorization of the syndrome [15]. Questionnaires utilized for OAB may be used both clinically and in the research arena for screening, symptom assessment, and disease impact or as a measure of health-related quality of life. The majority of instruments currently utilized as research tools are not OAB specific and are not generally used for diagnostic purposes. The specific details of each questionnaire are beyond the scope of this chapter (Table 2.3).

Voiding Diaries

As noted previously, urinary frequency and urgency can be assessed by patient recall at the time of interview or by self-monitoring using frequency/volume charts or voiding diaries. Urinary incontinence episodes can be captured in a likewise fashion. Although useful for quantifying symptoms, voiding diaries are not usually utilized as an initial diagnostic tool for OAB as the symptoms of OAB may be due to a variety of causes. However, voiding diaries are extremely useful in numerically

Table 2.2 Differentiating OAB from stress incontinence

Symptoms	OAB	Stress incontinence
Urgency (strong, sudden desire to void)	Yes	No
Frequency with urgency	Yes	Rarely
Leaking during physical activity, e.g., coughing, sneezing, lifting, etc.	No	Yes
Amount of urinary leakage with each episode of incontinence	Large if present	Usually small
Ability to reach the toilet in time following an urge to void	No or just barely	Yes
Nocturnal incontinence (presence of wet pads or undergarments in bed)	Yes	Rare
Nocturia (waking to pass urine at night)	Usually	Seldom

Adapted from Rovner and Wein [14]
OAB overactive bladder

Table 2.3 Examples of questionnaires utilized in the evaluation of individuals with lower urinary tract symptoms

Questionnaire	Acronym	Item
Incontinence Impact Questionnaire [16, 17]	IIQ-7	QoL
Urge Incontinence Impact Questionnaire [18]	Urge-IIQ	QoL
King's Health Questionnaire [19]	ICIQ-KHQ	QoL
Bristol Female Lower Urinary Tract Symptoms Questionnaire [20]	BFLUTS	QoL, symptoms, sexual function
Urinary Incontinence Quality of Life Instrument [21]	I-QoL	QoL
Overactive Bladder Questionnaire [22, 23]	OAB-q	QoL, symptoms

QoL quality of life

assessing patient symptoms and evaluating patient outcomes before and after the initiation of treatment regimens. In short, voiding diaries are simple and inexpensive ways to obtain reasonably objective information on voiding behavior in the patient's usual environment. It should be noted that although self-monitoring techniques may in themselves modify the behavior they are measuring, reported micturition frequency and number of incontinence episodes as recorded on a voiding diary have been found to be highly reproducible on a test-retest analysis [24].

One particular use of the dairy is to assess the contribution of nocturia to the patient's symptoms. Nocturia is a highly prevalent condition and generally is considered bothersome by most individuals if there are two or more episodes per night [25, 26]. OAB often coexists with nocturia; however, there are many individuals with isolated nocturia due to nocturnal polyuria (NP) without daytime symptoms. Such patients do not have OAB. NP is a completely different condition from OAB and requires directed therapy.

Multiple studies have been performed in assessing the reliability, reproducibility, and accuracy of voiding diaries as a tool in the evaluation of lower urinary tract symptoms. Voiding diary parameters, specifically urinary frequency and incontinent episodes, have been often utilized as primary and secondary outcome measures in efficacy studies of various agents for the treatment of OAB [27–33]. Most voiding diaries will include intake volume, voided volumes, incontinent and urgency episodes, as well as types of activities being performed during these episodes. Although 72-h micturition diaries have shown excellent reliability, 24-h micturition diaries are more convenient for the patient and seem to provide valid data [34, 35]. In those patients with access to electronic devices, electronic voiding diaries have been used as a good alternative to paper voiding diaries with potentially better data quality and compliance [36].

Pad Tests

If incontinence is present in the setting of OAB, there are a variety of pad tests available to quantitate the amount of urine loss. However, urinary incontinence is not necessary for the diagnosis of OAB and may only be present in a minority of such patients [7]. Thus, they have limited diagnostic utility. Nevertheless, they can be extremely helpful and serve as a baseline for outcome assessments under certain conditions [3].

Physical Examination

A directed physical exam is important in every patient presenting with lower urinary tract symptoms suggestive of OAB. There are no signs or findings on physical examination that are specific to OAB, and therefore, the goal of the abdominal, pelvic, rectal, and neurological examinations is to help the clinician in excluding many of the differential diagnostic possibilities.

The abdomen is examined for wounds suggestive of prior surgery, skin abnormalities (e.g., rashes), hernias, and masses. Percussion or palpation may be performed to evaluate for a distended bladder suggesting poor bladder emptying and chronic urinary retention as a cause of the patient's symptoms. The lower back is also examined for scars reflecting prior lower back surgery, as well as a dimple or hair tuft suggestive of spina bifida occulta. A directed neurological assessment should be performed. The presence of motor or sensory deficits of the patient's lower extremities or perineum should be identified. Knee and ankle reflexes are assessed, and the patient's gait is observed. A rectal exam should be performed in men and women specifically for examination of rectal tone and the integrity of the sacral reflex arc (anal wink, bulbocavernosus reflex, etc.). Objective neurological abnormalities found on physical examination may prompt a referral to a neurologist and/or appropriate imaging of the central nervous system. During the assessment of rectal tone, the patient's ability to perform pelvic floor exercises properly (Kegel exercises) can be assessed.

In men, the prostate should be evaluated for size, texture, symmetry, nodules, and tenderness. The male genital exam should specifically look for evidence of meatal stenosis, phimosis, urethral discharge, testicular abnormalities, and genital lesions.

Female pelvic exams include an evaluation for pelvic organ prolapse (cystocele, vault prolapse, enterocele, rectocele, and perineal laxity), urethral hypermobility, vaginal epithelial atrophy, vaginal dryness, and rugation. The vaginal walls and surrounding perineal skin are examined for lesions, excessive vaginal discharge, or evidence of maceration or ulceration implying chronic urinary incontinence. In some cases, urethral diverticula may be diagnosed by careful palpation of the anterior vaginal wall and digital stripping of the urethra. A cough stress test is performed to evaluate for the presence of stress urinary incontinence. A careful bimanual pelvic examination is performed for the evaluation of adnexal, uterine, or other pelvic masses.

Urine Analysis

It is widely accepted, and all of the guideline groups concur, that patients should be asked to provide a clean catch midstream urine specimen as part of their initial assessment. There is some disagreement, however, as to whether a urine dipstick is adequate or formal urinalysis should be required. Both the American Urological Association (AUA) and European Association of Urology (EAU) agree that a formal urinalysis should be obtained, while National Institute for Health and Care Excellence (NICE) recommends performing a urine dipstick testing in women presenting with OAB symptoms [12]. The utility of a screening dipstick is that it can be performed in the office and provides rapid information specifically looking for hematuria, proteinuria, glucosuria, and the presence of nitrates and leukocytes. Urine microscopy and culture are the diagnostic gold standard, but reagent strip testing of urine is a sensitive and cheaper screening method. Altered bladder sensation during urinary tract infections can cause symptoms similar to those of

OAB. Tumors of the lower urinary tract may likewise cause urgency, frequency, and urge incontinence. Hematuria mandates urologic referral and further urologic investigation. OAB symptoms should never be treated empirically in the setting of hematuria without a proper evaluation of the hematuria. Irritative symptoms may prompt a voided urine sent for cytology which, if positive for tumor or dysplastic cells, should likewise mandate further urologic evaluation. Significant glucosuria or proteinuria should prompt further medical or nephrologic evaluation.

Post-void Residual Urine Measurement

It remains a point of contention whether all patients presenting with symptoms of OAB require a post-void residual measurement prior to the initiation of treatment. Patients with incomplete bladder emptying (chronic urinary retention) may present with symptoms indistinguishable from OAB including urinary frequency, urgency, and nocturia, with or without urinary incontinence. A low post-void residual urine determination excludes chronic urinary retention as a cause of lower urinary tract symptoms. In thin female patients, a bimanual pelvic examination is a simple method of examining for a distended or incompletely emptied bladder. Males and obese females are more challenging. Pelvic ultrasound or urethral catheterization may be used to measure the volume of urine remaining in the bladder after voiding with distinct advantages to each method. It is desirable to measure post-void residual urine in some groups of patients, particularly in the elderly with voiding symptoms and/or recurrent or persistent urinary tract infections, in those with complicated neurological disease and voiding dysfunction, and in all those with symptoms that suggest poor bladder emptying.

Urodynamics

Urodynamics assess the activity of the bladder and bladder outlet during the filling/storage and emptying phases of micturition. When combined with fluoroscopy (i.e., videourodynamics), this study evaluates both the anatomy and function of the lower urinary tract simultaneously [37]. As stated previously, OAB is by definition a symptom-based diagnosis and, as such, the definition precludes the need for immediate cystometrogram and/or pressure-flow urodynamic studies. In fact, the general consensus among guideline groups regarding an index patient is that urodynamic testing is not recommended prior to initiating conservative therapy but should be considered only if it may alter the choice of surgical management [16–18].

It is important to emphasize that OAB and detrusor overactivity are not synonymous although it is widely believed that involuntary bladder contractions are the primary underlying pathophysiology of OAB in some such patients. The sine qua non of a well-done diagnostic urodynamic study is reproducing the patient's symptoms during the study [19]. The absence of detrusor overactivity on urodynamics does not exclude OAB, and the finding of detrusor overactivity in an otherwise asymptomatic individual does not make the diagnosis. Furthermore, urodynamics are invasive (requiring urethral or suprapubic catheterization of the bladder), can be associated with significant morbidity, are relatively expensive, and are not widely available outside of the industrialized world.

Although UDS are not necessary for a diagnosis or initial management of OAB, these studies certainly have a role in the evaluation of lower urinary tract symptoms in a variety of selected circumstances [20]. These include those who have failed previous therapy for OAB, or those who have OAB symptoms in the setting of neurologic disease, vaginal prolapse, suspected bladder outlet obstruction, prior lower urinary tract surgery, prior pelvic radiotherapy, radical pelvic surgery, or a number of other complicated clinical scenarios.

Cystourethroscopy

Cystourethroscopy has a limited role in the evaluation of uncomplicated lower urinary tract symptoms as well as in the diagnosis of OAB. There are no endoscopic findings diagnostic of OAB although bladder trabeculation may be suggestive of long-term detrusor overactivity in some patients [21]. In the presence of a normal urine analysis and physical examination, endoscopic examination probably provides little additional diagnostic information for the patient with OAB. Cystoscopy is typically performed in patients with hematuria and sterile pyuria and patients with refractory urgency and frequency and/or urgency incontinence (i.e., following failure of initial therapy). Cystoscopy can also be helpful in the diagnosis or evaluation of urethral diverticulum, ureteroceles, ureteral ectopia, radiation cystitis, interstitial cystitis, bladder stones, urethral strictures, bladder outlet obstruction, and bladder trabeculation.

Imaging

Similar to urodynamic and endoscopic examination of the lower urinary tract in patients with OAB, the role of radiographic imaging is limited. No radiographic findings are specific to OAB. The role of imaging in the evaluation of OAB primarily involves excluding other conditions such as urethral diverticula or vaginal prolapse. The limitations of static imaging are obvious when evaluating a dynamic condition such as OAB. Videourodynamics may provide some advantages in this setting by combining the static images during cystourethrography with the dynamic information obtained during pressure-flow urodynamics. As mentioned previously, imaging of the central nervous system may be indicated in some individuals with suspected relevant neurological conditions.

Other Studies

There are no specific serum studies necessary in the evaluation of overactive bladder. Diabetes and thyroid disorders can cause symptoms mimicking OAB, and thus, the use of serum chemistry, TSH, or HgbA1c could be useful. PSA is often checked as well, as a screening test for prostate cancer in selected individuals.

Novel Biomarkers

There has been much recent interest in the use of novel biomarkers for the detection of overactive bladder. Biomarkers constitute any objective measurable indicator of a biological process. They can be used to diagnose a disease and assess the severity of its progression or as an indicator of disease prognosis, including prediction of response to specific therapies [22]. Putative markers include urinary growth factors and cytokines, bladder wall thickness on imaging, and potential predisposing genetic polymorphisms. Most research interest to date has focused on prostaglandin E2 (PGE2) and nerve growth factor (NGF). PGE2 administration has been known to enhance detrusor muscle activity and has been widely used in rat models for detrusor overactivity [23]. Conversely, induction of detrusor overactivity has been shown to increase levels of PGE2 in the urine, making it a potential detectable marker for OAB [38]. However, although early reports noted increased levels of urinary PGE2 in humans with OAB, more recent studies have not consistently supported this [39]. NGF, on the other hand, has more reliably been detected in individuals with OAB [39]. It is a member of the neurotropic factors and is required for the maintenance of sensory, autonomic, and CNS neurons [40]. Increased endogenous levels of NGF have been shown to be present in both rat models for detrusor activity as well as in human bladder tissue from patients with bladder conditions, including OAB [41, 42]. Unfortunately, NGF as a potential urinary biomarker for OAB suffers from a relative lack of discrimination given that elevated levels are also seen in response to other inflammatory conditions such as UTI and bladder stones. In summary, although these current potential biomarkers may correlate with OAB severity in some cases, future work is still required to assess their prognostic value and role in clinical practice.

Conclusions

An *initial evaluation* of the patient with OAB should include, at a minimum, (1) an assessment of the patient's symptoms, (2) physical examination, and (3) urine analysis. A sequential, organized approach should be employed, in which confounding conditions are identified and addressed. Once urinary tract infection has been excluded, it is possible in most cases to establish a working diagnosis based on the patient's description of symptoms. In some patients being evaluated for OAB, it may be desirable to obtain a voiding diary and measure post-void residual urine by catheterization or ultrasound. In cases where there is uncertainty regarding the diagnosis, more advanced investigations, such as urodynamic assessment and/or cystoscopy, may be carried out, usually by the specialist.

References

1. Milsom I, Abrams P, Cardozo L, Roberts RG, Thoroff J, Wein AJ. How widespread are the symptoms of an overactive bladder and how are they managed? A population-based study. BJU Int. 2001;87(7):760–6.
2. Marinkovic S, Rovner E, Moldwin R, Stanton S, Gillen L, Marinkovic C. The management of overactive bladder syndrome. BMJ. 2012;344:e2365.
3. Abrams P, Cardozo L, Fall M, Griffiths D, Rosier P, Ulmsten U, et al. The standardisation of terminology of lower urinary tract function: report from the Standardisation Sub-committee of the International Continence Society. Neurourol Urodyn. 2002;21(2):167–78.
4. Abrams P, Wein AJ. The overactive bladder and incontinence: definitions and a plea for discussion. Neurourol Urodyn. 1999;18(4):413–6.
5. Abrams P, Blaivas JG, Stanton SL, Andersen JT. The standardisation of terminology of lower urinary tract function. The International Continence Society Committee on Standardisation of Terminology. Scand J Urol Nephrol. 1988;114(Suppl):5–19.
6. Haylen BT, de Ridder D, Freeman RM, Swift SE, Berghmans B, Lee J, et al. An international Urogynecological Association (IUGA)/International Continence Society (ICS) joint report on the terminology for female pelvic floor dysfunction. Neurourol Urodyn. 2010;29(1):4–20.
7. Wein AJ, Rackley R. Overactive bladder: a better understanding of pathophysiology, diagnosis and management. J Urol. 2006;175(3 Pt w):S5–S10. Review.
8. Abrams P, Chapple C, Juneemann KP, Sharpe S. Urinary urgency: a review of its assessment as the key symptoms of the overactive bladder syndrome. World J Urol. 2012;30(3):385–92.
9. Stav K, Dwyer PL, Rosamilia A. Women overestimate daytime urinary frequency: the importance of the bladder diary. J Urol. 2009;181(5):2176–80.
10. Cardozo L, Coyne KS, Versi E. Validation of the urgency perception scale. BJU Int. 2005;95(4):591–6.
11. Freeman R, Hill S, Millard R, Slack M, Sutherst J; Tolterodine Study Group. Reduced perception of urgency in treatment of overactive bladder with extended-release tolterodine. Obstet Gynecol. 2003;102(3):605–11.
12. Zinner N, Harnett M, Sabounjian L, Sandage B Jr, Dmochowski R, Staskin D. The overactive bladder-symptom composite score: a composite symptom score of toilet voids, urgency severity and urge urinary incontinence in patients with overactive bladder. J Urol. 2005;173(5):1639–43.
13. Thurmon KL, Breyer BN, Erickson BA. Association of bowel habits with lower urinary tract symptoms in men: findings from the 2005–2006 and 2007–2008 National Health and Nutrition Examination Survey. J Urol. 2013;189(4):1409–14.
14. Rovner ES, Wein AJ. Today's treatment of overactive bladder and urge incontinence. Women's Health in Prim Care. 2000;3(3):179–92.
15. Nambiar A, Lucas M. Chapter 4: guidelines for the diagnosis and treatment of overactive bladder (OAB) and neurogenic detrusor overactivity (NDO). Neurourol Urodyn. 2014;33(Suppl):S21–5.
16. Gormley EA, Lightner DJ, Burgio KL, Chai TC, Clemens JQ, Culkin DJ, et al; American Urological Association; Society of Urodynamics, Female Pelvic Medicine & Urogenital Reconstruction. Diagnosis and treatment of overactive bladder (non-neurogenic) in adults:

AUA/SUFU guideline. 2012; amended 2014. http://www.auanet.org/guidelines/overactive-bladder-(oab)-(aua/sufu-guideline-2012-amended-2014. Accessed 27 Apr 2018.
17. Thuroff JW, Abrams P, Andersson KE, Artibani W, Chapple CR, Drake MJ, et al. EUA guidelines on urinary incontinence. Eur Urol. 2011;59(3):387–400.
18. National Institute of Clinical Excellence (NICE). CG171 urinary incontinence in women: full guideline. 2013.
19. Colhoun A, Goudelocke C, Rovner ES. Reproduction of female lower urinary tract symptoms on urodynamics. Low Urin Tract Symptoms. 2012;4(2):59–62.
20. Rovner E, Goudeloke C. Urodynamics in the evaluation of overactive bladder. Curr Urol Rep. 2010;11(5):343–7.
21. Gowda M, Danford JM, Slaughter JC, Zimmerman CW, Ward RM. Clinical findings associated with bladder trabeculations in women. Int Urogynecol J. 2013;24(7):1167–71.
22. Cartwright R, Afshan I, Derpapas A, Vijaya G, Khullar V. Novel biomarkers for overactive bladder. Nat Rev Urol. 2011;8(3):139–45.
23. Klarskov P, Gerstenberg T, Ramirez D, Christenson P, Hald P. Prostaglandin type E activity dominates in urinary tract smooth muscle in vitro. J Urol. 1983;129(5):1071–4.
24. Bradley CS, Brown JS, Van Den Eeden SK, Schembri M, Ragins A, Thom DH. Urinary incontinence self-report questions: reproducibility and agreement with bladder diary. Int Urogynecol J. 2011;22(12):1565–71.
25. Coyne KS, Sexton CC, Thompson CL, Milsom I, Irwin D, Kopp ZS, Chapple CR, et al. The prevalence of lower urinary tract symptoms (LUTS) in the USA, the UK and Sweden: results from the Epidemiology of LUTS (EpiLUTS) study. BJU Int. 2009;104(3):352–60.
26. Kupelian V, Wei JT, O'Leary MP, Norgaard JP, Rosen RC, McKinlay JB. Nocturia and quality of life: results from the Boston area community health survey. Eur Urol. 2012;61(1):78–84.
27. Appell RA, Sand P, Dmochowski R, Anderson R, Zinner N, Lama D, et al. Prospective randomized controlled trial of extended-release oxybutynin chloride and tolterodine tartrate in the treatment of overactive bladder: results of the OBJECT study. Mayo Clin Proc. 2001;76(4):358–63.
28. Burgio KL. Influence of behavior modification on overactive bladder. Urology. 2002;60(5 Suppl 1):72–6.
29. Chapple CR, Rechberger T, Al Shukri S, Meffan P, Everaert K, Huang M, et al. Randomized, double-blind placebo- and tolterodine-controlled trial of the once-daily antimuscarinic agent solifenacin in patients with symptomatic overactive bladder. BJU Int. 2004;93(3):303–10.
30. Diokno AC, Appell RA, Sand PK, Dmochowski RR, Gburek BM, Klimberg IW, et al. Prospective, randomized, double-blind study of the efficacy and tolerability of the extended-release formulations of oxybutynin and tolterodine for overactive bladder: results of the OPERA trial. Mayo Clin Proc. 2003;78(6):687–95.
31. Dmochowski RR, Sand PK, Zinner NR, Gittelman MC, Davila GW, Sanders SW, et al. Comparative efficacy and safety of transdermal oxybutynin and oral tolterodine versus placebo in previously treated patients with urge and mixed urinary incontinence. Urology. 2003;62(2):237–42.
32. Haab F, Stewart L, Dwyer P. Darifenacin, an M3 selective receptor antagonist, is an effective and well tolerated once-daily treatment for overactive bladder. Eur Urol. 2004;45(4):420–9. discussion 429
33. Van Kerrebroeck P, Kreder K, Jonas U, Zinner N, Wein A; Tolterodine Study Group. Tolterodine once-daily: superior efficacy and tolerability in the treatment of the overactive bladder. Urology. 2001;57(3):414–21.
34. Mazurick CA, Landis JR. Evaluation of repeat daily voiding measures in the national interstitial cystitis data base study. J Urol. 2000;163(4):1208–11.
35. Brown JS, McNaughton KS, Wyman JF, Burgio KL, Harkaway R, Bergner D, et al. Measurement characteristics of a voiding diary for use by men and women with overactive bladder. Urology. 2003;61(4):802–9.
36. Sussman RD, Richter L, Tefera E, Park A, Sokol A, Gutman R, Iglesia C. Utilizing technology in assessment of lower urinary tract symptoms: a randomized trial of electronic versus paper voiding diaries. Female Pelvic Med Reconstr Surg. 2016;22(4):224–8.

37. Homma Y, Batista JE, Bauer SB, Griffiths DJ, Hilton P, Kramer G, et al. Urodynamics. In: Abrams P, Wein A, Schussler B, Kawabi K, Bump R, Melchior H, et al., editors. Incontinence. First international consultation on incontinence. Recommendations of the International Scientific Committee: the evaluation and treatment of urinary incontinence. Plymouth: Health Publication Ltd; 1999. p. 317–72.
38. Masunaga K, Yoshida M, Inadome A, Iwashita H, Miyamae K, Ueda S. Prostaglandin E2 release from isolated bladder strips in rats with spinal cord injury. In J Urol. 2006;13(3):271–6.
39. Liu H, Tyagi p CMB, Kuo HC. Urinary nerve growth factor but not prostaglandin E2 increases in patients with interstitial cystitis/bladder pain syndrome and detrusor overactivity. BJU Int. 2010;106(11):1681–5.
40. Fry CH, Sahai A, Vahabi B, Kanai A, Birder L. What is the role for biomarkers for lower urinary tract disorders? ICI-RS 2013. Neurourol Urodyn. 2017;33(5):602–5.
41. Oddiah D, Anand P, McMahon SB, Rattray M. Rapid increase of NGF, BDNF and NT-3 mRNAs in inflamed bladder. Neuroreport. 1998;9(7):1455–8.
42. Yokoyama T, Kumon H, Nagai A. Correlation of urinary nerve growth factor level with pathogenesis of overactive bladder. Neurourol Urodyn. 2008;27(5):417–20.

Chapter 3
The Placebo Effect in Overactive Bladder Syndrome

Svjetlana Lozo and Peter K. Sand

Initially seen as a nuisance variable, the placebo effect has been widely recognized as a distinct determinant of health in a number of different diseases and conditions. Dr. Arthur K. Shapiro spent much of his career in psychiatry studying placebo effects, and in 1964 he described a placebo as "any therapeutic procedure which is given deliberately to have an effect or unknowingly has an effect on a symptom, syndrome, disease or patient, but which is objectively without specific activity for the condition being treated" [1]. The placebo effect became mainstream in medicine when placebos began to be used in clinical trials as a control. One of the first documented uses of a placebo dates back to 1784 in a trial conducted by Benjamin Franklin and Antoine Lavoisier. In this trial, Franklin and Lavoisier were commissioned by Louis XVI to test Franz Mesmer's claim that uncovered "animal magnetism" contained certain healing properties. Patients were exposed to "mesmerized" objects or untreated (placebo) objects without telling them which ones they had been exposed to. Results of the research showed that a patient's responses to objects were completely unrelated to whether or not the object had been "mesmerized," and therefore they concluded that "animal magnetism" had no scientific basis [2]. Nevertheless, it was not until the 1900s that the placebo effect emerged as a phenomenon on its own. One of the most influential studies to shine the light on the placebo effect was a meta-analysis done by Beecher in 1955 [2]. Combining the data from 15 different studies, Beecher was able to show a 35% improvement in the symptoms of pain, seasickness, cough, and anxiety in the placebo arms of the trials. This led him to argue that the placebo effect was significant and worthy of further study.

S. Lozo
Division of Urogynecology, Department of Obstetrics & Gynecology, NorthShore University HealthSystem, University of Chicago Pritzker School of Medicine, Skokie, IL, USA

P. K. Sand (✉)
Division of Urogynecology, Department of Obstetrics & Gynecology, NorthShore University HealthSystem, University of Chicago Pritzker School of Medicine, Winnetka, IL, USA

L. Cox, E. S. Rovner (eds.), *Contemporary Pharmacotherapy of Overactive Bladder*, https://doi.org/10.1007/978-3-319-97265-7_3

Explanations of the Placebo Effect

The recognition of a placebo phenomenon has led to the development of a number of different theories to explain the effect. Some of the classical theories and concepts discussed in the research literature include the regression to the mean, expectancy theory, described by Kirsch in 1985; classical conditioning effects, described Wickramasekera in 1980; context effects, described by Di Blasi in 2001; and meaning response, described by Moerman and Jonas in 2002 [2].

One popular explanation for a placebo effect in clinical trials is to suggest that it is due to a "regression to the mean." This hypothesis was first described by Sir Francis Galton in 1886, in his article entitled "Regression Toward Mediocrity in Hereditary Stature." Subsequently, scientists have consistently noticed that variability in bivariate distributions will be reduced on subsequent observations. Measured variables will tend to regress toward mean expected values on repetitive testing. One of the first examples that Galton used to illustrate this example was to examine the average height of parents and their children. He noted that parents who were noted to be tall had children who were shorter than them and short parents had children who on average were taller than them. In both examples, children with parents at the extreme end of the distribution had heights closer to the population mean height [3].

"Expectancy theory" and "classical conditioning" are often seen as competing theories to explain the placebo effect [4]. Expectancy theory rationalizes that the placebo produces certain effects because the recipient expects it to produce an effect. An interesting implication of this theory is that drug advertising may potentially lead to powerful placebo effects. So how does expectancy produce a placebo effect? Lundth et al. in 2000 described that expectancies affect anxiety levels and therefore taking a placebo could potentially reduce anxiety and lead to improvement in the immune system [5]. Another explanation is that the placebo influences changes in expectancy and those changes lead to the changes in the subject's behavior that have a direct influence on one's health outcomes [6, 7]. In order to explain how none of the theories above can account for the placebo effect in healthy individuals, Kirsch described the response expectancy theory. He reported that response expectancies represent an anticipation of the occurrence of responses such as pain, emotional responses, sexual arousal, and nausea. The bottom line is that the expectation of having a subjective experience leads directly to the expected subjective experience [8].

"Classical conditioning theory" approaches placebo as a conditioned response. In this theory, an unconditioned response (placebo medication) is paired with neural stimuli, such as pill casings and syringes, or – more generally – with certain places, people, and procedures. Initially these stimuli are neutral with respect to eliciting certain unconditioned effects of an active drug, but as they become repeatedly associated, the unconditioned stimulus becomes a conditioned stimulus eliciting a conditioned response. Therefore, placebo medication eventually becomes a conditioned stimulus producing a conditioned response, which is the placebo response in this case [4]. Most of the research of this theory has been produced in animal models. One of the most controversial studies was performed by Ader and Cohen in 1975, when they injected rats with a novel saccharine-flavored liquid with or without the immunosuppressant cyclophosphamide. They were able to show that rats that were injected with the saccharine solution alone had a decreased immune response as would be expected from treatment with cyclophosphamide [9]. Both classical conditioning and expectancy theory are extremely appealing explanations for the placebo effect and have often been pitted against each other.

The "context effect" described by Di Blasi et al. in 2001 centered mostly on the doctor-patient relationship as part of the placebo effect. Their systematic review noted inconsistencies regarding emotional and cognitive care in the doctor-patient relationship. They noted that patients taken care of by physicians who have a warm, reassuring, and friendly manner do better than patients attended by physicians who do not offer reassurance and keep consultations formal, providing another element that may add to the placebo effect [10].

"Meaning response" indicates that the meaning (the anticipated physiological or psychological response) is what the patient attributes to the placebo. Moerman and Jonas make the argument that even though we do not intend it, most of the elements of the physician-patient interaction are "meaningful." Physicians' manners, white coats, style and use of language have been shown to influence patient outcomes. Moerman and Jonas argue that clinically we should conceptualize meaning response as observation effect instead of placebo effect [11]. This is illustrated by a study in which 200 patients with symptoms, but no abnormal physical signs, were assigned to have either a negative or positive consultation with a physician. In the group that received a positive consultation, 64% reported feeling better after 2 weeks compared to only 39% of subjects who received a negative consultation [12].

The most recent theory regarding placebos was developed in 2011 by Colloca and Miller [13]. This theory is based on the idea that the placebo effect is a learned response in which different types of verbal, social, and physiological influences cue or trigger previously formed expectations that generate a placebo effect via the central nervous system (CNS). For example, when a patient encounters a treatment, the treatment presents cues that cause the individual to recollect sensations experienced in one or several prior situations. This recollection develops into an expectation of what is likely to be experienced in response to the current treatment. These prior experiences drive the placebo effect via their influence on the CNS. Placebo effects clearly rely, to some degree, on the patient's perception – as it is well known that informing a patient about the use of an inactive placebo consistently reduces its efficacy [13]. Nevertheless, further research is needed to fully understand and uncover the "cause" of the placebo phenomenon. This "cause" may well be different in different individuals and may vary in different situations for the same individual.

Meissner et al., in their 2007 review of clinical studies [14], noted that placebo treatments had significant effects on physical rather than on biochemical parameters. They noted that in comparison to the administration of active pharmacological medications, administration of a placebo improved physical parameters on average by one-third. However, the same efficacy was not found for the biochemical parameters. Their conclusion was that placebo interventions have a more significant effect on physical rather than on biochemical parameters.

The Placebo Effect and OAB Treatment

An extensive placebo effect has been observed throughout all of the overactive bladder (OAB) syndrome trials. OAB is a multifactorial disorder defined by International Continence Society's terminology committee as a syndrome characterized by urgency, with or without urinary incontinence, usually accompanied by frequency and nocturia in the absence of urinary tract infections or other obvious pathologies. The prevalence of the condition increases with age in both females and males, affecting approximately 30–40% of population aged 75 and older. The condition has a significant negative effect on a patient's QOL and presents a significant economic burden [15].

Patients with OAB symptoms are often encouraged to keep bladder diaries to assess the severity of their condition, as well as to gain better insight into their symptoms. The bladder diary measures OAB parameters such as the number of micturition episodes during the day and night, urgency episodes, the number of incontinence episodes, and the mean volume voided per micturition. Just this observation while recording these data has been shown to modify an individual's OAB symptoms and may contribute to any noted "placebo effect" found in clinical trials where bladder diaries are recorded. More objective measurement of the severity and etiology of OAB features may be accomplished with urodynamic testing [16, 17].

Conservative treatment strategies for OAB include weight loss, bladder training or timed voiding, bladder control strategies, pelvic floor muscle training, and fluid intake management [18]. Behavioral therapies are usually the initial treatment option, and they center on educating patients about lower urinary tract anatomy and physiology and specifically what happens during the storage and voiding phases of the micturition cycle. Patients are asked to keep a bladder diary and to decrease their fluid intake after dinner in order to decrease nocturia. They may be encouraged to modify their diet and what liquids they drink and when they drink them, to reduce incontinence or urgency episodes without affecting adequate hydration status. Timed voiding and bladder drill can also be implemented to defer voiding and inhibit detrusor overactivity by utilizing the vesico-inhibitory reflexes. This mechanism centers on patients contracting the levator muscles to inhibit involuntary detrusor contractions, voiding on a timed schedule, and gradually increasing the inter-voiding interval. Some patients can actually restore cortical control over their involuntary detrusor contractions and stop their urgency urinary incontinence (UUI) and urinary frequency with these interventions [19, 20].

Studies have shown that behavioral therapy has been effective in decreasing the number of incontinence episodes in the population affected by OAB. Fantl et al. performed a study in women aged 55 and older and noted that those women who underwent behavioral therapy experienced a 57% decrease in the number of urinary incontinence episodes (including stress urinary incontinence) [20]. Since pharmacological therapy is often the next step in the treatment algorithm, studies have noted that a combination of behavioral and pharmacological therapy might be more effective than monotherapy alone. The American Urological Association and the

Society of Urodynamics, Female Pelvic Medicine, and Urogenital Reconstruction suggest that initiating behavioral and drug therapy simultaneously may improve outcomes, including frequency, voided volume, urinary incontinence, and symptom distress [18].

Numerous studies have been designed as randomized, placebo-controlled trials to determine the efficacy and tolerability of medications used for treating OAB. Anticholinergics are the most commonly used class of medications for OAB and have been compared to placebo in numerous studies with a wide variety of placebo responses recorded.

Several hypotheses have been developed as possible explanations for the substantial placebo effect witnessed in the treatment of OAB. A significant percentage of patients suffering from OAB have experienced bothersome symptoms for a long time. Getting a diagnosis, as part of clinical trial, and finding that their current condition is not life-threatening and is treatable, may offer a significant degree of relief, which could possibly add to the placebo response [21]. Participating in OAB clinical trials usually involves completing bladder diaries and receiving education about the storage and voiding phases of the micturition cycle by trained medical professionals. This education process often tends to improve patients' OAB symptoms through a bladder training effect and eventually leads to modification of patients' fluid intake [22]. The International Consultation on Incontinence guidelines recommend fluid manipulation as one of the strategies for management of OAB [23]. Randomized, prospective trials in adults with OAB have shown that a reduction of 25% in fluid intake from baseline was effective in reducing OAB symptoms such as daytime urinary frequency, urgency, and nocturia [24].

The effect of placebo in OAB has been examined from a number of different perspectives. Zinner et al. in 2013 attempted to understand placebo and treatment effects in patients undergoing treatment with solifenacin succinate. The aim of the study was to identify the combination of variables that would help to determine which group of patients was more or less likely to respond to the active medication or placebo. The authors used data from two separate Phase IIIb clinical trials of solifenacin succinate versus placebo in subjects with OAB. Individual answers from OAB questionnaires were used to create predictive models for high placebo and high medication responders. Outcomes of interest examined were urinary urgency and UUI episodes. In the placebo group, 14 separate variables were identified to help distinguish those with significant reductions in urgency and those who did not have a significant improvement. These variables were low patient-perceived bladder control at baseline (PPBC), high values from questionnaire for nocturnal voids in combination with low number of nocturnal episodes, as well as high responses to questions 1, 2, 10, 11, 18, and 28 on the OAB-q. (Form OAB-q LF 4-week recall (Fig. 3.1) is available from www.pfizerpatientreportedoutcomes.com.) Patients who responded to placebo also had low scores on questions 3, 5, 7, 27, and 32 on the OAB-q. In the actively treated subjects, nine variables distinguishing between high and low responders were identified. Patients who were high responders to treatment were noted to have a low baseline PPBC; high responses to questions 1, 4, 16, 24, and 33 on the OAB-q; and low responses to questions 6.7 and 26. When these variables were combined, the authors were able to identify patients who were more likely to experience a strong placebo effect versus those who experienced a strong treatment response. This prediction model has not been prospectively tested with other medications. This is one of the limitations of the study. However, the study does provide some insight into distinguishing which patients may be more responsive to placebo treatment. Further study may help us to determine if a questionnaire can be used to categorize subjects into different groups, based on their predicted responsiveness to placebo or active treatment, for recruitment to clinical trials [25].

In order to examine the placebo effect in OAB, Lee et al. [26] performed a meta-analysis and systematic review looking at the placebo response in antimuscarinic trials for OAB (Table 3.1) [27–62]. They carefully examined the placebo arm data for incontinence episodes, micturition episodes, voided volume, and other study

OAB-q

This questionnaire asks about how much you have been bothered by selected bladder symptoms during the past 4 weeks. Please place a ✓ or × in the box that best describes the extent to which you were bothered by each symptom during the past 4 weeks. There are no right or wrong answers. Please be sure to answer every question.

During the past 4 weeks, how bothered were you by. . .	**Not at all**	**A little bit**	**Some-what**	**Quite a bit**	**A great deal**	**A very great deal**
1. Frequent urination during the daytime hours?	☐ 1	☐ 2	☐ 3	☐ 4	☐ 5	☐ 6
2. An uncomfortable urge to urinate?	☐ 1	☐ 2	☐ 3	☐ 4	☐ 5	☐ 6
3. A sudden urge to urinate with little or no warning?	☐ 1	☐ 2	☐ 3	☐ 4	☐ 5	☐ 6
4. Accidental loss of small amounts of urine?	☐ 1	☐ 2	☐ 3	☐ 4	☐ 5	☐ 6
5. Nighttime urination?	☐ 1	☐ 2	☐ 3	☐ 4	☐ 5	☐ 6
6. Waking up at night because you had to urinate?	☐ 1	☐ 2	☐ 3	☐ 4	☐ 5	☐ 6
7. An uncontrollable urge to urinate?	☐ 1	☐ 2	☐ 3	☐ 4	☐ 5	☐ 6
8. Urine loss associated with a strong desire to urinate?	☐ 1	☐ 2	☐ 3	☐ 4	☐ 5	☐ 6

The above questions asked about your feelings about individual bladder symptoms. For the following questions, please think about your overall bladder symptoms in the past 4 weeks and how these symptoms have affected your life. Please answer each question about how often you have felt this way to the best of your ability. Please place a ✓ or × in the box that best answers each question.

Fig. 3.1 Overactive bladder questionnaire long form 4-week recall. (From Pfizer (New York, NY, USA), with permission. Permission for any use must be granted by Pfizer; this measure is available at www.pfizerpatientreportedoutcomes.com)

During the past 4 weeks, how often have your bladder symptoms . . .	None of the time	A little of the time	Some of the time	A good bit of the time	Most of the time	All of the time
9. Made you carefully plan your commute?	☐ 1	☐ 2	☐ 3	☐ 4	☐ 5	☐ 6
10. Caused you to feel drowsy or sleepy during the day?	☐ 1	☐ 2	☐ 3	☐ 4	☐ 5	☐ 6
11. Caused you to plan "escape routes" to restrooms in public places?	☐ 1	☐ 2	☐ 3	☐ 4	☐ 5	☐ 6
12. Caused you distress?	☐ 1	☐ 2	☐ 3	☐ 4	☐ 5	☐ 6
13. Frustrated you?	☐ 1	☐ 2	☐ 3	☐ 4	☐ 5	☐ 6
14. Made you feel like there is something wrong with you?	☐ 1	☐ 2	☐ 3	☐ 4	☐ 5	☐ 6
15. Interfered with your ability to get a good night's rest?	☐ 1	☐ 2	☐ 3	☐ 4	☐ 5	☐ 6
16. Caused you to decrease your physical activities (exercising, sports, etc.)?	☐ 1	☐ 2	☐ 3	☐ 4	☐ 5	☐ 6
17. Prevented you from feeling rested upon waking in the morning?	☐ 1	☐ 2	☐ 3	☐ 4	☐ 5	☐ 6
18. Frustrated your family and friends?	☐ 1	☐ 2	☐ 3	☐ 4	☐ 5	☐ 6
19. Caused you anxiety or worry?	☐ 1	☐ 2	☐ 3	☐ 4	☐ 5	☐ 6
20. Caused you to stay home more often than you would prefer?	☐ 1	☐ 2	☐ 3	☐ 4	☐ 5	☐ 6
21. Caused you to adjust your travel plans so that you are always near a restroom?	☐ 1	☐ 2	☐ 3	☐ 4	☐ 5	☐ 6
22. Made you avoid activities away from restrooms (i.e., walks, running, hiking)?	☐ 1	☐ 2	☐ 3	☐ 4	☐ 5	☐ 6
23. Made you frustrated or annoyed about the amount of time you spend in the restroom?	☐ 1	☐ 2	☐ 3	☐ 4	☐ 5	☐ 6
24. Awakened you during sleep?	☐ 1	☐ 2	☐ 3	☐ 4	☐ 5	☐ 6

Fig. 3.1 (continued)

During the past 4 weeks, how often have your bladder symptoms . . .	None of the time	A little of the time	Some of the time	A good bit of the time	Most of the time	All of the time
25. Made you worry about odor or hygiene?	☐ 1	☐ 2	☐ 3	☐ 4	☐ 5	☐ 6
26. Made you uncomfortable while traveling with others because of needing to stop for a restroom?	☐ 1	☐ 2	☐ 3	☐ 4	☐ 5	☐ 6
27. Affected your relationships with family and friends?	☐ 1	☐ 2	☐ 3	☐ 4	☐ 5	☐ 6
28. Caused you to decrease participating in social gatherings, such as parties or visits with family or friends?	☐ 1	☐ 2	☐ 3	☐ 4	☐ 5	☐ 6
29. Caused you embarrassment?	☐ 1	☐ 2	☐ 3	☐ 4	☐ 5	☐ 6
30. Interfered with getting the amount of sleep you needed?	☐ 1	☐ 2	☐ 3	☐ 4	☐ 5	☐ 6
31. Caused you to have problems with your partner or spouse?	☐ 1	☐ 2	☐ 3	☐ 4	☐ 5	☐ 6
32. Caused you to plan activities more carefully?	☐ 1	☐ 2	☐ 3	☐ 4	☐ 5	☐ 6
33. Caused you to locate the closest restroom as soon as you arrive at a place you have never been?	☐ 1	☐ 2	☐ 3	☐ 4	☐ 5	☐ 6

Fig. 3.1 (continued)

characteristics from randomized placebo-controlled trials. They found 36 studies that met their inclusion criteria. The mean age of the subjects enrolled in the placebo arms was 58.9 years. The median study duration was 12 weeks (range 2–12 weeks), and the mean number of patients in the placebo arms of the trials was 164 (range 13–508). The most commonly published OAB trials studied tolterodine ($n = 15$), oxybutynin ($n = 8$), propiverine ($n = 5$), and solifenacin ($n = 5$). This meta-analysis noted that the number of subjects included in the placebo arm tended to increase in more recent studies and that there was a positive association between the probability of studies reporting statistically successful outcomes and the size of placebo arm for all reported end points.

The patient populations in these studies that were assigned to placebo were noted to have 3.16 (SD 1) incontinence episodes per day. At the study end point, mean incontinence episodes were reduced by 1.16 (SD 0.46). This change in incontinence episodes was highly associated with baseline values ($r = 0.69$). Using both a fixed effects model and a random effects model, point estimates were noted to be statistically significant at −1.09 (−1.17, −1.02) and −1.15 (−1.34, −0.96) for incontinence episodes, respectively (Fig. 3.2) [26].

Table 3.1 Results for placebo treatment in the studies included in the meta-analysis

Study	Placebo	Duration (week)	Mean micturitions/day			Mean incontinence episodes/day			Mean volume voided per micturition (ml)		
	n		Baseline	End of treatment	Change from baseline	Baseline	End of treatment	Change from baseline	Baseline	End of treatment	Change from baseline
Abrams, 1998 [27]	57	12	11.7	ND	−1.6	3.4	ND	−0.9	157	ND	6
Burgio, 1998 [28]	65	8	ND	ND	ND	2.2	1.2	−1.03	ND	ND	ND
Cardozo, 2004 [29]	301	12	ND	ND	−1.59	ND	ND	−1.25	ND	ND	10.67
Chapple, 2004 [30]	38	4	11.1	10.1	−1.03	1.7	1.4	−0.29	134.7	144.4	9.7
Chapple, 2004 [31]	267	12	12.2	11	−1.2	2.7	2	−0.76	143.8	151.2	7.4
Chapple, 2007 [32]	285	12	12	10.9	−1.02	3.7	2.5	−1.2	150.2	159.9	9.77
Dmochowski, 2002 [33]	132	12	ND	ND	−1.7	ND	ND	ND	ND	ND	ND
Dmochowski, 2003 [34]	117	12	12.3	10.9	−1.4	5	2.9	−2.1	175	182	9
Dmochowski, 2008 [35]	284	12	12.9	11.1	−1.8	4	2.4	−1.6	151.8	169.6	17.8
Dorschner, 2003 [36]	49	4	7.1	6.5	−0.6	0.4	0.2	−0.1	187	178	−8.4
Drutz, 1999 [37]	56	12	11.4	10.3	−1.1	3.6	2.6	−1	160	172	12
Halaska, 1994 [38]	47	4	ND	ND	ND	ND	ND	ND	195	221	26
Herschorn, 2007 [39]	204	12	11.8	10.1	−1.7	3.2	1.8	−1.4	ND	ND	ND
Homms, 2003 [40]	122	12	11.1	9.6	−1.5	2.7	1.6	−1.09	130.7	145.8	15.2
Jacquetin, 2001 [41]	51	4	11.7	10.5	−1.2	2.4	ND	−0.4	148	155	7
Jünemann, 2000 [42]	60	3	ND	ND	−1.9	ND	ND	ND	ND	ND	ND
Jünemann, 2006 [43]	202	4.57	13.4	10.3	−3.07	3.5	1.7	−1.78	144.2	173.5	29.3
Khullar, 2004 [44]	285	8	10.6	9.3	−1.3	3.1	ND	−1.14	167	185.9	18.9
Lee, 2006 [45]	79	12	13	10.4	−2.58	ND	ND	ND	ND	ND	ND
Madersbacher, 1999 [46]	72	4	11.5	10.5	−1	ND	ND	ND	ND	ND	ND
Malone-Lee, 2001 [47]	43	4	9.9	10.3	0.4	5.1	4.4	−0.7	152	162	10
Malone-Lee, 2002 [48]	73	12	ND	ND	ND	ND	ND	ND	ND	ND	15.91

Table 3.1 (continued)

Study	Placebo	Duration (week)	Mean micturitions/day			Mean incontinence episodes/day			Mean volume voided per micturition (ml)		
	n		Baseline	End of treatment	Change from baseline	Baseline	End of treatment	Change from baseline	Baseline	End of treatment	Change from baseline
Millard, 1999 [49]	64	12	11.3	9.9	−1.4	3.5	2.2	−1.3	158	168	10
Nitti, 2007 [50]	274	12	12.2	11.1	−1.08	3.7	2.7	−0.96	159	167.4	8.38
Rackley, 2006 [51]	421	12	12.6	ND	ND	0.72	ND	ND	140.1	ND	ND
Rentzhog, 1998 [52]	13	2	10.2	ND	−0.3	4.1	ND	−0.4	ND	ND	ND
Robinson, 2007 [53]	61	6	11.9	10.1	−1.81	2.9	2.2	−0.66	145.5	156.9	11.4
Rogers, 2008 [54]	211	12	12.5	10.3	−2.2	2.2	0.8	−1.3	ND	ND	ND
Rudy, 2006 [55]	329	12	13.2	11.4	−1.76	ND	ND	ND	154.6	164.1	9.44
Staskin, 2007 [56]	303	12	12.7	10.8	−1.99	4.1	2.2	−1.93	155.9	174.8	18.89
Thüroff, 1991 [57]	27	4	ND	ND	−0.3	ND	ND	ND	ND	ND	ND
Uchida, 2002 [58]	53	4	10.9	9.9	−1	2.3	1	−1.3	196	202	6
Van Kerrebroeck, 2001 [59]	508	12	11.3	9.1	−2.2	3.3	2.3	−0.99	136	150	14
Wang, 2006 [60]	21	12	ND	ND	ND	ND	ND	ND	350	340	10
Yamaguchi, 2007 [61]	405	12	11.4	10.3	−0.94	2	1.3	−0.72	152.8	164.5	11.67
Zinner, 2004 [62]	256	12	12.9	11.6	−1.29	4.3	2.4	−1.9	156.6	164.3	7.7

From Lee et al. [26], with permission
ND No data

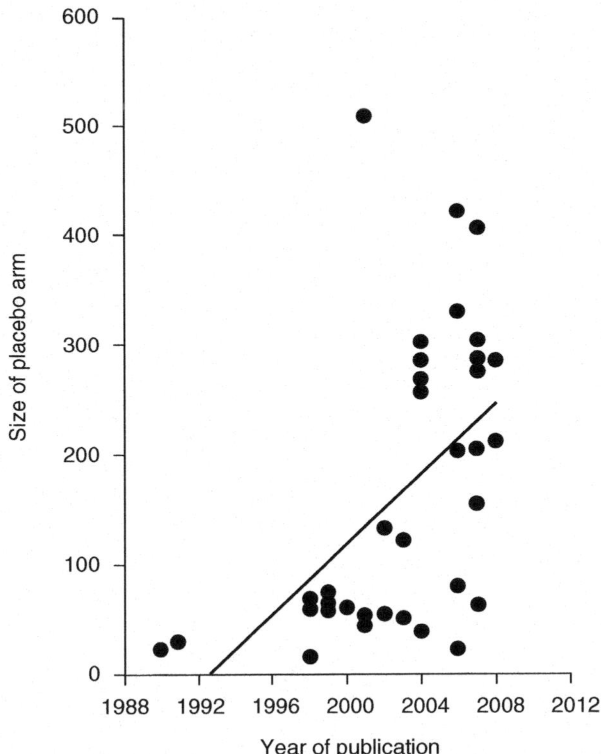

Fig. 3.2 Relationship between baseline and change score. (From Lee et al. [26], with permission)

Subjects in the placebo group were noted to have a mean of 11.8 (SD 0.9) micturition episodes per day at baseline. At the completion of the study, micturition episodes were reduced by 1.4 (SD 0.7) episodes per day in the placebo arm. Using a 95% confidence interval, point estimate change from baseline in micturition episodes per day was −1.29 (−1.38, −1,12) using a fixed effects model and −1.27 (−1.51, −1.03) using random effects model. Both results were noted to be statistically significantly changed from baseline.

Mean voided volume in the placebo group was noted to be 163.1 mL (SD 42.9) at baseline. Following treatment with placebo, the mean voided volume increased by 12.5 mL (SD 5.9). At the 95% confidence interval, point estimate change in voided volume from baseline was noted to be 18.6 (18.3,18.9) mL using a fixed effects model and 12.4 (9.3,15.5) mL using a random effects model. Both results were noted to be statistically significant.

This meta-analysis showed that individual studies utilized two approaches to manage the placebo response. The first approach of enrolling more severely affected patients was used in the more recent trials. This method was shown to be counterproductive because an increase in the response in the active treatment arms was offset with a larger response in the placebo patients. It was also noted that the probability of success of the study was unrelated to the magnitude of the placebo effect for any of the variables examined. The second method they observed being used to try to decrease the placebo response was the use of a larger study size. This assured successful study outcomes for the subjective study parameters, but was significantly less successful for objective study outcomes [26].

Mangera et al. performed a meta-analysis in 2011 and examined the placebo effect on OAB [17]. Their analysis included 62 trials, which included a placebo arm. Five commonly reported outcome parameters were identified: change in incontinence episodes per day, change in micturition episodes per day, change in urgency episodes per day, change in mean voided volume per micturition, and change in maximum cytometric capacity [17].

A total of 1847 patients in 12 studies reported changes in incontinence episodes per day. The mean reduction in incontinence episodes per day for the placebo cohort was 1.12 episodes (SD 0.59), and it was noted to be statistically significant. This study also examined if the study size affects the magnitude of change in the placebo group. They found no significant correlation between the study sample size and the degree of placebo effect on incontinence episodes (Table 3.2) [27, 29–31, 33, 34, 36, 37, 41, 44, 46, 49, 51, 53, 55, 58, 59, 61–67].

The change in micturition episodes per day within the placebo group was described in 11 studies including 1938 patients. Placebo patients experienced a mean reduction of −1.04 (SD 0.8) micturition episodes/day, which was noted to be statistically significant. Eleven studies examined the effect of placebo on the mean micturition volume. The weighted mean change in micturition volume was noted to be 10.61 ml (SD 12.9), which was noted to be statistically significant (Table 3.3) [27, 29, 31, 33, 34, 36, 37, 41, 43–46, 49, 51, 53, 55, 57–59, 61–63, 65–69].

This meta-analysis noted no changes in urgency episodes per day following placebo treatment. However, the data were pulled from only 3 studies that included 928 patients. The weighted mean change in urgency episodes/day was −1.15 (SD 1.74), which was not statistically significant. Another surprising finding in this meta-analysis was the effect of placebo on maximum cytometric capacity. Six studies with 208 patients showed statistically significant changes in maximum cytometric capacity following placebo treatment. The weighted change in maximum cytometric capacity was −16.87 ml (SD 9.99). Further analysis noted that the smaller studies were more likely to have decreased cytometric capacity following placebo treatment, while larger studies tended to show an increase in maximum cytometric capacity.

Magnera and his team found that placebo led to statistically significant improvement in four out of five commonly reported OAB parameters. Findings reported in this study were similar to the results found by Lee and colleagues. Lack of statistically significant findings in urinary urgency episodes per day following placebo treatment was likely affected by the small number of trials examining this parameter [17, 26].

Table 3.2 Incontinence episodes per day after placebo in patients with OAB

Study	Study duration (week)	Patients receiving placebo (*n*)	Change in mean number of incontinence episodes per day (SD)
Abrams et al. 1998 [27]	12	57	−0.9 (1.5)
Cardozo et al. 2004 [29]	12	301	−1.25 (NA)
Chapple et al. 2004 [63]	12	183	−1.45 (NA)
Chapple et al. 2004 [31]	12	267	−0.76 (2.26)
Chapple et al. 2004 [30]	6	38	−0.29 (NA)
Dmochowski et al. 2002 [33]	12	132	−2.74 (3.01)
Dmochowski et al. 2003 [34]	12	117	−2.1 (3)
Dorschner et al. 2003 [36]	4	49	−0.1 (NA)
Drutz et al. 1999 [37]	12	56	−1 (2.2)
Homma et al. 2006 [64]	8	167	−1.44 (1.74)
Jacquetin et al. 2001 [41]	4	51	−0.4 (1.9)
Jonas et al. 1997 [65]	4	44	−1.5 (2)
Khullar et al. 2004 [44]	8	285	−1.1 (2.1)
Madersbacher et al. 1999 [46]	4	72	−0.7 (NA)
Millard et al. 1999 [49]	12	64	−1.3 (2.5)
Rackley et al. 2006 [51]	12	421	−0.01 (NA)
Robinson et al. 2007 [53]	8	61	−0.66 (NA)
Rudy et al. 2006 [55]	12	329	−1.7 (NA)
Cardozo et al. 2008 [66]	16	224	−1.4 (NA)
Uchida et al. 2002 [58]	6	53	−1.3 (NA)
Van Kerrebroeck et al. 2001 [59]	13	508	−0.99 (NA)
Yamaguchi et al. 2007 [61]	12	406	−0.72 (1.95)
Zinner et al. 2004 [62]	12	261	−1.9 (NA)
Zinner et al. 2005 [67]	2	76	−0.91 (NA)

From Mangera et al. [17], with permission

When examining the effect of placebo in the treatment of OAB, it is important to determine the role of neurophysiology and the brain in the development of the disease. Magnetic resonance imaging scans have showed increased brain activity associated with the urge to void and suppression of that urge [70]. One can wonder if the significant placebo effect in the treatment of OAB points toward the brain's role in OAB. First desire to void has also been noted to be associated with increased oxyhemoglobin concentrations in both frontal lobes; it is therefore possible that placebo may play a role in modulating the CNS component of OAB [71]. This idea can be extended to examining the role of bladder training and bladder drill in managing OAB. A behavioral effect on the CNS may explain why some patients respond better to this treatment modality than others [71].

Table 3.3 Micturition episodes per day after placebo treatment in patients with OAB

Study	Study duration (week)	Patients receiving placebo (*n*)	Change in mean number of incontinence episodes per day (SD)
Abrams et al. 1998 [27]	12	57	−1.6 (3.6)
Cardozo et al. 2004 [29]	12	301	−1.59 (NA)
Chapple et al. 2004 [63]	12	183	−1.42 (NA)
Chapple et al. 2004 [31]	12	267	−1.2 (3.26)
Dmochowski et al. 2002 [33]	12	132	−1.7 (3)
Dmochowski et al. 2003 [34]	12	117	−1.4 (2.7)
Dorschner et al. 2003 [36]	4	49	−0.06 (NA)
Drutz et al. 1999 [37]	12	56	−1.1 (2.9)
Jacquetin et al. 2001 [41]	4	51	−1.2 (2.7)
Jonas et al. 1997 [65]	4	44	−0.6 (NA)
Jünemann et al. 2000 [43]	3	79	−1.9 (NA)
Khullar et al. 2004 [44]	8	285	−1.3 (2.3)
Lee et al. 2006 [45]	12	88	−2.58 (NA)
Madersbacher et al. 1999 [46]	4	72	−1 (NA)
Millard et al. 1999 [49]	12	64	−1.4 (2.3)
Moore et al.1990 [68]	>78	25	1.2 (NA)
Rackley et al. 2006 [51]	12	421	−1.46 (NA)
Riva et al. 1984 [69]	2.86	30	−0.79(NA)
Robinson et al. 2007 [53]	8	61	−1.81
Rudy et al. 2006 [55]	12	329	−1.76 (NA)
Cardozo et al. 2008 [66]	16	224	−1.3(NA)
Thüroff et al. 1991 [57]	4	52	−0.3 (NA)
Uchida et al. 2002 [58]	6	53	−1 (NA)
Van Kerrebroeck et al. 2001 [59]	13	508	2.2 (4)
Yamaguchi et al. 2007 [61]	12	406	−0.94 (2.29)
Zinner et al. 2004 [62]	12	261	−1.29 (NA)
Zinner et al. 2005 [67]	2	76	−0.85 (NA)

From Mangera et al. [17], with permission

From this review, it is clear that we can only postulate why placebo treatment has shown such a large effect on the parameters usually examined in OAB. One of the possible trial designs to control the placebo effect was proposed by Staskin et al. They proposed that an emphasis be placed on a "non-drug" group: a cohort of patients involved in the trial would be given the same information, bladder training, and tests to complete, as the group given medication [72]. Another idea proposed by these authors was the use of a nocebo group, balancing the placebo group and presenting information to subjects to suggest that the treatment could "make them better, not affect them or make them worse." This would be one way to counteract the positive expectation bias noted in placebo groups.

When looking at the data, it is important to distinguish between statistically significant findings and findings that are clinically meaningful for one's treatment of

OAB. Both the meta-analyses by Lee et al. and Magnera et al. reported an average decrease in micturition episodes by one void/day. Even though it is statistically significant, it is unlikely to have a large impact on one's QOL. QOL parameters are extremely important to keep in mind when examining OAB data, because this is primarily a quality-of-life disorder. However, it is important to keep in mind that QOL assessments are generally performed on self-administered questionnaires, and those measurements are more prone to a placebo effect than classical, more objective measurements. Eickhoff et al. in 2006 described statistical modeling that can be used to account for a placebo effect in QOL responses. This statistical model can be used for analysis of a variety of QOL instruments to provide meaningful interpretation of specific items and the suspected placebo effect [73].

Conclusion

Placebo effects play a significant role in the treatment of OAB. This stems from the fact that treatment of OAB is complex and involves significant behavioral and physiological changes. While placebo effects have a greater impact on subjective versus objective outcome measures, they seem to significantly influence both in OAB. Some of the strategies that may be used in the development of clinical trials to minimize a strong placebo effect are longer experimental periods, stricter patient selection, larger number of subjects, and better-defined objective and subjective outcome measures. A strong placebo effect is a double-edged sword that may lead to the development of a poorly powered clinical trial but may also add to the treatment benefit of therapies for OAB.

References

1. Shapiro AK. Factors contributing to the placebo effect: their implications for psychotherapy. Am J Psychother. 1964;18(Suppl 1):73–88.
2. Colagiuri B, Schenk LA, Kessler MD, Dorsey SG, Colloca L. The placebo effect: from concepts to genes. Neuroscience. 2015;307:171–90.
3. Galton F. Regression towards mediocrity in hereditary stature. J Anthropol Inst G B Irel. 1886;15:246–63.
4. Stewart-Williams S, Podd J. The placebo effect: dissolving the expectancy versus conditioning debate. Psychol Bull. 2004;130(2):324–40.
5. Lundh LG. Suggestion, suggestibility, and the placebo effect. Hypn Int Monogr. 2000;4:71–90.
6. Bootzin R. The role of expectancy in behavior change. In: White L, Tursky B, Schwartz GE, editors. Placebo: theory, research, and mechanisms. New York: Guilford Press; 1985. p. 196–210.
7. Turner JA, Deyo RA, Loeser JD, Von Korff M, Fordyce WE. The importance of placebo effects in pain treatment and research. JAMA. 1994;271(20):1609–14.
8. Kirsch I, Lynn SJ, Vigorito M, Miller RR. The role of cognition in classical and operant conditioning. J Clin Psychol. 2004;60(4):369–92.
9. Ader R, Cohen N. Behaviorally conditioned immunosuppression. Psychosom Med. 1975;37(4):333–40.

10. Di Blasi Z, Harkness E, Ernst E, Georgiou A, Kleijnen J. Influence of context effects on health outcomes: a systematic review. Lancet. 2001;357(9258):757–62.
11. Moerman DE, Jonas WB. Toward a research agenda on placebo. Mind Body Med. 2000;16(1):33–46.
12. Thomas KB. General practice consultations: is there any point in being positive? Br Med J (Clin Res Ed). 1987;294(6581):1200–2.
13. Colloca L, Miller FG. How placebo responses are formed: a learning perspective. Philos Trans R Soc Lond Ser B Biol Sci. 2011;366(1572):1859–69.
14. Meissner K, Distel H, Mitzdorf U. Evidence for placebo effects on physical but not on biochemical outcome parameters: a review of clinical trials. BMC Med. 2007;5:3.
15. Abrams P, Artibani W, Cardozo L, Dmochowski R, van Kerrebroeck P, Sand P; International Continence Society. Reviewing the ICS 2002 terminology report: the ongoing debate. Neurourol Urodyn. 2009;28(4):287.
16. Wein AJ, Rackley RR. Overactive bladder: a better understanding of pathophysiology, diagnosis and management. J Urol. 2006;175(3 Pt 2):S5–10.
17. Mangera A, Chapple CR, Kopp ZS, Plested M. The placebo effect in overactive bladder syndrome. Nat Rev Urol. 2011;8(9):495–503.
18. Gormley EA, Lightner DJ, Burgio KL, Chai TC, Clemens JQ, Culkin DJ, et al.; American Urological Association; Society of Urodynamics, Female Pelvic Medicine & Urogenital Reconstruction. Diagnosis and treatment of overactive bladder (non-neurogenic) in adults: AUA/SUFU guideline. J Urol. 2012;188(6 Suppl):2455–63.
19. Nicolson P, Kopp Z, Chapple CR, Kelleher C. It's just the worry about not being able to control it! A qualitative study of living with overactive bladder. Br J Health Psychol. 2008;13(Pt 2):343–59.
20. Fantl JA, Wyman JF, McClish DK, Harkins SW, Elswick RK, Taylor JR, Hadley EC. Efficacy of bladder training in older women with urinary incontinence. JAMA. 1991;265(5):609–13.
21. Nabi G, Cody JD, Ellis G, Herbison P, Hay-Smith J. Anticholinergic drugs versus placebo for overactive bladder syndrome in adults. Cochrane Database Syst Rev. 2006;4:CD003781.
22. Herschorn S, Chapple CR, Snijder R, Siddiqui E, Cardozo L. Could reduced fluid intake cause the placebo effect seen in overactive bladder clinical trials? Analysis of a large solifenacin integrated database. Urology. 2017;106:55–9.
23. Haylen BT, de Ridder D, Freeman RM, Swift SE, Berghmans B, Lee J, et al.; International Urogynecological Association; International Continence Society. An International Urogynecological Association (IUGA)/International Continence Society (ICS) joint report on the terminology for female pelvic floor dysfunction. Neurourol Urodyn. 2010;29(1):4–20.
24. Hashim H, Abrams P. How should patients with an overactive bladder manipulate their fluid intake? BJU Int. 2008;102(1):62–6.
25. Zinner NR, Ammann LP, Haas GP, Janning SW, He W, Bukofzer S. Finding unrecognized information in overactive bladder clinical trial data: a new approach to understanding placebo and treatment effects. Neurourol Urodyn. 2013;32(4):308–13.
26. Lee S, Malhotra B, Creanga D, Carlsson M, Glue P. A meta-analysis of the placebo response in antimuscarinic drug trials for overactive bladder. BMC Med Res Methodol. 2009;9:55.
27. Abrams P, Freeman R, Anderström C, Mattiasson A. Tolterodine, a new antimuscarinic agent: as effective but better tolerated than oxybutynin in patients with an overactive bladder. Br J Urol. 1998;81(6):801–10.
28. Burgio KL, Locher JL, Goode PS, Hardin JM, McDowell BJ, Dombrowski M, Candib D. Behavioral vs drug treatment for urge urinary incontinence in older women: a randomized controlled trial. JAMA. 1998;280(23):1995–2000.
29. Cardozo L, Lisec M, Millard R, van Vierssen TO, Kuzmin I, et al. Randomized, double-blind placebo controlled trial of the once daily antimuscarinic agent solifenacin succinate in patients with overactive bladder. J Urol. 2004;172(5 Pt 1):1919–24.
30. Chapple CR, Araño P, Bosch JL, De Ridder D, Kramer AE, Ridder AM. Solifenacin appears effective and well tolerated in patients with symptomatic idiopathic detrusor overactivity in a placebo- and tolterodine-controlled phase 2 dose-finding study. BJU Int. 2004;93(1):71–7.

31. Chapple CR, Rechberger T, Al-Shukri S, Meffan P, Everaert K, Huang M, Ridder A; YM-905 Study Group. Randomized, double-blind placebo-and tolterodine-controlled trial of the once-daily antimuscarinic agent solifenacin in patients with symptomatic overactive bladder. BJU Int. 2004;93(3):303–10.
32. Chapple C, Van Kerrebroeck P, Tubaro A, Haag-Molkenteller C, Forst HT, et al. Clinical efficacy, safety, and tolerability of once-daily fesoterodine in subjects with overactive bladder. Eur Urol. 2007;52(4):1204–12.
33. Dmochowski RR, Davila GW, Zinner NR, Gittelman MC, Saltzstein DR, Lyttle S, Sanders SW; Transdermal Oxybutynin Study Group. Efficacy and safety of transdermal oxybutynin in patients with urge and mixed urinary incontinence. J Urol. 2002;168(2):580–6.
34. Dmochowski RR, Sand PK, Zinner NR, Gittelman MC, Davila GW, Sanders SW; Transdermal Oxybutynin Study Group. Comparative efficacy and safety of transdermal oxybutynin and oral tolterodine versus placebo in previously treated patients with urge and mixed urinary incontinence. Urology. 2003;62(2):237–42.
35. Dmochowski R, Sand P, Zinner NR, Staskin DR. Trospium chloride 60 mg once daily (QD) for overactive bladder syndrome: results of a placebo-controlled interventional study. Urology. 2008;71(3):449–54.
36. Dorschner W, Stolzenburg JU, Griebenow R, Halaska M, Brünjes R, Frank M, Wieners F. The elderly patient with urge incontinence or urge-stress incontinence–efficacy and cardiac safety of propiverine. Aktuelle Urol. 2003;34(2):102–8. (Article in German).
37. Drutz HP, Appell RA, Gleason D, Klimberg I, Radomski S. Clinical efficacy and safety of tolterodine compared to oxybutynin and placebo in patients with overactive bladder. Int Urogynecol J Pelvic Floor Dysfunct. 1999;10(5):283–9.
38. Halaska M, Dorschner W, Frank M. Treatment of urgency and incontinence in elderly patients with propiverine hydrochloride. Neurourol Urodyn. 1994;13:428–30.
39. Herschorn S, Heessakkers J, Castro-Diaz D, Brodsky M. Tolterodine extended release (TER) improves objective and subjective outcomes after 1 week of treatment in patients with overactive bladder (OAB) (abstract). Int Urogynecol J. 1994;18(Suppl 1):S78.
40. Homma Y, Paick JS, Lee JG, Kawabe K. Clinical efficacy and tolerability of extended-release tolterodine and immediate release oxybutynin in Japanese and Korean patients with an overactive bladder: a randomized, placebo-controlled trial. BJU Int. 2003;92(7):741–7.
41. Jacquetin B, Wyndaele J. Tolterodine reduces the number of urge incontinence episodes in patients with an overactive bladder. Eur J Obstet Gynecol Reprod Biol. 2001;98(1):97–102.
42. Jünemann KP, Al-Shukri S. Efficacy and tolerability of trospium chloride and tolterodine in 234 patients with urge syndrome: a double-blind, placebo-controlled, multicentre clinical trial. Neurourol Urodyn. 2000;19(4):488–90.
43. Jünemann KP, Hessdörfer E, Unamba-Oparah I, Berse M, Brünjes R, Madersbacher H, Gramatté T. Propiverine hydrochloride immediate and extended release: comparison of efficacy and tolerability in patients with overactive bladder. Urol Int. 2006;77(4):334–9.
44. Khullar V, Hill S, Laval KU, Schiøtz HA, Jonas U, Versi E. Treatment of urge-predominant mixed urinary incontinence with tolterodine extended release a randomized, placebo-controlled trial. Urology. 2004;64(2):269–74. discussion 274–5
45. Lee KS, Choo MS, Paick JS, Lee JG, Seo JT, Lee JZ, et al. Propiverine hydrochloride reduced frequency and perception of urgency in treatment of overactive bladder: a 12 week prospective, randomized, double-blind, placebo controlled study (Abstract 279). International Continence Society; 29 Nov–1 Dec 2006; Christchurch, New Zealand.
46. Madersbacher H, Halaska M, Voigt R, Alloussi S, Hofner K. A placebo-controlled, multicentre study comparing the tolerability and efficacy of propiverine and oxybutynin in patients with urgency and urge incontinence. BJU Int. 1999;84(6):646–51.
47. Malone-Lee JG, Walsh JB, Maugourd MF. Tolterodine: a safe and effective treatment for older patients with overactive bladder. J Am Geriatr Soc. 2001;49(6):700–5.
48. Malone-Lee J, Whately-Smith C. A study of the significance of identifying detrusor instability in the treatment of overactive bladder symptoms (abstract 228). International Continence Society 2002; Heidelberg, Germany; 28–30 Aug 2002.

49. Millard R, Tuttle J, Moore K, Susset J, Clarke B, Dwyer P, Davis BE. Clinical efficacy and safety of tolterodine compared to placebo in detrusor overactivity. J Urol. 1999;161(5):1551–5.
50. Nitti VW, Dmochowski R, Sand PK, Forst HT, Haag-Molkenteller C, Massow U, et al. Efficacy, safety, and tolerability of fesoterodine in subjects with overactive bladder. J Urol. 2007;178(6):2488–94.
51. Rackley R, Weiss JP, Rovner ES, Wang JT, Guan Z; 037 STUDY GROUP. Nighttime dosing with tolterodine reduces overactive bladder-related nocturnal micturitions in patients with overactive bladder and nocturia. Urology. 2006;67(4):731–6.
52. Rentzhog L, Stanton SL, Cardozo L, Nelson E, Fall M, Abrams P. Efficacy and safety of tolterodine in patients with detrusor instability. Br J Urol. 1998;81(1):42–8.
53. Robinson D, Cardozo L, Terpstra G, Bolodeoku J. A randomized double-blind placebo-controlled multicentre study to explore the efficacy and safety of tamsulosin and tolterodine in women with overactive bladder syndrome. BJU Int. 2007;100(4):840–5.
54. Rogers R, Bachmann G, Jumadilova Z, Sun F, Morrow JD, Guan Z, Bavendam T. Efficacy of tolterodine on overactive bladder symptoms and sexual and emotional quality of life in sexually active women. Int Urogynecol J Pelvic Floor Dysfunct. 2008;19(11):1551–7.
55. Rudy D, Cline K, Harris R, Goldberg K, Dmochowski R. Multicenter phase III trial studying trospium chloride in patients with overactive bladder. Urology. 2006;67(2):275–80.
56. Staskin D, Sand P, Zinner N, Dmochowski R. Once daily trospium chloride is effective and well tolerated for the treatment of overactive bladder: results from a multicenter phase III trial. J Urol. 2007;178(3 Pt 1):978–83.
57. Thüroff JW, Bunke B, Ebner A, Faber P, de Geeter P, Hannappel J, et al. Randomized, double-blind, multicenter trial on treatment of frequency, urgency and incontinence related to detrusor hyperactivity: oxybutynin versus propantheline versus placebo. J Urol. 1991;145(4):813–6; discussion 816–7.
58. Uchida T, Tempel D, Ridge S, Grimes I, Smith N. US PII study results: efficacy and safety of YM905, a bladder-selective treatment for OAB (abstract). Int Urogynecol J. 2002;13:S12.
59. Van Kerrebroeck P, Kreder K, Jonas U, Zinner N, Wein A; Tolterodine Study Group. Tolterodine once-daily: superior efficacy and tolerability in the treatment of the overactive bladder. Urology. 2001;57(3):414–21.
60. Wang A, Chih S, Chen M. Comparison of electric stimulation and oxybutynin chloride in management of overactive bladder with special reference to urinary urgency: a randomized placebo-controlled trial. Urology. 2006;68(5):999–1004.
61. Yamaguchi O, Marui E, Kakizaki H, Itoh N, Yokota T, Okada H, et al.; Japanese Solifenacin Study Group. Randomized, double-blind, placebo-and propiverine-controlled trial of the once-daily antimuscarinic agent solifenacin in Japanese patients with overactive bladder. BJU Int. 2007;100(3):579–87.
62. Zinner N, Gittelman M, Harris R, Susset J, Kanellos A, Auerbach S. Trospium chloride improves overactive bladder symptoms: a multicenter phase III trial. J Urol. 2004;171(6 Pt 1):2311–5. quiz 2435
63. Chapple C. Fesoterodine a new effective and well-tolerated antimuscarinic for the treatment of urgency-frequency syndrome: results of a phase 2 controlled study (Abstract 142). International Continence Society 2004; Paris, France; 27 Aug 2004.
64. Homma Y, Koyama N. Minimal clinically important change in urinary incontinence detected by a quality of life assessment tool in overactive bladder syndrome with urge incontinence. Neurourol Urodyn. 2006;25(3):228–35.
65. Jonas U, Höfner K, Madersbacher H, Holmdahl TH. Efficacy and safety of two doses of tolterodine versus placebo in patients with detrusor overactivity and symptoms of frequency, urge incontinence, and urgency: urodynamic evaluation. The International Study Group. World J Urol. 1997;15(2):144–51.
66. Cardozo L, Hessdörfer E, Milani R, Arañó P, Dewilde L, et al.; SUNRISE Study Group. Solifenacin in the treatment of urgency and other symptoms of overactive bladder: results from a randomized, double-blind, placebo-controlled, rising-dose trial. BJU Int. 2008;102(9):1120–7.

67. Zinner N, Tuttle J, Marks L. Efficacy and tolerability of darifenacin, a muscarinic M3 selective receptor antagonist (M3 SRA), compared with oxybutynin in the treatment of patients with overactive bladder. World J Urol. 2005;23(4):248–52.
68. Moore KH, Hay DM, Imrie AE, Watson A, Goldstein M. Oxybutynin hydrochloride (3 mg) in the treatment of women with idiopathic detrusor instability. Br J Urol. 1990;66(5):479–85.
69. Riva D, Casolati E. Oxybutynin chloride in the treatment of female idiopathic bladder instability. Results from double blind treatment. Clin Exp Obstet Gynecol. 1984;11(1–2):37–42.
70. Kuhtz-Buschbeck JP, van der Horst C, Pott C, Wolff S, Nabavi A, Jansen O, Jünemann KP. Cortical representation of the urge to void: a functional magnetic resonance imaging study. J Urol. 2005;174(4 Pt 1):1477–81.
71. Matsumoto S, Ishikawa A, Matsumoto S, Homma Y. Brain response provoked by different bladder volumes: a near infrared spectroscopy study. Neurourol Urodyn. 2011;30(4):529–35.
72. Staskin D, Dmochowski R, Serels S, Andoh M, Smith M. Report from a randomized, placebo-controlled study showing significant improvement in urgency and patient-reported outcomes in over-active bladder patients treated with solifenacin. Int Urogynecol J. 2007;18:S73–4.
73. Eickhoff JC. Placebo effect-adjusted assessment of quality of life in placebo-controlled clinical trials. Stat Med. 2008;27(9):1387–402.

Chapter 4
Outcome Measures and Patient Expectations for Overactive Bladder

Gary E. Lemack and Rena D. Malik

Introduction

Several studies have attempted to elucidate the most impactful symptom of OAB on patients' quality of life (Table 4.1) [1–6]. In the National Overactive Bladder Evaluation (NOBLE) Program Survey, an assessment of 919 participants with OAB in the USA, urgency urinary incontinence (UUI) was found to result in significant worse health-related quality of life in women, worse depression and sleep disturbance in men, and overall significantly worse bother [1]. Similarly in the EPIC study, a cross-sectional survey of adults with OAB, lower urinary tract symptoms (LUTS), and urinary incontinence (UI) in five countries, 1434 participants with OAB, both men and women, with UUI experienced significantly more bother than those without any incontinence [3].

Similarly, the FINNO study found that health-related quality of life (HRQoL) was significantly impacted by UUI of any severity and frequency [4] and that patients with UUI can experience social isolation, psychological distress, and fear of leaving home or avoidance of public settings [7]. Elderly women are especially susceptible to impairment in quality of life (QoL) with reports of decrease in energy, increase in pain, emotional and sleep disturbances, social isolation, and mobility problems compared to that of their age-matched peers [8].

While UUI is undoubtedly bothersome, other OAB symptoms have been found to be impactful in other populations. In analysis of the Epidemiology of Lower Urinary Tract Symptoms (EpiLUTS), a cross-sectional population study conducted in the UK, Sweden, and the USA, urinary urgency was significantly associated with OAB symptom bother. In Sweden and the UK, urgency increased the odds of reporting symptom bother by 7.47 in men and 4.83 in women, while frequency, nocturia, and UUI were less impactful [5]. In the US population, urinary urgency was also

G. E. Lemack (✉) · R. D. Malik
Department of Urology, UT Southwestern Medical Center, Dallas, TX, USA
e-mail: gary.lemack@utsouthwestern.edu

L. Cox, E. S. Rovner (eds.), *Contemporary Pharmacotherapy of Overactive Bladder*, https://doi.org/10.1007/978-3-319-97265-7_4

Table 4.1 Trials describing the most bothersome overactive bladder symptom

Trial/author	Study design	*N*	Outcomes	Most bothersome OAB symptom
NOBLE, 2004 [1]	Nested case control study of national cross-sectional survey in the USA	919	OAB-q, SF-36, CES-D, MOS-sleep	Urgency urinary incontinence
IMPACT, 2006 [2]	Multicenter, open-label tx with tolterodine ER x 3 weeks	863	3-day bladder diary, OAB-q, PPBC, AUA-SI	Daytime frequency
EPIC, 2008 [3]	Case-controlled analysis of a population-based, cross-sectional survey of adults in five countries	1,434	PPBC, OAB-V8	Urgency urinary incontinence
FINNO, 2011 [4]	Population-based, cross-sectional survey in Finland	6,000	DAN-PSS, 15D sore	Urgency urinary incontinence
EpiLUTS, 2011 [5]	Population-based, cross-sectional, Internet survey in the Sweden and the UK	10,000	PPBC, OAB-q-SF, SF-12, HADS, overall health rating	Urinary urgency
EpiLUTS, 2012 [6]	Population-based, cross-sectional, Internet survey in the USA	12,374	PPBC, OAB-q-SF, SF-12, HADS, overall health rating	Urinary urgency

AUA-SI American Urological Association Symptom Index, *OAB-V8* Overactive Bladder Awareness Tool, *CES-D* Center for Epidemiologic Studies Depression Scale, *HADS* Hospital Anxiety and Depression Scale, *DAN-PSS* Danish Prostate Symptom Score

strongly correlated with symptom bother in both men (r = 0.65) and women (r = 0.70) [6]. In a review of the Improvement in Patients: Assessing Symptomatic Control with Tolterodine (IMPACT) trial, the most bothersome symptom reported by patients with continent and incontinent OAB was daytime frequency (47.3% and 27.6%, respectively) followed closely by nocturnal frequency (41.8% and 26.3%, respectively) [2]. Nocturia in patients with OAB is highly prevalent; however, its impact on QoL is significantly associated with increasing number of voids per night [9]. Ultimately, OAB symptoms can be associated with a significant degree of bother, but it remains important to elucidate patients' perception of bother associated with their specific symptoms.

Outcome Measures for OAB

A variety of measures have been used to quantify or assess patient symptoms and outcomes following intervention for OAB. Traditional measures include those that can be elicited via patient interview. Specifically, patients are asked to quantify their daily number of voids, incontinence episodes, number of pads used per day, and urgency episodes. This is a commonly utilized outcome measure as it is expeditious and can be completed during taking of the history of the patient. While there may exist some discrepancy in actual incontinence episodes and those reported by the patient, it is likely to reflect the patient's own perception of their incontinence and help guide their expectations in management [10].

Bladder Diaries

For further objective assessment of patient symptoms, patients are often asked to complete a bladder diary (sometimes called a voiding diary or frequency/micturition chart). A bladder diary is a form completed by the patient with instructions to document the time and volume of their fluid intake and voids throughout a 24-h period. Additionally, patients are asked to document sensation of urgency proceeding voids, the presence of incontinence, and the use of incontinence pads or catheterization if needed. Diaries are typically utilized to assess micturition frequency, the number of urinary incontinence episodes and categorization of incontinence as stress or urge, mean voided volume (functional bladder capacity), and number and volume of nocturnal voids [11]. Additionally, bladder diaries will give an accurate assessment of total urine production (and the relative urine excretion during the day and at night) which may help in counseling and treatment.

Typically, bladder diaries are completed for a period of 1 to 7 days, utilizing longer diaries for patients with inconsistent symptoms or fewer daily episodes of urgency or UUI or variable nocturia. While reliability for bladder diaries improves with increasing length of documentation, patient compliance decreases. Hence typically a 3-day diary is deemed sufficient for most patients [12, 13]. These can be completed prior to initiating intervention and at varying time points during treatment to objectively assess improvement in patient symptoms. In addition to serving as a diagnostic tool, bladder diaries can also be therapeutic in increasing patient awareness of the timing of fluid intake and associated frequency, urgency, incontinence, or nocturia. However, bladder diaries can be challenging and inconvenient for patients to complete, particularly those with cognitive, physical or learning disabilities, poor health literacy, or poor fluency in the language in which they are written [14]. Additionally, there is no validated form for the bladder diary; hence they can vary considerably in content, format, duration, and recall period [15].

Patient-Reported Outcomes

While objective measures have an important place in the management of OAB, subjective patient-reported outcome measures have become favored largely as they are more representative of treatment success, particularly with a condition such as OAB which impacts patients largely by affecting QoL. Additionally, while objective measures may show a biologic response, they do not necessarily correlate with patient perception or bother (i.e., Urodynamic evaluation) [16]. Patient-reported outcomes (PROs) define treatment outcomes that are subjectively reported by the patient [17, 18]. They are designed specifically to assess the patient's perception of the impact of disease and/or treatment on overall health and QoL. Over the last several years, PROs have progressively been utilized by regulatory bodies to evaluate new pharmaceuticals either alone or in combination with clinician – reported outcomes – or combined with more objective physiological measures [18]. With regard to OAB, it has become increasingly clear that defining patient expectations prior to intervention can influence subjective outcomes [19]. The use of PROs has thus become commonplace in the management of OAB to assess the patient perception of severity of disease, impact on QoL, symptom frequency, and treatment satisfaction. Furthermore, it has been recommended that a comprehensive evaluation should include, at a minimum, symptoms, patient satisfaction, adverse events, and HRQoL [20].

Patient Questionnaires

A variety of validated surveys, categorized as patient-reported outcomes (PROs), have been used to better characterize patient outcomes related to OAB. There are two major types of PROs: generic and disease-specific. Generic PROs are not specific to one disease type but aim to be applicable to a variety of conditions across a diverse demographic of patients. They are typically well-studied, reliable, and readily available; however, they may not capture all details relevant to a specific condition [21]. Condition-specific PROs are created for one specific condition or diagnosis and typically include questions that are more inclusive of problems cited by patients with that diagnosis. When selecting an appropriate PRO, it's important to select one that is valid, reliable, and responsive for your intended patient population that will measure the outcomes that are valuable to the clinician and patient alike [17, 22, 23].

In 2009, a systematic review of 39 relevant publications was conducted to assess the impact of urinary incontinence and overactive bladder on QoL. Of those assessed, ten included patients with OAB and utilized the SF-12, OAB-q, MOS-SF36, EQ-5d, KHQ, I-QoL, IIQ, and EQ VAS. We have included these and other relevant PROs in our discussion below (Table 4.2) [24–53].

Disease Specific

Questionnaires Focusing on OAB (+/− Incontinence). King's Health Questionnaire (KHQ) The KHQ has undergone a number of revisions with the most current version [25] validated and reliable in both genders and in culturally diverse cohorts. It specifically targets patients with lower urinary tract symptoms

Table 4.2 Patient-reported outcome measures for overactive bladder (OAB)

Name of instrument	Target population	No of items	Recall period	Languages	MCID (points)	Subscales
Questionnaires focusing on OAB						
King's Health Questionnaire (KHQ) [25]	M/F,UI, and OAB	21	Current	Afrikaans, Bulgarian, Cantonese, Czech, Danish, Dutch, English, Estonian, Finnish, French, German, Greek, Hebrew, Hindi, Italian, Japanese, Korean, Latvian, Lithuanian, Malay, Mandarin, Norwegian, Polish, Portuguese, Romanian, Russian, Slovak, Spanish, Swedish, Tagalog, Tamil, Thai, Ukrainian	5	Role limitations, physical limitations, social limitations, personal limitations, emotional problems, sleep/energy disturbance, coping measures, symptom severity, incontinence impact, general health perception
Overactive Bladder questionnaire (OAB-q) [26]	M/F, OAB	33	4 weeks	Afrikaans, Chinese, Danish, English, French, Italian, German, Korean, Norwegian, Polish, Portuguese, Romanian, Slovak, Swedish, and Turkish [27]	10 [28]	Symptom bother, coping, concern, social interaction, sleep
OAB-SF [29]	M/F,OAB	19	4 weeks		–	Symptom bother, HRQoL
Patient Perception of Bladder Condition [30]	M/F, LUTS, and OAB	1	Current	Afrikaans, Chinese, Czech, English, French, Korean, Lithuanian, Slovak, Spanish [31]	–	Global assessment
Primary OAB Symptom questionnaire (POSQ) [32]	M/F, OAB	5	2 weeks	English	–	Symptom bother
Urgency Questionnaire (UQ) [33]	M/F, OAB	19	1 week	English, Portuguese [34]	–	Nocturia, fear of incontinence, time to control urge, impact on daily activities, UU severity, intensity, impact, and discomfort
ICIQ-OAB [35, 36]	M/F, OAB	4	4 weeks	Danish, Dutch, English, Finnish, French, German, Israeli, Italian, Japanese, Korean, Norwegian, Portuguese, Spanish, Swedish, Taiwanese, Tamil, Turkish	–	Frequency, nocturia, urgency, UUI

(continued)

Table 4.2 (continued)

Name of instrument	Target population	No of items	Recall period	Languages	MCID (points)	Subscales
Questionnaires focusing on urinary incontinence						
ICIQ-UI SF [37]	M/F, UI	4	4 weeks	Afrikaans, Arabic, Bulgarian, Czech, Danish, Dutch, English, Estonian, Finnish, French, German, Greek, Hungarian, Icelandic, Italian, Japanese, Norwegian, Polish, Portuguese, Romanian, Russian, Slovakian, Swedish, Turkish, Ukrainian	2.5 [38]	Frequency of UI, amount of leakage, overall impact of UI, self-diagnostic item
Incontinence Impact Questionnaire (IIQ) [39]	F, UI	30	Current	English, Italian, Turkish	–	Physical, activity, travel, social, emotional
IIQ-7 (short form) [40]	F, UI	7	Current	Arabic, Chinese, Dutch, English, French, Malaysian, Polish, Portuguese, Spanish, Turkish	–	Physical, activity, travel, social, emotional
UDI [39]	F, LUTS/prolapse	19	NS	Arabic, English, Swedish	35 [41]	Irritative, stress, obstructive/discomfort
UDI-6 [40]	F, LUTS/prolapse	6	NS	Arabic, Chinese, Dutch, English, French, Malaysian, Polish, Portuguese, Spanish, Turkish	–	Irritative, stress, obstructive/discomfort
Incontinence Quality of Life Questionnaire (I-QoL) [42]	M/F, UI	22	Today	Afrikaans, Danish, Dutch, English, Finnish, French, German, Greek, Hebrew, Italian, Japanese, Korean, Mandarin, Norwegian, Polish, Portuguese, Slovak, Spanish, Swedish	12.1[a] [43]	Avoidance/limiting behaviors, social embarrassment, psychological

Patient satisfaction instruments						
OAB Satisfaction Questionnaire OAB-S [44]	M,F, OAB	21/41	Current	Afrikaans, Chinese, Czech, Danish, English, French, Italian, Lithuanian, Korean, Norwegian, Slovak, Spanish, Swedish, Turkish [27]	–	OAB control expectations, impact on daily living, control, satisfaction with control, medication tolerability, fulfillment of expectations, interruption of day-to-day life, willingness to continue treatment, improvement of life with treatment
Benefit, Satisfaction, and Willingness Questionnaire(BSW) [45]	M/F, OAB	3	Current	English, Korean, Spanish	–	Benefit, satisfaction, willingness to continue with treatment
Treatment Benefit Scale (TBS) [46]	M/F, OAB	1	–	English, Spanish	–	Patient perception of outcome
Subject's Assessment of Treatment Tolerance (SATT) [47]	M/F, OAB	1	–	English	–	Patient tolerance of treatment
Subject's Assessment of Treatment Satisfaction (SATS) [47]	M/F, OAB	1	–	English	–	Patient satisfaction with treatment
Self-Assessment Goal Achievement (SAGA) [48, 49]	M/F, OAB	14	Current	Danish, Dutch, English, Finnish, French, German, Greek, Icelandic, Italian, Norwegian, Spanish, Swedish [50]	–	Importance of symptoms (baseline), goal achievement (follow-up) for lower urinary tract symptoms

(continued)

Table 4.2 (continued)

Name of instrument	Target population	No of items	Recall period	Languages	MCID (points)	Subscales
Generic HRQoL instruments						
Medical Outcomes Study Short Form-36 (SF-36) [51]	Generic QoL	36	4 weeks	121 languages	5	Physical activities, social activities, usual role activities due to physical and emotional problems, bodily pain, general mental health, vitality, and general health perception
MOS 12-Item Health Survey (SF-12)	Generic QoL	12	4 weeks	121 languages	–	Physical activities, social activities, usual role activities due to physical and emotional problems, bodily pain, general mental health, vitality, and general health perception
EQ-5D [52]	Generic QoL	5	Current	170 languages	0.074 [53]	Mobility, self-care, usual activity, social relationships, pain, mood

Adapted from Bartoli et al. [24], with permission

MCID minimal clinically important difference, *HRQoL* health-related quality of life, *UU* urinary urgency, *UUI* urgency urinary incontinence, *UI* urinary incontinence

[a]Mean change in lower responder threshold for improvement in I-QoL total summary score associated with a >50% reduction in incontinence episodes in OAB patients

and overactive bladder [54]. It consists of questions in domains of role limitations, physical limitations, social limitations, personal relationships, emotions, sleep, energy, and severity (coping) measures. It also assesses symptom severity, incontinence impact, and general health perception. It has been translated in 33 languages and validated in culturally appropriate populations in several of the 33 translations.

Overactive Bladder Questionnaire (OAB-q) OAB-q is a 33-item questionnaire that is made up of 8 questions related to symptom bother and 25 specific to HRQoL [26]. Symptom items address both the frequency and bother of frequency, urgency, nocturia, and incontinence symptoms. HRQoL items addressed include coping behaviors, work, commuting and travel, sleep, physical activities, social activities, self-esteem/psychological well-being, relationships, and sexual function. Items are answered using 6-point Likert scales for frequency ranging from "none of the time" to "all of the time" and "not at all" to "a very great deal" for the symptom bother items (in response to how "bothered" were you). The OAB-q is notable for its ability to capture both incontinent and continent OAB and has been validated in diverse populations. It has good psychometric properties including internal consistency, reliability, test-rest reliability, construct validity, and responsiveness to change.

The *Overactive Bladder Questionnaire-Short Form (OAB-SF)* is a shortened version of the OAB-q created to reduce the burden of patients completing the assessment. It includes 19 items, 6 of which evaluate symptom bother and the remaining 13 assess HRQoL [29]. This was recently validated in both community and clinical samples with both incontinent and continent OAB.

Patient Perception of Bladder Condition (PPBC) This is a single-item global bladder questionnaire. On a 6-point scale, patients are asked to rate their perceived bladder condition as 0 = no problems at all to 6 = many severe problems. The PPBC is considered to have good test-retest reliability, and construct validity, as it correlated well with bladder diary variables, the KHQ and OAB-q questionnaires, and reliability. It provides a short and quick assessment of patient perceptions that can ultimately help discussions regarding expectations with treatment of OAB.

Primary OAB Symptom Questionnaire (POSQ) This is a five-item questionnaire, also called the OAB Bother Rating Scale, which aims to delineate the degree of bother associated with OAB symptoms and identify which of the symptoms is most bothersome. While this does not delve into QoL measures, it does allow a validated form for patients to express their most bothersome symptom and therefore allow the clinician to choose a treatment paradigm focused at reducing the impact of that particular symptom [32].

Urgency Questionnaire (UQ) This questionnaire was developed in order to assess the severity of urinary urgency and its impact on HRQoL with a designated recall period of 1 week [33]. It includes four subscales including nocturia, fear of incontinence, time to control urge, and impact on daily activities which are assessed using a 5-point Likert scale as well as four visual analog scales which aim to quantify urinary urgency's severity, intensity, impact, and discomfort. This can be particularly useful in patients with continent OAB as it focuses on urgency and fear of incontinence which can be predominant in this population.

International Consultation on Incontinence Questionnaire-Overactive Bladder (ICIQ-OAB) The International Continence Society (ICS) and International Consultation on Urological Diseases organized the first International Consultation on Incontinence (ICI), in part, in order to develop a universally applicable questionnaire that could be utilized by a variety of populations to assess urinary tract symptoms, named the ICIQ [55]. The ICIQ developed numerous modules relating to specific urinary, vaginal, and bowel symptoms, one of which is the ICIQ-OAB. This is a four-item validated instrument created from two existing validated questionnaires: the ICSmale [36] and the Bristol Female Lower Urinary Tract Symptoms (BFLUTS) Questionnaire [35]. It aims to assess the presence of and bother related to urinary frequency, nocturia, urgency, and incontinence. It is scored from 0 to 16 with greater values indicating worse severity of symptoms.

Questionnaires Focusing on Incontinence

There are numerous available PRO measures for incontinence, varying from those that are generic in terms of impact on QoL and others which specifically address particular features associated with incontinence (i.e., male incontinence, stress urinary incontinence, etc.) We selected those that are commonly used for patients with OAB to review in this chapter.

International Consultation on Incontinence Questionnaire-Urinary Incontinence-Short Form (ICIQ-UI-SF) This is a three-item questionnaire with one self-assessment that assesses the degree and impact of urinary incontinence [37]. This has been shown to be associated with the KHQ and number of UUI episodes on bladder diary and subsequently useful for patients with incontinent OAB. This may however not be ideal for "dry" OAB patients.

Incontinence Impact Questionnaire (IIQ) The IIQ consists of 30 items, 24 of which relate to the impact on UI on a number of daily activities (i.e., shopping, recreation, activity) and 6 of which assess patient feelings associated with UI (i.e., frustration, fear, anger). Each item is answered on a scale of 0 to 4 in relation to how greatly UI impacts the activity or feeling (0 = not at all to 4 = greatly). The IIQ divides the questions into four subscales including activity (six items), travel (six items), social relationships (ten items), and emotional health (eight items). Total scoring of the IIQ is on a scale of 400 points similar to that of the UDI (see below) [39]. The *IIQ-7* is shortened version which includes the same subscales in a shortened format of seven questions to reduce patient burden and convenience in a clinical setting [40].

Urogenital Distress Inventory (UDI) The UDI consists of 19 items which assesses the presence and degree of bother associated with urinary incontinence. The items are graded on a Likert scale associated with degree of bother (0 = not at all to 4 = greatly). The items are subcategorized into three subscales including irritative symptoms (6 items), obstructive/discomfort (11 items), and stress symptoms (2 items). When calculated, the total score of all three subscales is summed to give a value on a scale of 0–300 and provides equal weighting to all subscales [39]. The *UDI-6* is a shortened form utilizing the same subscales (two questions per category) which has good psychometric properties [40].

Both the UDI and IIQ were validated utilizing a relatively homogenous group of women that were predominantly Caucasian and high school graduates, considered mentally competent (MMSE >23) with at least one episode of urinary incontinence a week. Both were scientifically confirmed to be reliable, valid, and sensitive to change.

Incontinence-Specific Quality of Life Measure (I-QoL) This validated PRO was created to assess QoL of both men and women with all subtypes and severities of urinary incontinence [42]. It includes 22 items addressing 3 major subscales including avoidance and limiting behaviors (8 items), psychosocial impacts (9 items), and social embarrassment (5 items) on a 4-point Likert scale utilizing language created by patient interviews. It has been further utilized in a variety of patient populations and specifically demonstrated as reliable, valid, and responsive in patients with OAB and UI, particularly in patients who have failed first-line anticholinergic therapy [43].

Patient Satisfaction Instruments

Overactive Bladder Treatment Satisfaction Questionnaire [44] (OAB-S). The OAB-S was developed to evaluate patient satisfaction with pharmacologic and non-pharmacologic treatment of OAB. It was developed in the USA utilizing English- and Spanish-speaking patients with a diagnosis of OAB undergoing treatment with antimuscarinics. It consists of five subscales including OAB control expectations (ten items), impact on daily living with OAB (ten items), OAB control (ten items), satisfaction with control (ten items), and OAB medication tolerability (six items) in addition to five stand-alone items regarding fulfillment of expectations, interruption of day-to-day life, willingness to continue treatment, and improvement of life with treatment. The questionnaire can be administered pretreatment (21 items) or post-treatment (41 items).

Several, single-item patient-reported outcomes have been developed to assess patient satisfaction of treatment. Those include the *Treatment Benefit Scale (TBS)*, the *Subject's Assessment of Treatment Tolerance (SATT)*, and the *Subject's Assessment of Treatment Satisfaction (SATS)*. The TBS is a single-item question which assesses the patient perception of their treatment outcome. It is a validated OAB-specific measure which asks patients to evaluate their change in condition from prior assessment after undergoing treatment on a scale of 1, greatly improved, to 4, worsened during treatment [46]. The SATT asks patients to rate their tolerance of the treatment provided from 1, inadequate, to 4, excellent [47]. While this does not relate specifically to patient outcomes with treatment, it discriminated between patients who did or did not experience adverse events with medication treatment for OAB. The SATS allows the patient to rate their overall satisfaction with treatment on a range from 1, extremely satisfied, to 4, not satisfied [47].

Benefit, Satisfaction, and Willingness Questionnaire (BSW) The BSW is an investigator/clinician-administered tool that can be utilized to evaluate patients' perceptions of treatment outcomes [45]. It is comprised of three items: (1) perceived benefit with a response of no/little/much benefit, (2) treatment satisfaction with a yes or no response followed by a qualification of little or very satisfied/dissatisfied, and (3) willingness to continue with responses similar to that of satisfaction question. While not specifically asked, the assumption is that the patient will consider the risks and benefits associated with treatment to provide a response including side effects, cost, convenience in addition to symptom relief, and impact on QoL.

Self-Assessment Goal Achievement (SAGA) The SAGA was developed as a means to create a validated instrument which providers can utilize to allow patients to clearly identify their treatment goals in both clinical and research practice [48]. It is designed with the intention to allow patients to selectively answer questions regarding symptoms or complaints which are of importance to them and provide open-ended answers to individualize their goals for treatment. The SAGA consists of two modules, the first made up of nine questions relating the symptoms of frequency; sensation of pressure leading to use the bathroom; voiding; starting or maintaining a urine stream; urine loss when coughing, exercising, and sneezing; urine leakage; and urgency. Additionally, it includes five open-ended questions. On the baseline and follow-up modules, patients are asked to specify the importance of the goal and level of goal achievement, respectively, on a 5-point Likert scale [49]. Goal achievement on the follow-up module of the SAGA was shown to be associated with better HRQoL and fewer symptoms. However, follow-up goal achievement had low-to-moderate correlation with other validated surveys which assess patients' impression of the impact of their symptoms and their HRQoL at baseline.

Generic HRQoL Instruments

Generic measures are widely available and utilized for application in a wide range of patient populations and conditions. They are often unable to assess the true impact on QoL of patients with UI with lacking detail on social embarrassment, avoidance behavior, psychosocial impact, sleep, and impact on sexuality [56]. Therefore, they are often used in combination with condition-specific measures for patient assessment.

Short Form Health Survey (SF-36) This generic HRQoL assessment was created to produce a comprehensive evaluation of patient well-being and perception of general health [51, 57, 58]. It evaluates eight domains to assess limitation in physical activities (ten items), social activities (two items), usual role activities due to physical (four items) and emotional problems (three items), bodily pain (two items), general mental health (five items), vitality (four items), and general health perception (five items). From those, two aggregate summary measures are created: the physical component summary (PCS) and the mental component summary (MCS). It has been tested in patients with a spectrum of socioeconomic characteristics, diagnoses, and disease severity. The *SF-12* is an abbreviated version with only 12 questions of the same 8 domains selected to reproduce the PCS and MCS subscales. The PCS and MCS subscales are scored from 0 to 100 with higher scores indicating better health status.

EuroQol EQ-5D This is an instrument which measures general HRQoL in six dimensions, mobility, self-care, usual activity, pain, and mood [52]. For each item, the respondent is asked to rate the degree of problems as no problems, mild/moderate problems, or severe problems. It provides a composite index score which ranges from 0 to 100 or worst to best imaginable health state. While it was initially created and validated in multiple European countries, it has since been validated in the adult US populations. The *EQ VAS* is a part of the EQ-5d, which records the patient's self-perceived health on a visual analog scale.

International Consortium for Health Outcomes Measurement (ICHOM) Core Measures for OAB Treatment

The ICHOM is a nonprofit organization that convenes international working groups with clinicians, researchers, and patients to define standardized outcomes for medical conditions [59]. Recently, the ICHOM published a core group of outcome measures to recommend as standard in management of OAB patients [60]. These were determined by systematic literature review and structured patient group discussions and scored using the Grades of Recommendation, Assessment, Development, and Evaluation (GRADE) scale [61] and reviewed according to the International Society for Quality of Life Research (ISOQOL) guidelines [62]. Recommendations were the inclusion of case-mix factors, specifically, age, sex, BMI, presence of comorbid bowel conditions, diabetes, cognitive impairment, pelvic organ prolapse, BPH or prostatitis, history of pelvic surgery, and current use of estrogens or OAB treatments. Patient-reported outcome measurements (PROMs) included in the standard set are the ICIQ-OAB, OAB-Q SF, ICIQ-FLUTSsex or ICIQ-MLUTSsex, and the TBS. They include a suggested follow-up timeline with case-mix factors and PROMs collected at baseline and follow-up with PROMs and treatment satisfaction and tolerance measures at intervals based on clinician judgment. Success is suggested to be determined by patient definition and positive responses on the TBS.

ICIQ-Female/Male Sexual Matters Associated with Lower Urinary Tract Symptoms (ICIQ-FLUTSsex/ICIQ-MLUTSsex) These are four-item questionnaires as part of the ICIQ module aimed to evaluate sexual matters associated with lower urinary tract symptoms in men and women. In women, it is derived from the previously published BFLUTS [35] and assesses the impact of urinary symptoms, presence of pain or urinary leakage from sexual intercourse, and pain or discomfort due to "dry vagina." In men, it is derived from the ICSmale short form [63] and includes items regarding the possibility of erections/orgasms, presence of pain or discomfort during ejaculation, and the impact of urinary symptoms.

Urodynamics

Multichannel urodynamic evaluation, while not required, can sometimes be undertaken in patients with OAB providing details on evidence of detrusor overactivity, early bladder sensation, and reduced maximum cystometric capacity. While previously considered mandatory, evidence of detrusor overactivity is not seen in patients with symptoms suggestive of OAB in up to 20–46% of urodynamic evaluations completed [64, 65]. When completed for usual standard of care, urodynamic evaluation (UDS) prior to and after treatment of OAB, improvement in previous parameters can be utilized as an outcome measure for OAB. In patients with detrusor overactivity, resolution of detrusor overactivity or increase in bladder volume prior to the presence of an involuntary detrusor contraction can be considered improvement. Additionally, increased volume at first sensation or sense of urgency and increase in maximum cystometric capacity can also be used to demonstrate physiological changes that are considered to be consistent with overall improvements in OAB. While UDS does provide quantitative measurement of physiological "improvement," these findings clearly do not always correlate with patient satisfaction. Thus failure to show urodynamic improvement does not necessarily imply failure of an intervention, and thus incorporating its use into routine outcome assessment may be unnecessary and unfruitful.

Cost

Costs associated with the management of OAB are significant – with direct costs related to medical consultations, diagnostics, medications, and incontinence pads. In addition, there are numerous indirect costs related to loss of productivity at work, work absenteeism, associated clinical depression, and resulting falls and injuries related to rushing to the restroom. In the aforementioned EPIC study, direct costs ranged from 333 million to 1.2 billion per country and 4.7 billion for associated nursing home costs and 1.1 billion related to work absenteeism [66]. In 2000, the cost associated with OAB was estimated to be 12.02 billion [67].

Reduction in cost (economic or specific to the patient) with treatment can be viewed as an outcome measure. Limited data exists on this topic. An analysis of 275 elderly OAB patients was done to assess anticholinergic adherence utilizing administrative claims data and its association with healthcare costs. These authors found that increased adherence was associated with a significant decrease in cost [68]. However, this finding may be due to worse OAB disease severity resulting in non-response to anticholinergics and subsequent nonadherence. The use of intravesical onabotulinumtoxinA for overactive bladder was assessed in a cost-consequence analysis of 101 patients in the UK in comparison to standard of care (i.e., physician visits, relevant diagnostic tests, continuation of anticholinergics, as well as costs incurred by patients/employers due to loss of work and transportation). These authors found the cost-effectiveness ratio (CER), or cost per quality-adjusted life year gained (QALY), of £510 for patients with idiopathic OAB per improved patient-year relative to standard care [69]. This is significantly lower than the CER threshold defined by the National Institute for Health and Care Excellence of £20,000–£30,000 per QALY proving the cost-effectiveness of treatment [70].

Patient Pre-set Expectations

Despite the variety of tools available to provide qualitative and quantitative measures of improvement in patient outcomes, arguably the most valuable is determination of patient's expectations prior to treatment. They have been described as "powerful predictors of treatment outcomes" as they are largely related to the placebo effect [19]. Patient expectations can have a significant impact on their perception of symptoms as patients fixate on certain symptoms and ignore others with waxing and waning intensity based on motivation, anxiety, or other coexisting factors. Patient expectations can be variable depending on patient subjective desires (i.e., to sleep through the night versus to reduce incontinent episodes during the day) and their comorbid conditions and baseline health and QoL. It is vital to clearly identify this on the first patient encounter and utilize shared decision-making to determine a treatment that will aim to meet their expectations to a reasonable degree. Ultimately it remains the provider's responsibility to assess if that selected treatment is meeting the patient expectations. This certainly is an area for future exploration.

Conclusions

With a variety of outcome measures available to the practicing clinician, it is challenging to select one that is expeditious, easy to understand, and complete and provides a thorough assessment of the patient satisfaction or outcome.

Still, to optimize patient care and satisfaction, it is imperative to assess patient expectations in order to provide appropriate counseling focusing on realistic outcomes the patient can expect following intervention. Choosing a practical outcome measure for one's own particular practice, focusing on at least one PRO, seems reasonable in order to improve overall patient satisfaction.

References

1. Coyne KS, Payne C, Bhattacharyya SK, Revicki DA, Thompson C, Corey R, Hunt TL. The impact of urinary urgency and frequency on health-related quality of life in overactive bladder: results from a national community survey. Value Health. 2004;7(4):455–63.
2. Artibani W. Outcomes in overactive bladder treatment: patient perception – a key to success. Eur Urol Suppl. 2007;6:17–22.
3. Irwin DE, Milsom I, Kopp Z, Abrams P; EPIC Study Group. Symptom bother and health care–seeking behavior among individuals with overactive bladder. Eur Urol. 2008;53(5):1029–39.
4. Vaughan CP, Johnson TM 2nd, Ala-Lipasti MA, Cartwright R, Tammela TL, Taari K, et al. The prevalence of clinically meaningful overactive bladder: bother and quality of life results from the population-based FINNO study. Eur Urol. 2011;59(4):629–36.
5. Coyne KS, Sexton CC, Kopp ZS, Ebel-Bitoun C, Milsom I, Chapple C. The impact of overactive bladder on mental health, work productivity and health-related quality of life in the UK and Sweden: results from EpiLUTS. BJU Int. 2011;108(9):1459–71.
6. Milsom I, Kaplan SA, Coyne KS, Sexton CC, Kopp ZS. Effect of bothersome overactive bladder symptoms on health-related quality of life, anxiety, depression, and treatment seeking in the United States: results from EpiLUTS. Urology. 2012;80(1):90–6.
7. Norton PA, MacDonald LD, Sedgwick PM, Stanton SL. Distress and delay associated with urinary incontinence, frequency, and urgency in women. BMJ. 1988;297(6657):1187–9.
8. Grimby A, Milsom I, Molander U, Wiklund I, Ekelund P. The influence of urinary incontinence on the quality of life of elderly women. Age Ageing. 1993;22(2):82–9.
9. Coyne KS, Zhou Z, Bhattacharyya SK, Thompson CL, Dhawan R, Versi E. The prevalence of nocturia and its effect on health-related quality of life and sleep in a community sample in the USA. BJU Int. 2003;92(9):948–54.
10. Kenton K, FitzGerald MP, Brubaker L. What is a clinician to do – believe the patient or her urinary diary? J Urol. 2006;176(2):633–5.
11. Lose G, Fantl JA, Victor A, Walter S, Wells TL, Wyman J, Mattiasson A. Outcome measures for research in adult women with symptoms of lower urinary tract dysfunction. Neurourol Urodyn. 1998;17(3):255–62.
12. van Haarst EP, Bosch JL. The optimal duration of frequency-volume charts related to compliance and reliability. Neurourol Urodyn. 2014;33(3):296–301.
13. Dmochowski RR, Sanders SW, Appell RA, Nitti VW, Davila GW. Bladder-health diaries: an assessment of 3-day vs 7-day entries. BJU Int. 2005;96(7):1049–54.
14. Ku JH, Jeong IG, Lim DJ, Byun SS, Paick JS, Oh SJ. Voiding diary for the evaluation of urinary incontinence and lower urinary tract symptoms: prospective assessment of patient compliance and burden. Neurourol Urodyn. 2004;23(4):331–5.
15. Bright E, Drake MJ, Abrams P. Urinary diaries: evidence for the development and validation of diary content, format, and duration. Neurourol Urodyn. 2011;30(3):348–52.
16. Abrams P, Artibani W, Gajewski JB, Hussain I. Assessment of treatment outcomes in patients with overactive bladder: importance of objective and subjective measures. Urology. 2006;68(2 Suppl):17–28.
17. Acquadro C, Berzon R, Dubois D, Leidy NK, Marquis P, Revicki D, Rothman M; PRO Harmonization Group. Incorporating the patient's perspective into drug development and

communication: an ad hoc task force report of the Patient-Reported Outcomes (PRO) harmonization group meeting at the food and drug administration, February 16, 2001. Value Health. 2003;6(5):522–31.

18. Willke RJ, Burke LB, Erickson P. Measuring treatment impact: a review of patient-reported outcomes and other efficacy endpoints in approved product labels. Control Clin Trials. 2004;25(6):535–52.
19. Marschall-Kehrel D, Roberts RG, Brubaker L. Patient-reported outcomes in overactive bladder: the influence of perception of condition and expectation for treatment benefit. Urology. 2006;68(2 Suppl):29–37.
20. Cotterill N, Goldman H, Kelleher C, Kopp Z, Tubaro A, Brubaker L. What are the best outcome measures when assessing treatments for LUTD? – achieving the most out of outcome evaluation: ICI-RS 2011. Neurourol Urodyn. 2012;31(3):400–3.
21. Abrams P, Kelleher CJ, Kerr LA, Rogers RG. Overactive bladder significantly affects quality of life. Am J Manag Care. 2000;6(11 Suppl):S580–90.
22. Wiklund I. Assessment of patient-reported outcomes in clinical trials: the example of health-related quality of life. Fundam Clin Pharmacol. 2004;18(3):351–63.
23. Chassany O, Sagnier P, Marquis P, Fullerton S, Aaronson N; European Regulatory Issues on Quality of Life Assessment Group. Patient-reported outcomes: the example of health-related quality of life – a European guidance document for the improved integration of health-related quality of life assessment in the drug regulatory process. Drug Inf J. 2002;36: 209–38.
24. Bartoli S, Aguzzi G, Tarricone R. Impact on quality of life of urinary incontinence and overactive bladder: a systematic literature review. Urology. 2010;75(3):491–500.
25. Kelleher CJ, Cardozo LD, Khullar V, Salvatore S. A new questionnaire to assess the quality of life of urinary incontinent women. Br J Obstet Gynaecol. 1997;104(12):1374–9.
26. Coyne K, Revicki D, Hunt T, Corey R, Stewart W, Bentkover J, et al. Psychometric validation of an overactive bladder symptom and health-related quality of life questionnaire: the OAB-q. Qual Life Res. 2002;11(6):563–74.
27. McKown S, Abraham L, Coyne K, Gawlicki M, Piault E, Vats V. Linguistic validation of the N-QOL (ICIQ), OAB-q (ICIQ), PPBC, OAB-S and ICIQ-MLUTSsex questionnaires in 16 languages. Int J Clin Pract. 2010;64(12):1643–52.
28. Coyne KS, Matza LS, Thompson CL, Kopp ZS, Khullar V. Determining the importance of change in the overactive bladder questionnaire. J Urol. 2006;176(2):627–32.
29. Coyne KS, Thompson CL, Lai JS, Sexton CC. An overactive bladder symptom and health-related quality of life short-form: validation of the OAB-q SF. Neurourol Urodyn. 2015;34(3):255–63.
30. Coyne KS, Matza LS, Kopp Z, Abrams P. The validation of the patient perception of bladder condition (PPBC): a single-item global measure for patients with overactive bladder. Eur Urol. 2006;49(6):1079–86.
31. Reilly K, McKown S, Gawlicki M, Coyne KS. Linguistic validation of the patient perception of bladder condition questionnaire (PPBC) in 10 languages (abstract PUK25). Value Health. 2006;9(6):A392.
32. Matza LS, Thompson CL, Krasnow J, Brewster-Jordan J, Zyczynski T, Coyne KS. Test-retest reliability of four questionnaires for patients with overactive bladder: the overactive bladder questionnaire (OAB-q), patient perception of bladder condition (PPBC), urgency questionnaire (UQ), and the primary OAB symptom questionnaire (POSQ). Neurourol Urodyn. 2005;24(3):215–25.
33. Coyne KS, Sexton CC, Thompson C, Bavendam T, Brubaker L. Development and psychometric evaluation of the urgency questionnaire for evaluating severity and health-related quality of life impact of urinary urgency in overactive bladder. Int Urogynecol J. 2015;26(3): 373–82.
34. Moraes RP, Silva JLD, Calado AA, Cavalcanti GA. Validation of the urgency questionnaire in Portuguese: a new instrument to assess overactive bladder syndrome. Int Braz J Urol. 2018;44(2):338–47.

35. Jackson S, Donovan J, Brookes S, Eckford S, Swithinbank L, Abrams P. The Bristol female lower urinary tract symptoms questionnaire: development and psychometric testing. Br J Urol. 1996;77(6):805–12.
36. Donovan JL, Abrams P, Peters TJ, Kay HE, Reynard J, Chapple C, et al. The ICS-'BPH' study: the psychometric validity and reliability of the ICS male questionnaire. Br J Urol. 1996;77(4):554–62.
37. Avery K, Donovan J, Peters TJ, Shaw C, Gotoh M, Abrams P. ICIQ: a brief and robust measure for evaluating the symptoms and impact of urinary incontinence. Neurourol Urodyn. 2004;23(4):322–30.
38. Nyström E, Sjöström M, Stenlund H, Samuelsson E. ICIQ symptom and quality of life instruments measure clinically relevant improvements in women with stress urinary incontinence. Neurourol Urodyn. 2015;34(8):747–51.
39. Shumaker SA, Wyman JF, Uebersax JS, McClish D, Fantl JA. Health-related quality of life measures for women with urinary incontinence: the Incontinence Impact Questionnaire and the Urogenital Distress Inventory. Continence Program in Women (CPW) Research Group. Qual Life Res. 1994;3(5):291–306.
40. Uebersax JS, Wyman JF, Shumaker SA, McClish DK, Fantl JA. Short forms to assess life quality and symptom distress for urinary incontinence in women: the Incontinence Impact Questionnaire and the Urogenital Distress Inventory. Continence Program for Women Research Group. Neurourol Urodyn. 1995;14(2):131–9.
41. Dyer KY, Xu Y, Brubaker L, Nygaard I, Markland A, Rahn D, et al.; Urinary Incontinence Treatment Network (UITN). Minimum important difference for validated instruments in women with urge incontinence. Neurourol Urodyn. 2011;30(7):1319–24.
42. Wagner TH, Patrick DL, Bavendam TG, Martin ML, Buesching DP. Quality of life of persons with urinary incontinence: development of a new measure. Urology. 1996;47(1):67–72.
43. Patrick DL, Khalaf KM, Dmochowski R, Kowalski JW, Globe DR. Psychometric performance of the incontinence quality-of-life questionnaire among patients with overactive bladder and urinary incontinence. Clin Ther. 2013;35(6):836–45.
44. Piault E, Evans CJ, Espindle D, Kopp Z, Brubaker L, Abrams P. Development and validation of the overactive bladder satisfaction (OAB-S) questionnaire. Neurourol Urodyn. 2008;27(3):179–90.
45. Pleil AM, Coyne KS, Reese PR, Jumadilova Z, Rovner ES, Kelleher CJ. The validation of patient-rated global assessments of treatment benefit, satisfaction, and willingness to continue – the BSW. Value Health. 2005;8(Suppl 1):S25–34.
46. Colman S, Chapple C, Nitti V, Haag-Molkenteller C, Hastedt C, Massow U. Validation of treatment benefit scale for assessing subjective outcomes in treatment of overactive bladder. Urology. 2008;72(4):803–7.
47. Coyne KS, Margolis MK, Vats V, Nitti VW. Psychometric evaluation of brief patient-reported outcome measures of overactive bladder: the ICIQ-SF, SAC, SATS, SATT, and TBS. Health Outcomes Res Med. 2011;2(2):e61–9.
48. Brubaker L, Khullar V, Piault E, Evans CJ, Bavendam T, Beach J, et al. Goal attainment scaling in patients with lower urinary tract symptoms: development and pilot testing of the Self-Assessment Goal Achievement (SAGA) questionnaire. Int Urogynecol J. 2011;22(8):937–46.
49. Brubaker L, Piault EC, Tully SE, Evans CJ, Bavendam T, Beach J, et al. Validation study of the Self-Assessment Goal Achievement (SAGA) questionnaire for lower urinary tract symptoms. Int J Clin Pract. 2013;67(4):342–50.
50. Piault E, Doshi S, Brandt BA, Angün Ç, Evans CJ, Bergqvist A, Trocio J. Linguistic validation of translation of the Self-Assessment Goal Achievement (SAGA) questionnaire from English. Health Qual Life Outcomes. 2012;10:40.
51. Ware JE, Sherbourne CD. The MOS 36-item short-form health survey (SF-36). I. Conceptual framework and item selection. Med Care. 1992;30(6):473–83.
52. EuroQol Group. EuroQol – a new facility for the measurement of health-related quality of life. Health Policy. 1990;16(3):199–208.

53. Walters SJ, Brazier JE. Comparison of the minimally important difference for two health state utility measures: EQ-5D and SF-6D. Qual Life Res. 2005;14(6):1523–32.
54. Reese PR, Pleil AM, Okano GJ, Kelleher CJ. Multinational study of reliability and validity of the King's health questionnaire in patients with overactive bladder. Qual Life Res. 2003;12(4):427–42.
55. Abrams P, Avery K, Gardener N, Donovan J; ICIQ Advisory Board. The international consultation on incontinence modular questionnaire: www.iciq.net. J Urol. 2006;175(3 Pt 1):1063–6.
56. Haywood KL, Garratt AM, Lall R, Smith JF, Lamb SE. EuroQol EQ-5D and condition-specific measures of health outcome in women with urinary incontinence: reliability, validity and responsiveness. Qual Life Res. 2008;17(3):475–83.
57. McHorney CA, Ware JE Jr, Lu JF, Sherbourne CD. The MOS 36-item short-form health survey (SF-36): III. Tests of data quality, scaling assumptions, and reliability across diverse patient groups. Med Care. 1994;32(1):40–66.
58. McHorney CA, Ware JE Jr, Raczek AE. The MOS 36-item short-form health survey (SF-36): II. Psychometric and clinical tests of validity in measuring physical and mental health constructs. Med Care. 1993;31(3):247–63.
59. The International Consortium for Health Outcomes Measurement (ICHOM). http://www.ichom.org/. Accessed 5 Jan 2018.
60. Foust-Wright C, Wissig S, Stowell C, Olson E, Anderson A, Anger J, et al. Development of a core set of outcome measures for OAB treatment. Int Urogynecol J. 2017;28(12):1785–93.
61. Guyatt GH, Oxman AD, Kunz R, Atkins D, Brozek J, Vist G, et al. GRADE guidelines: 2. Framing the question and deciding on important outcomes. J Clin Epidemiol. 2011;64(4):395–400.
62. Reeve BB, Wyrwich KW, Wu AW, Velikova G, Terwee CB, Snyder CF, et al. ISOQOL recommends minimum standards for patient-reported outcome measures used in patient-centered outcomes and comparative effectiveness research. Qual Life Res. 2013;22(8):1889–905.
63. Frankel SJ, Donovan JL, Peters TI, Abrams P, Dabhoiwala NF, Osawa D, Lin AT. Sexual dysfunction in men with lower urinary tract symptoms. J Clin Epidemiol. 1998;51(8):677–85.
64. Aitchison M, Carter R, Paterson P, Ferrie B. Is the treatment of urgency incontinence a placebo response? Results of a five-year follow-up. Br J Urol. 1989;64(5):478–80.
65. Digesu GA, Khullar V, Cardozo L, Salvatore S. Overactive bladder symptoms: do we need urodynamics? Neurourol Urodyn. 2003;22(3):105–8.
66. Irwin DE, Milsom I, Hunskaar S, Reilly K, Kopp Z, Herschorn S, et al. Population-based survey of urinary incontinence, overactive bladder, and other lower urinary tract symptoms in five countries: results of the EPIC study. Eur Urol. 2006;50(6):1306–14; discussion 1314–5.
67. Hu TW, Wagner TH, Bentkover JD, LeBlanc K, Piancentini A, Stewart WF, et al. Estimated economic costs of overactive bladder in the United States. Urology. 2003;61(6):1123–8.
68. Balkrishnan R, Bhosle MJ, Camacho FT, Anderson RT. Predictors of medication adherence and associated health care costs in an older population with overactive bladder syndrome: a longitudinal cohort study. J Urol. 2006;175(3 Pt 1):1067–71; discussion 1071–2. Erratum in J Urol. 2006;175(5):1967.
69. Kalsi V, Popat RB, Apostolidis A, Kavia R, Odeyemi IA, Dakin HA, et al. Cost-consequence analysis evaluating the use of botulinum neurotoxin-A in patients with detrusor overactivity based on clinical outcomes observed at a single UK centre. Eur Urol. 2006;49:519–27.
70. Appleby J, Devlin N, Parkin D. NICE's cost effectiveness threshold. BMJ. 2007;335(7616):358–9.

Chapter 5
National and International Guidelines for Overactive Bladder

Lindsey Cox

Introduction

Overactive bladder syndrome (OAB) is an extremely prevalent and bothersome condition [1–3]. There are several clinical guidelines for OAB, as there are for many common prevalent conditions. Clinical guidelines have become a major part of medical practice. Guidelines attempt to synthesize the available best evidence to answer common clinical questions and to provide a framework for treatment of common conditions. There are so many guidelines that there are guideline clearinghouses that summarize and appraise the content of the available guidelines, as well as published "Guideline of Guidelines" [4]. This chapter will review the major guidelines that have recommendations for pharmacotherapy of OAB.

It is imperative that clinicians recognize that guidelines are not the legal "standard of care" and that clinical expertise is not supplanted by guidelines. Guidelines can help streamline decision-making, but not every patient is the index patient that the committee had in mind when developing a guideline, and, furthermore, personal preferences and individual values should be elicited and taken into account when making clinical decisions for individual patients. All providers who care for OAB patients should be familiar with the major guidelines that apply to the workup and treatment of this highly prevalent condition.

There is a specific framework set out by each guideline-producing entity on how the document was created, which is commonly described at the beginning of the guideline. There are general steps for guideline production, including convening a panel or committee for guideline development, defining specific questions to be answered by the guideline, determining a search strategy for systematic reviews of the evidence, screening items for relevance, determining how the evidence will be evaluated, and creating recommendations that answer the questions based on the

L. Cox
Department of Urology, Medical University of South Carolina, Charleston, SC, USA
e-mail: coxli@musc.edu

L. Cox, E. S. Rovner (eds.), *Contemporary Pharmacotherapy of Overactive Bladder*, https://doi.org/10.1007/978-3-319-97265-7_5

evidence, often with a rating of both the level of evidence that contributed and the strength of the recommendation. Some documents use previously published guidelines as a basis for recommendations. Most guideline committees use a grading system to determine the level of evidence for each included item.

Systems that define levels of evidence were initially developed by various groups to assess the evidence used to answer specific questions. The first report of this type of system was published by the Canadian Task Force on the Periodic Health Examination in 1979 and was developed to qualify the literature used to generate recommendations about what to include in the periodic health exam [5]. Other groups modified or expanded on this type of system to assess the evidence they used for various purposes, including creating guidelines; however, not every purpose uses the same grading system. For example, when looking at evidence for disease prognosis, prospective cohorts or systematic reviews of prospective cohorts would have the highest level of evidence, not randomized controlled trials (RCTs), which typically are assigned the highest level. Some guideline committees use existing systems, and some modify or create their own systems. The Oxford system is commonly used and is outlined in Table 5.1 [6]. The Oxford system was developed to help clinicians assess the evidence used to answer questions about treatments, and the 2011 version has been revised and simplified from the widely used first version that was put forth in 2009 [7]. The description of the individual guideline's creation and use of the systems for defining levels of evidence and grading recommendations is a good resource for understanding the context of the recommendations and the basis from which they were formulated.

Each guideline discussed below contains some recommendations related to pharmacotherapy of OAB, although many of the guidelines present these recommendations in the context of more general clinical entities, such as "Lower Urinary Tract Symptoms" or "Incontinence." The guidelines contain far more comprehensive information than is presented here, and further reading of the guidelines in their entirety is recommended.

American Urological Association/Society of Urodynamics, Female Pelvic Medicine and Urogenital Reconstruction (AUA/SUFU)

The Society of Urodynamics, Female Pelvic Medicine and Urogenital Reconstruction (SUFU) and the American Urological Association (AUA) came together to formulate a guideline for the diagnosis and treatment of OAB. This guideline was first published in 2012 and amended in 2014 [8]. The AUA, for all of its guideline documents, categorizes evidence strength as Grade A, "well-conducted RCTs or exceptionally strong observational studies"; Grade B, "RCTs with some weaknesses of procedure or generalizability or generally strong observational studies"; or Grade C, "observational studies that are inconsistent, have small sample sizes or have other

Table 5.1 Oxford Centre for Evidence-Based Medicine 2011 levels of evidence

Question	Step 1 (level 1[a])	Step 2 (level 2[a])	Step 3 (level 3[a])	Step 4 (level 4[a])	Step 5 (level 5)
How common is the problem?	Local and current random sample surveys (or censuses)	Systematic review of surveys that allow matching to local circumstances[b]	Local nonrandom sample[b]	Case series[b]	n/a
Is this diagnostic or monitoring test accurate? (diagnosis)	Systematic review of cross-sectional studies with consistently applied reference standard and blinding	Individual cross-sectional studies with consistently applied reference standard and blinding	Nonconsecutive studies or studies without consistently applied reference standards[b]	Case-control studies or poor or nonindependent reference standard[b]	Mechanism-based reasoning
What will happen if we do not add a therapy? (prognosis)	Systematic review of inception cohort studies	Inception cohort studies	Cohort study or control arm of randomized trial[a]	Case series or case-control studies or poor-quality prognostic cohort study[b]	n/a
Does this intervention help? (treatment benefits)	Systematic review of randomized trials or *n*-of-1 trials	Randomized trial or observational study with dramatic effect	Nonrandomized controlled cohort/follow-up study[b]	Case series, case-control, or historically controlled studies[b]	Mechanism-based reasoning
What are the COMMON harms? (treatment harms)	Systematic review of randomized trials, systematic review of nested case-control studies, *n*-of-1 trial with the patient you are raising the question about, or observational study with dramatic effect	Individual randomized trial or (exceptionally) observational study with dramatic effect	Nonrandomized controlled cohort/follow-up study (post-marketing surveillance) provided there are sufficient numbers to rule out a common harm (for long-term harms, the duration of follow-up must be sufficient)[b]	Case series, case-control, or historically controlled studies[b]	Mechanism-based reasoning

(continued)

Table 5.1 (continued)

Question	Step 1 (level 1[a])	Step 2 (level 2[a])	Step 3 (level 3[a])	Step 4 (level 4[a])	Step 5 (level 5)
What are the RARE harms? (treatment harms)	Systematic review of randomized trials or *n*-of-1 trial	Randomized trial or (exceptionally) observational study with dramatic effect			
Is this (early detection) test worthwhile? (screening)	Systematic review of randomized trials	Randomized trial	Nonrandomized controlled cohort/follow-up study[b]	Case series, case-control, or historically controlled studies[b]	Mechanism-based reasoning

[a]Level may be graded down on the basis of study quality, imprecision, and indirectness (study PICO does not match questions PICO), because of inconsistency between studies or because the absolute effect size is very small; level may be graded up if there is a large or very large effect size

[b]As always, a systematic review is generally better than an individual study

problems that potentially confound interpretation of data." The AUA guideline nomenclature links the guideline statement type to the evidence strength: "*Standards* are directive statements that an action should (benefits outweigh risks/burdens) or should not (risks/burdens outweigh benefits) be undertaken based on Grade A (high level of certainty) or Grade B (moderate level of certainty) evidence. *Recommendations* are directive statements that an action should (benefits outweigh risks/burdens) or should not (risks/burdens outweigh benefits) be undertaken based on Grade C (low level of certainty) evidence. *Options* are non-directive statement that leaves the decision regarding an action up to the individual clinician and patient because the balance between benefits and risks/burdens appears equal or appears uncertain based on Grade A (high quality; high certainty), B (moderate quality; moderate certainty), or C (low quality; low certainty) evidence. *Clinical Principles* are statements about a component of clinical care that is widely agreed upon by urologists or other clinicians for which there may or may not be evidence in the medical literature. *Expert Opinions* are statements, achieved by consensus of the Panel, that are based on members' clinical training, experience, knowledge, and judgment for which there is no evidence" [8].[8]

Table 5.2 summarizes the AUA/SUFU guideline statements that pertain to pharmacologic therapy. Overall, the AUA/SUFU guideline makes strong statements for the use of antimuscarinics, β_3-agonists, and botulinum toxin for treatment, but none of the recommendations are based on Grade A evidence. Several of the guideline recommendations are "Clinical Principles" that help the clinician navigate the use

Table 5.2 American Urological Association; Society of Urodynamics, Female Pelvic Medicine and Urogenital Reconstruction. Guideline statements pertaining to pharmacotherapy of overactive bladder [8]

	Statement	Category	Evidence strength
Guideline Statement 7	Behavioral therapies may be combined with pharmacologic management	Recommendation	Grade C
Guideline Statement 8	Clinicians should offer oral antimuscarinics or oral β_3-adrenoceptor agonists as second-line therapy	Standard	Grade B
Guideline Statement 9	If immediate-release (IR) and extended-release (ER) formulations are available, then ER formulations should preferentially be prescribed over IR formulations because of lower rates of dry mouth	Standard	Grade B
Guideline Statement 10	Transdermal (TDS) oxybutynin (patch [now available to women ages 18 years and older without a prescription] or gel) may be offered	Recommendation	Grade C
Guideline Statement 11	If a patient experiences inadequate symptom control and/or unacceptable adverse drug events with one antimuscarinic medication, then a dose modification or a different antimuscarinic medication or a β_3-adrenoceptor agonist may be tried	Clinical principle	
Guideline Statement 12	Clinicians should not use antimuscarinics in patients with narrow-angle glaucoma unless approved by the treating ophthalmologist and should use antimuscarinics with extreme caution in patients with impaired gastric emptying or a history of urinary retention	Clinical principle	
Guideline Statement 13	Clinicians should manage constipation and dry mouth before abandoning effective antimuscarinic therapy. Management may include bowel management, fluid management, dose modification, or alternative antimuscarinics	Clinical principle	
Guideline Statement 14	Clinicians must use caution in prescribing antimuscarinics in patients who are using other medications with anticholinergic properties	Expert opinion	
Guideline Statement 15	Clinicians should use caution in prescribing antimuscarinics or β_3-adrenoceptor agonists in the frail OAB patient	Clinical principle	
Guideline Statement 16	Patients who are refractory to behavioral and pharmacologic therapy should be evaluated by an appropriate specialist if they desire additional therapy	Expert opinion	

(continued)

Table 5.2 (continued)

	Statement	Category	Evidence strength
Guideline Statement 17	Clinicians may offer intradetrusor onabotulinumtoxinA (100 U) as third-line treatment in the carefully selected and thoroughly counseled patient who has been refractory to first- and second-line OAB treatments. The patient must be able and willing to return for frequent post-void residual evaluation and able and willing to perform self-catheterization if necessary	Standard option	Grade B C
Guideline Statement 20	Practitioners and patients should persist with new treatments for an adequate trial in order to determine whether the therapy is efficacious and tolerable. Combination therapeutic approaches should be assembled methodically, with the addition of new therapies occurring only when the relative efficacy of the preceding therapy is known. Therapies that do not demonstrate efficacy after an adequate trial should be ceased	Expert opinion	

of pharmacotherapy.SUFU has also put forth a "Clinical Care Pathway" alongside the guideline that contains resources to help both clinicians and patients navigate OAB treatment (Fig. 5.1).

International Consultation on Incontinence (ICI): 6th Edition

The International Consultation on Urologic Diseases (ICUD) is a nongovernmental organization that is registered under the World Health Organization. The ICUD has produced several consultations on urinary incontinence, most recently the Sixth International Consultation on Incontinence (ICI) [6]. The sixth edition of the ICI book, produced with the support of the International Continence Society, is essentially an extended guideline that analyzes the evidence and makes recommendations based on a modification of the Oxford Centre for Evidence-Based Medicine system discussed earlier [9]. The chapter "Pharmacological Treatment of Urinary Incontinence" addresses drugs used for the treatment of OAB (Table 5.3).

Most of the antimuscarinics (darifenacin, fesoterodine, imidafenacin, solifenacin, tolterodine, trospium, oxybutynin, and propiverine) were given Grade A recommendations based on consistent level 1 evidence. Mirabegron was also given a Grade A recommendation. Phosphodiesterase 5 inhibitors sildenafil, tadalafil, and vardenafil were given a Grade B recommendation. Botulinum toxin was given a Grade A recommendation for both neurogenic and idiopathic bladder dysfunction.

No antidepressants (imipramine or darifenacin) or alpha blockers had higher than a Grade C recommendation specifically for the treatment of OAB and urinary

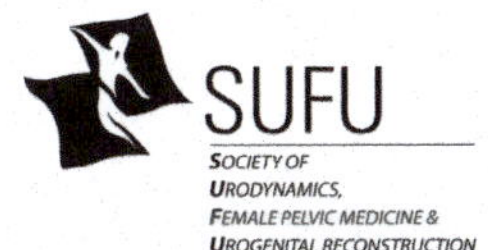

Society of Urodynamics, Female Pelvic Medicine & Urogenital Reconstruction Foundation

Overactive Bladder Clinical Care Pathway

Overactive Bladder Syndrome (OBA)

A clinical syndrome characterized by the presence of urinary urgency, usually accompanied by frequency and nocturia, with or without urgency urinaryincontinence in the absence of obvious pathology

Diagnostic Apprioach

Goal:
To document symptoms and signs that characterize OAB and to exclude other disorders that could be cause of patient's symptoms

Required Evaluation:
- History/Assessment of Lower Urinary Tract Symptoms (LUTS)– onset, duration, and degree of brother
- Contributing comobidities
- Fluid Intake
- PE
- Urinalysis

Optional Evaluation: performed at provider's discretion
- Post void residual urine *(if retention is suspected)*
- Bladder diary
- Urodynamics, cystoscopy and diagnostic renal/ bladder ultrasound should *not* be used in the initial work-up of the uncomplicated patient, but may be used in complicated or refractory patients at provider's discreation

Patients Education

Patient Discussion:
- Discuss healthy bladder habits
- Review normal bladder function
- Discuss normal uid intake and voided volumes
- What is normal vs. abnormal frequency?

Establish Treatment Plan/Expectations:
- OAB is variable and chronic symptom complex, with bo single ideal treatment
- Available treatments vary in required patient effort, invasiveness, risk, and reversibility
- Most OAB treatments can improve but do not eliminate symptoms

1st Line or Initial Treatment

Behavior/Lifestyle:
Sholud be discussed and offered as first line therapy to all patients

- Urge suppression, PFMT, bladder training
- Dietary modification
- Therapies may be instituted at any time and combined with pharmacotherapy
- Optimal treatment duration/trial 4-8 weeks

2nd Line Treatment (medication)

Pharmacotherapy:
Initiate if inadequate improvement with conservative management or at provider's discretion if the symptoms warranted to be bothersome enough

- Current classes of medications include: Antimuscarinics, Beta-3 agonist
- Choice of class or medication depends on age, comorbidities, concomitant medications, formulary restriction
  - Trial of pharmacotherapy should be at least 4-8 weeks
  - Manage side effects (if present)
    - Avoid costiopation
    - Adjust uids, drymouth aids
    - *Patient medication aid tool**
    - Medication change or dose adjustment

Reassess After 4 – 8 Weeks

If at any point during treatment the patient is satisfied, continue present treatment. If inadequate symptom relief, consider adding medication, dose escalation, change in medication, combination antimuscarinic and Beta-3 agonist medication, consider 3rd line treatments or refer to specialist.

**Coming Soon*

Fig. 5.1 Society of Urodynamics, Female Pelvic Medicine and Urogenital Reconstruction (SUFU) Foundation. The SUFU Foundation Overactive Bladder Clinical Care Pathway. (Courtesy and with permission of SUFU www.sufu.org.com)

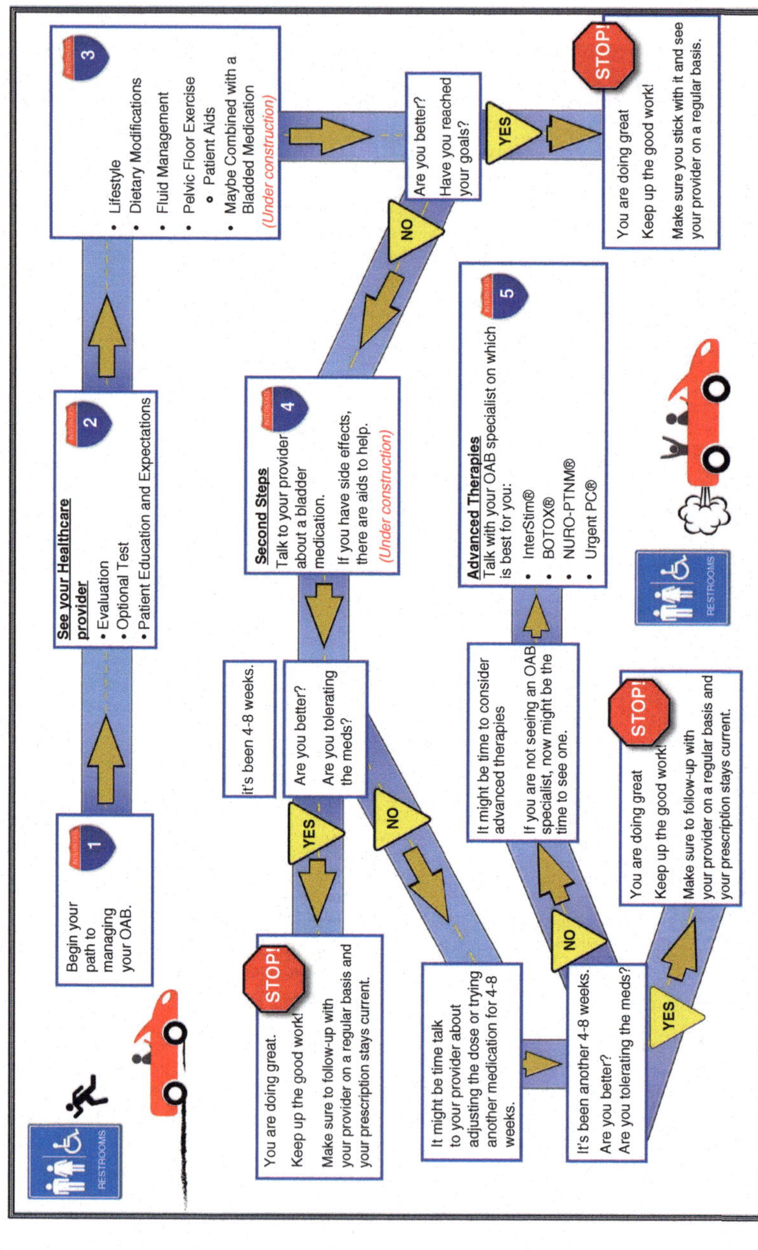

Fig. 5.1 (continued)

Table 5.3 International Consultation on Incontinence (ICI) recommendations regarding drug therapy for overactive bladder and urinary incontinence

	Level of evidence	Grade of recommendation
Antimuscarinic drugs		
Atropine, hyoscyamine	3	C
Darifenacin	1	A
Fesoterodine	1	A
Imidafenacin	1	A
Propantheline	2	B
Solifenacin	1	A
Tolterodine	1	A
Trospium	1	A
Drugs with mixed actions		
Oxybutynin	1	A
Propiverine	1	A
Flavoxate	2	D
Drugs acting on membrane channels		
Calcium antagonists	2	D
K-channel openers	2	D
Antidepressants		
Imipramine	3	C
Duloxetine	2	C
Alpha-AR antagonists		
Alfuzosin	3	C
Doxazosin	3	C
Prazosin	3	C
Terazosin	3	C
Tamsulosin	3	C
Silodosin	3	C
Naftopidil	3	C
Beta-AR antagonists		
Terbutaline (β_2)	3	C
Salbutamol (β_2)	3	C
Mirabegron (β_3)	1	A
PDE-5 inhibitors[e]		
(sildenafil, tadalafil, vardenafil)	1	B
COX inhibitors		
Indomethacin	2	C
Flurbiprofen	2	C

(continued)

Table 5.3 (continued)

	Level of evidence	Grade of recommendation
Toxins		
Botulinum toxin (neurogenic)[c]	1	A
Botulinum toxin (idiopathic)[c]	1	A
Capsaicin (neurogenic)[b]	2	C
Resiniferatoxin (neurogenic)[b]	2	C
Other drugs		
Baclofen[a]	3	C
Hormones		
Estrogen	2	C
Desmopressin[d]	1	A

From Abrams et al. [9], with permission of the International Continence Society
[a]Intrathecal
[b]Intravesical
[c]Bladder wall
[d]Nocturia (nocturnal polyuria), caution hyponatremia, especially in the elderly.
[e](Male LUTS/OAB)

incontinence (UI). (Grade C recommendation usually depends on level 4 studies or "majority evidence" from level 2/level 3 studies or Delphi-processed expert opinion.) Estrogens were also evaluated as treatments for OAB symptoms, with a description of the evidence for both systemic and local (topical) therapy. These drugs were assessed as having a level of evidence of 2 and were given an overall grade of recommendation C regarding the treatment of OAB and UI. The authors note that systemic therapy has not been proven to be effective in reducing OAB symptoms in a meta-analysis and that the evidence suggests that local therapy reduces incontinence.

The chapter authors also provide extensive safety information regarding use of all of these treatments in the older adult, which is a very useful summary of the evidence for cognitive and cardiac safety in pharmacotherapy for OAB. No specific recommendations are made in this section, but this review is recommended reading for all providers who treat these conditions.

UK National Institute for Care and Clinical Excellence (NICE)

There are two guidelines produced by the UK National Institute for Health and Care Excellence (NICE) organization that pertain to pharmacotherapy of OAB. The first is Urinary Incontinence in Women: Management. This guideline from 2013 replaces the first version from 2006; it was most recently updated in November 2015 [10]. The guideline reports detailed recommendations for counseling patients on OAB pharmacotherapy and choosing OAB drugs. These recommendations include discussing adverse events and expected benefits of treatment prior to initiating pharmacotherapy for OAB. The guideline also recommends starting with the lowest dose of a medication, then offering either a face-to-face or telephone review in 4 weeks. If there is suboptimal improvement or intolerable side effects, the recommendations are to offer dose escalation or another drug with the lowest cost, with transdermal treatment reserved for patients unable to tolerate oral medication. The guideline also addresses desmopressin use for nocturia, with recommendations to use with caution in women with cystic fibrosis and to avoid use in patients over 65 with hypertension or cardiovascular disease. The guideline also addresses hormone therapy, recommending against the use of systemic hormone therapy but offering intravaginal estrogen for the treatment of OAB symptoms in postmenopausal women with vaginal atrophy.

NICE also has a guideline specifically regarding the use of mirabegron [11]. This is a separate document outlining recommendations for the use of mirabegron in OAB. The major recommendation includes consideration for clinical effectiveness and cost-effectiveness and recommends mirabegron as an "option" for patients in whom antimuscarinics are contraindicated or ineffective or have side effects that are not tolerable.

American College of Obstetricians and Gynecologists (ACOG) and the American Urogynecologic Society (AUGS)

A joint document of the American College of Obstetricians and Gynecologists and the American Urogynecologic Society by the Committee on Practice Bulletins was published in 2015 [12]. This document is essentially more of a review than a guideline. There is a summary of conclusions and recommendations graded level A for "good and consistent scientific evidence," level B for "limited or inconsistent scientific evidence," and level C "based primarily on consensus and expert opinion" at the end of the document, but pharmacotherapy, other than botulinum toxin injection, is not addressed in these conclusions. Antimuscarinic therapy and mirabegron are both described as improving continence in OAB, and topical, but not systemic, estrogen therapy is also described as having "some benefit" for decreasing incontinence. The recommendation that "intradetrusor onabotulinumtoxinA may be a treatment option for OAB in appropriate patients, and consideration of its use requires shared decision-making between the patient and physician" was also graded level A.

American Urogynecologic Society

The AUGS Guidelines Committee also produced a consensus statement regarding the use of anticholinergics. The committee recommends that providers counsel patients on increased risks of cognitive impairment and dementia, prescribe the lowest effective dose, and consider alternative medications when possible. The committee also recommends consideration of third-line therapies in patients who do not wish to use medications for OAB due to adverse events.

European Association of Urology (EAU)

The European Association of Urology has two guidelines that address pharmacotherapy for OAB: the EAU Guidelines on Assessment and Nonsurgical Management of Urinary Incontinence [13] and EAU Non-neurogenic Male Lower Urinary Tract Symptoms (LUTS) Guidelines [14]. Standard procedure for EAU guidelines includes annual updates.

The EAU Guidelines on Assessment and Nonsurgical Management of Urinary Incontinence addresses incontinence generally but does have specific recommendations for pharmacotherapy for urgency UI in index patients and in the elderly. The recommendations for drugs for urgency UI all come with a strength rating of "Strong" and include the following: (1) offer antimuscarinics or mirabegron for patients who have failed conservative therapy, (2) consider the use of extended-release formulations of antimuscarinics when possible, (3) consider dose escalation or alternative antimuscarinic or mirabegron or combination therapy if initial antimuscarinic is ineffective, and (4) encourage the early review of efficacy and side effects for patients on antimuscarinics. They also offer a recommendation on the cautious use of antimuscarinics in the elderly, also with a "Strong" strength rating.

The EAU Non-neurogenic Male Lower Urinary Tract Symptoms (LUTS) Guidelines were first published in 2000. The 2017 document presented a comprehensive update of the 2016 publication. The guideline authors address antimuscarinic use in men with LUTS including OAB. Recommendations are based on level 2 evidence. A "Strong" recommendation was made for using antimuscarinics in men with "moderate to severe LUTS who mainly have bladder storage symptoms," and a "Weak" recommendation is made, suggesting not using antimuscarinics in men with post-void residual (PVR) >150 cc, based on evidence that antimuscarinic monotherapy can increase PVR, noting that acute retention is a rare event with PVR below this threshold.

Canadian Urological Association (CUA)

The Canadian Urological Association Guideline on Adult Overactive Bladder was published in 2017 [15]. The guidelines note their use of primary literature searches as well as evidence from other guidelines and used the Oxford grading system. The guideline addresses pharmacotherapy of OAB in the sections labeled "Second-line treatment," "Special considerations in frail older people," and "Third-line treatment." The guideline recommends that "Second-line treatment of OAB should include the use of oral AMs *[antimuscarinics*], transdermal oxybutynin or oral β_3

adrenoceptor agonist (Evidence strength Grade A)." The guideline also recommends starting with lowest recommended dose, considering contraindications and adverse events when prescribing, and offering an alternative if the initial prescribed therapy is ineffective. The guideline states, "Immediate release formulations of AMs should be avoided if other formulations are available (Evidence strength Grade A)," and notes that combination therapy with solifenacin and mirabegron is an option with evidence strength Grade C.

The guideline has a large section that describes considerations for treating OAB in frail older persons. The summary recommendations include "Age-related changes in pharmacokinetics affect AM drugs for UI and these factors should be incorporated into treatment planning (Evidence strength Grade B)" and "Drugs may be effective at lower doses in frailer compared with healthier older persons (Evidence strength Grade C)." The guideline authors also note that polypharmacy is a common issue in this population and can lead to drug-drug interactions and that antimuscarinics are potentially inappropriate medications for frail older people, with particular attention to counseling patients on cholinesterase inhibitors, used for dementia, prior to using an antimuscarinic for OAB.

The guideline recommends that "OnabotulinumtoxinA (100 U) may be offered as long-term therapy to carefully selected patients with symptoms of frequency, urgency, and urgency incontinence who have had an inadequate response to or are intolerant of OAB pharmacotherapy (Evidence strength Grade A)." The guideline goes on to state that careful counseling must occur regarding the need for repeated injection, the likelihood of needing catheterization, and the need for follow-up.

Society of Obstetricians and Gynaecologists of Canada (SOGC)

The Society of Obstetricians and Gynaecologists of Canada developed a Clinical Practice Guideline on "Treatments for Overactive Bladder: Focus on Pharmacotherapy," which was published in 2012 [16]. The guideline has been "reaffirmed for current use" per their website. The recommendations were made using the grading of recommendation ranking described by the Canadian Task Force on Preventive Health Care.

Recommendations with a I-A ranking, meaning "evidence obtained from at least one properly randomized controlled trial" with "good evidence to recommend the clinical ... action," include recommendations for oxybutynin, tolterodine, trospium, solifenacin, and darifenacin as treatment for OAB with similar objective efficacy. Oxybutynin is specifically noted to have superior cost-effectiveness but more side effects than the other oral options, and transdermal oxybutynin is noted to have fewer adverse events than oral. The guidelines also recommend offering patients a choice among bladder training and functional electric and anticholinergic therapy. Vaginal estrogen, not oral or transdermal, is recommended for OAB symptoms with level III-B ranking (opinions of authorities, based on clinical experience or reports of expert committees; fair evidence to recommend clinical action). Intravesical botulinum toxin injection, sacral nerve stimulation, and percutaneous tibial nerve stimulation are recommended for patients with refractory symptoms with a I-A ranking.

Conjoint Urological Society of Australia and New Zealand (USANZ) and Urogynaecological Society of Australasia (UGSA)

The USANZ/USGA Guidelines on the management of adult non-neurogenic OAB were published in 2016 [17]. The recommendations were formulated based on the Oxford Level of Evidence Scale. The guidelines address pharmacotherapy for OAB along with diagnosis and surgical management. Medical therapy for OAB with antimuscarinics (oxybutynin, tolterodine, solifenacin, and darifenacin) was given a Grade A recommendation based on level 1a evidence. Topical estrogens are recommended with a Grade A recommendation based on level 1b evidence for postmenopausal women with UI and vaginal atrophy. Desmopressin is recommended with a Grade B recommendation based on level 1b evidence for patients with bothersome nocturnal frequency or nocturnal polyuria with serum sodium and blood pressure monitoring, using the lowest dosage possible on initiation of therapy. Mirabegron is recommended with a Grade A recommendation based on level 1b evidence, and the guideline notes that the cardiovascular side effects appear to be clinically insignificant and the drug is well tolerated in the older adult. The use of botulinum toxin for third-line treatment received a Grade A recommendation based on level 1 evidence, with recommendation of offering this therapy after two or more pharmacological therapies.

American College of Physicians

The American College of Physicians (ACP) published a Clinical Practice Guideline on the Nonsurgical Management of Urinary Incontinence in Women in 2014 [18]. This guideline's target audience includes all clinicians and is based on an Agency for Healthcare Research and Quality systematic evidence review.

There are two main recommendations that apply to pharmacotherapy for UI/lower urinary tract symptoms: "The ACP recommends against treatment with systemic pharmacologic therapy for stress UI. (Grade: strong recommendation, low-quality evidence)" and "The ACP recommends pharmacologic treatment in women with urgency UI if bladder training was unsuccessful. Clinicians should base the choice of pharmacologic agents on tolerability, adverse effect profile, ease of use, and cost of medication. (Grade: strong recommendation, high-quality evidence)."

American Geriatrics Society

The American Geriatrics Society Beers Criteria document is one of the most frequently consulted sources for prescribing medications for older adults [19]. The 2015 update includes recommendations on medications used for the treatment of UI and lower urinary tract symptoms. The guideline also reviews other medications that prescribers should be aware of when utilizing certain classes of drugs in the elderly.

Desmopressin is listed as a "potentially inappropriate medication (PIM)" in older adults due to the risk of hyponatremia. This was given a "Strong" recommendation with a "Moderate" level of evidence. A "Strong" recommendation with a "Moderate" quality of evidence was given to avoid or minimize the number of anticholinergic drugs in elderly patients due to the increased risk of cognitive decline.

Cochrane

Cochrane is a nonprofit, nongovernmental organization based out of the United Kingdom that conducts systematic reviews of evidence to answer clinical questions. While not a guideline, the Cochrane Reviews are a helpful collection of resources for the clinician. Notably, many of the guideline committees utilize these systematic reviews during the creation of the guidelines above; however, the reviews are also useful as stand-alone documents that review the evidence for individual treatments.

There are several Cochrane Reviews that are germane to the topic of pharmacotherapy of OAB:

1. Anticholinergic drugs versus other medications for OAB syndrome in adults [20]
2. Anticholinergic drugs versus placebo for OAB syndrome in adults [21]
3. Botulinum toxin injections for adults with OAB syndrome [22]
4. Which anticholinergic drug for OAB symptoms in adults [23]
5. Anticholinergic drugs versus non-drug active therapies for non-neurogenic overactive bladder syndrome in adults [24]
6. Desmopressin for treating nocturia in men [25]

Conclusions

Clinical guidelines are an invaluable resource for the practicing clinician treating patients with OAB. Pharmacotherapy for OAB is addressed in numerous clinical guidelines, which tend to agree on the use of antimuscarinics and mirabegron for second-line therapy, after conservative management. The guidelines also generally agree that there is good quality evidence for the use of botulinum toxin in patients who are refractory to oral pharmacotherapy.

References

1. Liberman JN, Hunt TL, Stewart WF, Wein A, Zhou Z, Herzog AR, et al. Health-related quality of life among adults with symptoms of overactive bladder: results from a U.S. community-based survey. Urology. 2001;57(6):1044–50.
2. Stewart WF, Van Rooyen JB, Cundiff GW, Abrams P, Herzog AR, Corey R, et al. Prevalence and burden of overactive bladder in the United States. World J Urol. 2003;20(6):327–36.
3. Abrams P, Kelleher CJ, Kerr LA, Rogers RG. Overactive bladder significantly affects quality of life. Am J Manag Care. 2000;6(11 Suppl):S580–90.
4. Syan R, Brucker BM. Guideline of guidelines: urinary incontinence. BJU Int. 2016;117(1):20–33.
5. The periodic health examination. Canadian Task Force on the Periodic Health Examination. Can Med Assoc J. 1979;121(9):1193–254.
6. OCEBM Levels of Evidence Working Group. The Oxford levels of evidence 2. Oxford Centre for Evidence-Based Medicine. http://www.cebm.net/index.aspx?o=5653. Accessed 19 June 2018.
7. Howick J, Chalmers I, Glasziou P, Greenhalgh T, Heneghan C, Liberati A, et al. Explanation of the 2011 Oxford Centre for Evidence-Based Medicine (OCEBM) levels of evidence (background document). Oxford Centre for Evidence-Based Medicine. https://www.cebm.net/index.aspx?o=5653 (2011). Accessed 19 June 2018.
8. Gormley EA, Lightner DJ, Burgio KL, Chai TC, Clemens JQ, Culkin DJ; American Urological Association; Society of Urodynamics, Female Pelvic Medicine & Urogenital Reconstruction, et al. Diagnosis and treatment of overactive bladder (non-neurogenic) in adults: AUA/SUFU guideline. 2012; amended 2014. http://www.auanet.org/guidelines/overactive-bladder-(oab)-(aua/sufu-guideline-2012-amended-2014). Accessed 19 June 2018.
9. Abrams P, Cardozo L, Wagg A, Wein A, editors. Incontinence. 6th ed. Bristol: ICI-ICS. International Continence Society; 2017.
10. National Institute for Health and Care Excellence. Urinary incontinence in women: the management of urinary incontinence in women. CG171. Published 2013; last updated 2015. http://www.ncbi.nlm.nih.gov/pubmed/25340217. Accessed 19 June 2018.
11. National Institute for Health and Care Excellence. Mirabegron for treating symptoms of overactive bladder. Technology appraisal guidance (TA290). Published 26 June 2013. https://www.nice.org.uk/guidance/ta290. Accessed 19 June 2018.
12. Committee on Practice Bulletins—Gynecology and the American Urogynecologic Society. Urinary incontinence in women. Female Pelvic Med Reconstr Surg. 2015;21(6):304–14.
13. Nambiar AK, Bosch R, Cruz F, Lemack GE, Thiruchelvam N, Tubaro A, et al. EAU guidelines on assessment and nonsurgical Management of Urinary Incontinence. Eur Urol. 2018;73(4):596–609.
14. European Association of Urology. Guidelines. Gravas S, Cornu JN, Drake MJ, Gacci M, Gratzke C, Hermann TRW, et al. Treatment of Non-neurogenic Male LUTS. First published in 2000; updated in 2017. http://uroweb.org/guideline/treatment-of-non-neurogenic-male-luts/#1_4. Accessed 19 June 2018.
15. Corcos J, Przydacz M, Campeau L, Gray G, Hickling D, Honeine C, et al. CUA guideline on adult overactive bladder. Can Urol Assoc J. 2017;11(5):E142–73.
16. Geoffrion R; Urogynaecology Committee. Treatments for overactive bladder: focus on pharmacotherapy. J Obstet Gynaecol Can. 2012;34(11):1092–1101.
17. Tse V, King J, Dowling C, English S, Gray K, Millard R, et al. Conjoint Urological Society of Australia and New Zealand (USANZ) and Urogynaecological Society of Australasia (UGSA) guidelines on the management of adult non-neurogenic overactive bladder. Br J Urol. 2016;117(1):34–47.

18. Qaseem A, Dallas P, Forciea MA, Starkey M, Denberg TD, Shekelle P. Clinical guidelines Committee of the American College of Physicians. Nonsurgical management of urinary incontinence in women: a clinical practice guideline from the American College of Physicians. Ann Intern Med. 2014;161(10):429–40.
19. American Geriatrics Society 2015 Beers Criteria Update Expert Panel. American Geriatrics Society 2015 updated Beers criteria for potentially inappropriate medication use in older adults. J Am Geriatr Soc. 2015;63(11):2227–46.
20. Roxburgh C, Cook J, Dublin N. Anticholinergic drugs versus other medications for overactive bladder syndrome in adults. Cochrane Database Syst Rev. 2007;(4):CD003190.
21. Nabi G, Cody JD, Ellis G, Herbison P, Hay-Smith J. Anticholinergic drugs versus placebo for overactive bladder syndrome in adults. Cochrane Database Syst Rev. 2006;(4):CD003781.
22. Duthie JB, Vincent M, Herbison GP, Wilson DI, Wilson D. Botulinum toxin injections for adults with overactive bladder syndrome. Cochrane Database Syst Rev. 2011;(12):CD005493.
23. Madhuvrata P, Cody JD, Ellis G, Herbison GP, Hay-Smith EJ. Which anticholinergic drug for overactive bladder symptoms in adults. Cochrane Database Syst Rev. 2012;1:CD005429.
24. Rai BP, Cody JD, Alhasso A, Stewart L. Anticholinergic drugs versus non-drug active therapies for non-neurogenic overactive bladder syndrome in adults. Cochrane Database Syst Rev. 2012;12:CD003193.
25. Han J, Jung JH, Bakker CJ, Ebell MH, Dahm P. Desmopressin for treating nocturia in men. Cochrane Database Syst Rev. 2017;10:CD012059.

Chapter 6
Antimuscarinic Pharmacotherapy for Overactive Bladder

Ariana L. Smith and Alan J. Wein

Abbreviations

5-HMT	5-Hydroxymethyl tolterodine
ACET	Antimuscarinic clinical effectiveness trial
Ach	Acetylcholine
CIC	Clean intermittent catheterization
CNS	Central nervous system
CYP	Cytochrome
DEO	N-desethyl-oxybutynin
DO	Detrusor overactivity
ER	Extended release
HRQoL	Health-related quality of life
IMPACT	Improvement in patients: assessing symptomatic control with tolterodine extended-release study
IR	Immediate release
LUT	Lower urinary tract
M	Muscarinic receptor
OAB	Overactive bladder
OPERA	Overactive bladder: performance of extended-release agents trial
OXY	Oxybutynin
OXY-TDS	Oxybutynin transdermal delivery system
PDE	Phosphodiesterase
PVRs	Post-void residuals
QTc	Corrected QT interval
RCT	Randomized controlled trial

A. L. Smith (✉) · A. J. Wein
University of Pennsylvania, Philadelphia, PA, USA
e-mail: ariana.smith@uphs.upenn.edu

L. Cox, E. S. Rovner (eds.), *Contemporary Pharmacotherapy of Overactive Bladder*, https://doi.org/10.1007/978-3-319-97265-7_6

SCI	Spinal cord injury
STAR	Solifenacin and tolterodine as an active comparator in a randomized trial
TDS	Transdermal delivery system
TOLT	Tolterodine
UUI	Urgency urinary incontinence

Introduction

The lower urinary tract (LUT) includes the bladder, the urethra, the prostate in men, and the surrounding nerves, muscles, and fascias and serves two basic functions: storage of urine and emptying of urine. Failure of the LUT to adequately store urine may be secondary to pathology in the bladder, the outlet (urethra and prostate), or the surrounding structures. The most common etiology is overactive bladder (OAB), a syndrome of urgency, with or without urgency urinary incontinence (UUI), usually associated with frequency and nocturia [1].

OAB may be the result of increased bladder sensation during bladder filling or result from involuntary bladder contractions, termed detrusor overactivity (DO). Heightened or altered sensation of the bladder may manifest as urinary urgency, with or without DO, and is commonly associated with neurologic disease, inflammatory processes of the bladder, bladder outlet obstruction, aging, and psychosocial stress or may be idiopathic [2]. Therapy is aimed at decreasing sensory (afferent) input, decreasing involuntary (efferent) contractions, and increasing bladder capacity.

Uropharmacology

Pharmacology of the LUT or "uropharmacology" addresses the neural innervation and receptor contents of the bladder, urethra, and surrounding structures. The targets of pharmacologic intervention include not only these structures but also the peripheral nerves and ganglia that supply these tissues and the central nervous system (CNS), including the spinal cord and supraspinal areas [3]. Specifically, pharmacologic targets include nerve terminals, which alter the release of neurotransmitters, receptor subtypes, cellular second messenger systems, and ion channels [4]. The autonomic nervous system assumes primary control over the two functions of the LUT; however, due to its lack of specificity and ubiquitous nature of its receptors, there are no pharmacologic agents that are purely selective for the LUT. Consequently, side effects of treatment are common and are the result of collateral effects on organ systems that share some of the same neurophysiologic or pharmacologic characteristics as the bladder and urethra [2].

Our approach to pharmacologic management of OAB is to start with the simplest and least expensive form of treatment first. Continued use of behavioral and dietary modifications is encouraged. After assessment of efficacy and side effects, appropriate dose escalation and/or substitution with another, potentially more costly, therapeutic option can be offered. Alternatively, a combination of agents or drugs can be used, ideally with synergistic mechanisms of action and non-synergistic side effects. In our experience, although great improvement can occur with rational pharmacologic therapy, a perfect result, i.e., the restoration to normal function, is seldom achieved.

Antimuscarinic Agents

Physiologic bladder contractions are thought to be primarily triggered by acetylcholine (ACh)-induced stimulation of postganglionic parasympathetic muscarinic cholinergic receptor sites on bladder smooth muscle [3, 5]. Atropine and other antagonists of ACh, which bind these receptor sites, will depress normal bladder contractions and involuntary bladder contractions of any cause [3, 6]. In addition, these agents increase the volume to first involuntary contraction and the total bladder capacity and decrease the amplitude of the contraction [7].

The commonly held belief regarding antimuscarinic drugs is that they competitively bind to receptors on the detrusor during the filling/storage phase, that are otherwise stimulated by ACh during micturition, thereby decreasing contraction of the bladder. During normal bladder filling and storage, there is no sacral parasympathetic outflow [8]; therefore, it is likely that alternative mechanisms are responsible for the antimuscarinic effects on the filling/storage phase of the micturition cycle. Antimuscarinics have been found to increase bladder capacity and decrease urgency. Muscarinic receptors are also present in bladder urothelium and suburothelium [9], and there is a basal acetylcholine release in human detrusor muscle, which may be produced, at least partly, by the urothelium and suburothelium [10]. This suggests that detrusor tone may be affected by ongoing acetylcholine-mediated stimulation. There is now good direct experimental evidence that the antimuscarinics decrease activity in both C and A-delta afferent nerve fibers during bladder filling/storage [2, 11].

Acetylcholine acts on both nicotinic and muscarinic receptors. Muscarinic receptors are responsible for signal transduction between parasympathetic nerves and smooth muscle of the detrusor [4]. Five different muscarinic receptor subtypes have been identified in the human body and are designated M1 to M5. The majority of muscarinic receptors in human smooth muscle are of the M2 subtype; however, the M3 receptor subtype mediates most smooth muscle contraction, including that of the bladder. Muscarinic receptors are found not only on smooth muscle cells of the bladder but also on urothelial cells, on suburothelial nerves, and on suburothelial structures such as interstitial cells with M2 and M3 preponderance [9]. Studies in animals have implicated the M2 receptors in the contraction of diseased bladders [11].

Available antimuscarinic agents differ in molecular size, molecular charge, and lipophilicity and can be can be categorized as tertiary or quaternary amines [4]. Tertiary compounds have higher lipophilicity and less molecular charge than quaternary agents. Small molecular size with little molecular charge and greater lipophilicity increases the passage through the blood-brain barrier with the theoretical potential of greater CNS side effects. Quaternary compounds have greater molecular charge and less lipophilicity resulting in limited passage into the CNS and theoretically a low incidence of CNS side effects [12].

Meta-analysis of antimuscarinic use found that these agents are more effective than placebo in improving urinary frequency, urgency, continent days, and mean voided volume [13]. Health-related quality of life (HRQoL) is improved with use of these agents. All of the currently available antimuscarinic agents improve symptoms with comparable efficacy, but some measurable differences in tolerability exist [14]. Since the biochemical profile of each drug and the dosing schedule differ, these pharmacologic properties along with medical comorbidities and concomitant medication use should be considered when individualizing treatment for patients.

The currently available antimuscarinic agents lack selectivity for the bladder and as a result produce side effects on other organ systems. The most common adverse effects include dry mouth, blurred vision, constipation, pruritis, tachycardia, somnolence, impaired cognition, and headache. Constipation is reported as the most burdensome side effect [13]. This class of drug is contraindicated in patients with untreated urinary retention, gastric retention, severe decreased gastrointestinal motility conditions, and uncontrolled narrow-angle glaucoma. The concomitant use with other medications with anticholinergic properties may increase the frequency and/or severity of side effects. Patients with impairment in renal or liver metabolism and those with genetic heterogeneity in drug-metabolizing enzymes may experience increased side effects due to altered pharmacokinetic behavior of a given drug [14]. Several antimuscarinics should not be used with potent cytochrome (CYP) p450 3A4 inhibitors, including ritonavir, ketoconazole, itraconazole, verapamil, and cyclosporine [15–18].

It is estimated that approximately one-third of all patients with OAB have at least one risk factor for altered drug metabolism [14]. In addition, while relative muscarinic receptor selectivity exists for some agents, there is no uroselective option that avoids unpleasant systemic side effects. As a result, patient adherence is extremely poor with this class of drug and the search for uroselectivity continues. Intravesical administration in the absence of systemic absorption would greatly diminish the antimuscarinic side effects; however, this is only practical in patients who perform clean intermittent catheterization (CIC) and could administer the drug via the catheter.

Antimuscarinic agents together with beta-3 agonists (see Chap. 7) are considered first-line pharmacotherapy for OAB [19]. Several antimuscarinic agents are available for use in the United States and abroad with varying quality and quantity of research performed on them. The International Consultation on Incontinence has assessed and made recommendations on many of the available agents (Table 6.1) [2]. The clinical drug recommendations are based on evaluations made using a modification of the Oxford system.

Specific antimuscarinic agents are listed below with available data on efficacy and comparative efficacy with other drugs in class.

Table 6.1 Antimuscarinic drugs used in the treatment of overactive bladder. Assessments according to the modified Oxford system [2]

	Level of evidence	Grade of recommendation
Antimuscarinic drugs		
Atropine	3	C
Darifenacin	1	A
Fesoterodine	1	A
Hyoscyamine	3	C
Imidafenacin	1	B
Propantheline bromide	2	B
Scopolamine	3	C
Solifenacin	1	A
Tolterodine	1	A
Trospium	1	A
Drugs with mixed actions		
Flavoxate	2	D
Oxybutynin	1	A
Propiverine	1	A
Levels of evidence		
Level 1: Systematic reviews, meta-analyses, good quality randomized controlled trials		
Level 2: Randomized controlled trials, good quality prospective cohort studies		
Level 3: Case-control studies, case series		
Level 4: Expert opinion		
Grades of recommendation		
Grade A: Based on level 1 evidence (highly recommended)		
Grade B: Consistent level 2 or 3 evidence l (recommended)		
Grade C: Level 4 evidence (optional)		
Grade D: Evidence inconsistent/inconclusive (no recommendation or not recommended)		

Atropine

Atropine, along with hyoscyamine and scopolamine (both described below), are active belladonna alkaloids, derived from the toxic belladonna plant and possess anticholinergic properties [2]. Atropine has significant systemic side effects including ventricular fibrillation, tachycardia, dizziness, nausea, blurred vision, loss of balance, dilated pupils, photophobia, extreme confusion, and dissociative hallucinations which limit its use for the treatment of OAB. Intravesical atropine at a dose of 6 mg four times per day was shown to be as effective as intravesical oxybutynin (OXY; see below) for increasing bladder capacity with minimal systemic side effects in patients with multiple sclerosis in a double-blind, randomized placebo-controlled trial (RCT) with crossover design [20]. Its mention in this chapter is more of a historic one.

Darifenacin

Darifenacin is a tertiary amine with moderate lipophilicity and is a relatively selective M3 receptor antagonist. At least theoretically, darifenacin's advantage over other antimuscarinic agents is the ability to relatively selectively block the M3 receptor which although less prevalent than the M2 receptor, appears to be more important in bladder contraction. This selectivity is expected to increase efficacy in patients with OAB while reducing adverse events related to the blockade of other muscarinic subtypes [21]. Darifenacin has been developed as a controlled release formulation to allow once-daily dosing and is available at 7.5 and 15 mg/day, which allows dose escalation when needed.

Several RCTs have documented the efficacy of darifenacin. Haab et al. performed a multicenter, double-blind RCT comparing darifenacin 3.75 mg, 7.5 mg, and 15 mg and placebo once daily for 12 weeks [22]. The study enrolled 561 patients (85% female) aged 19–88 years with at least 6 months of OAB symptoms and included patients with prior use of antimuscarinic therapy. The 7.5 and 15 mg doses of darifenacin had rapid onset of effect with significant improvement in OAB symptoms over placebo at 2-week follow-up. Patients experienced improvement in micturition frequency, bladder capacity, urgency episodes, urgency severity, and number of incontinence episodes. No significant change in nocturia was seen. The most common side effects were mild-to-moderate dry mouth and constipation. The CNS and cardiac safety profiles were similar to placebo and discontinuation of the drug while on study was rare. Chapple et al. performed a review of the pooled data from three phase III, multicenter, double-blind RCTs in 2005 [23]. A total of 1,059 patients (again 85% female) with urinary frequency, urgency, and UUI were treated with darifenacin 7.5 mg, 15 mg, or placebo once daily for 12 weeks. A significant dose-related improvement in the number of weekly incontinence episodes was seen: 8.8 fewer incontinence episodes per week with the 7.5 mg dose and 10.6 fewer incontinence episodes per week with the 15 mg dose. Improvements in micturition frequency, bladder capacity, and urgency severity were also seen. The most common side effects were dry mouth and constipation; however, this resulted in few discontinuations in therapy during the trial.

One of the most notable patient-reported effects of antimuscarinic therapy is the ability to postpone urination. This is often reported as "warning time" and is defined as the time from first sensation of urgency to the time of voluntary micturition or incontinence. Improvement in warning time often translates into the ability to postpone urination a few extra minutes and can be the difference between wet and dry. Cardozo and Dixon performed a multicenter, double-blind RCT looking at improvement in warning time with darifenacin [24]. Overall, 47% of the darifenacin group compared to 20% of the placebo group achieved a >30% increase in mean warning time. The patients in this study received a 30 mg dose of darifenacin, which is higher than the clinically recommended dose. These results have not been replicated using the 15 mg dose.

Darifenacin has been shown to have sustained beneficial effects on HRQoL at 2 years of treatment [25]. The effects of darifenacin on cognitive function in older volunteers were tested in a randomized, double-blind, crossover study with 129 patients 65 years of age or older [26]. After 2 weeks of daily treatment, no change from baseline in cognitive function was found. The authors hypothesized that this was related to its M3 receptor selectivity. Chancellor et al. performed studies on the passage of antimuscarinic agents across the blood-brain barrier and found that darifenacin, along with trospium and fesoterodine, is actively transported away from the brain as the result of a protein-mediated transporter system [27]. Darifenacin has not been found to have any effect on QT/QTc intervals or heart rate compared to placebo [28, 29].

Fesoterodine

Fesoterodine is a newer antimuscarinic drug that like tolterodine (TOLT, see below) is a non-subtype selective muscarinic receptor antagonist [30]. It is metabolized rapidly and extensively to 5-hydroxymethyl tolterodine (5-HMT), the same active metabolite of TOLT [31]. Fesoterodine relies on nonspecific esterases to produce a rapid and complete conversion to 5-HMT with little pharmacokinetic variability. 5-HMT is further metabolized in the liver, but a modest percentage undergoes renal excretion without additional metabolism, raising the possibility that 5-HMT could also work from the luminal side of the bladder [32]. Whether this contributes to clinical efficacy in human remains unknown at this time. Fesoterodine is indicated for the treatment of OAB at doses of 4 and 8 mg daily allowing for dose escalation. The 4 mg per day dose can be used in patients with moderately impaired renal or hepatic function since there is dual metabolism of 5-HMT by both organ systems [33, 34].

In a multicenter, double-blind RCT with TOLT extended release (ER), 1132 patients were enrolled and received treatment [31]. The trial showed that both the 4 mg and 8 mg doses of fesoterodine were effective in improving symptoms of OAB with the 8 mg dose having a greater effect at the expense of a higher rate of dry mouth. One subject from the fesoterodine 8 mg group and one subject from the TOLT ER 4 mg group withdrew from the study due to bothersome dry mouth. The dose response relationship was confirmed in another study that pooled data from two phase III RCTs [35]. Fesoterodine 8 mg performed better than the 4 mg dose in improving urinary urgency and UUI as recorded by a 3-day bladder diary, supporting the use of dose titration. A study on the effect of fesoterodine on HRQoL in patients with OAB demonstrated improvement for both the 4 and 8 mg dose of the drug [36]. A head-to-head placebo-controlled trial comparing fesoterodine 8 mg to tolterodine ER 4 mg ($n = 1{,}590$) showed greater improvements in urgency incontinence episodes, completely dry rates, voided volume, and patient perception of improvement with fesoterodine [37]. No difference was noted in frequency of micturition and urgency episodes. Significantly greater side effects (dry mouth, headache, constipation, and discontinuation) were reported with fesoterodine. This study suggests that fesoterodine 8 mg can provide improved symptom control over tolterodine ER 4 mg at the expense of greater side effects. In a large double-blind, phase III study (*n* = 2,417), fesoterodine 8 mg showed greater improvement in urgency incontinence episodes, frequency of micturition, urgency episodes, and patient perception of improvement than tolterodine ER 4 mg or placebo [38]. No difference in voided volume or nocturia was noted. Dry mouth, constipation, and discontinuation rates were greater with fesoterodine 8 mg. Fesoterodine has not been found to prolong QT/QTc or produce other cardiac abnormalities [39].

The sustained effects of fesoterodine on OAB were analyzed using pooled analysis of two open-label extension studies [40]. About half of the study population (51%) was on fesoterodine for >24 months, and mean duration of exposure was 21 months. While 77% of patients elected to remain on the drug during the open-label extension, discontinuation was seen in 51% by the 24-month visit, generally as a result of insufficient clinical response and/or adverse events. Significant improvements in micturition episodes, urgency, urgency incontinence, and quality of life were seen at both 12 and 24 months compared to baseline. In addition, treatment satisfaction was reported in 96% at 12 months and 97% at 24 months [41].

The use of fesoterodine in the elderly was investigated in the SOPHIA trial which recruited patients >65 years of age [42]. Micturition episodes (day and night), urgency, urgency incontinence, and pad use significantly improved in the fesoterodine group compared to placebo at 12 weeks. However, in 46% of patients with urgency incontinence, no change in incontinence episodes was seen. The effects on mental status were assessed using the mini mental state examination, and no change from baseline or between age groups less than or older than age 75 was seen. Dry mouth was reported in 33.9% of the fesoterodine group (vs. 5.3% of the placebo group), and constipation was seen in 8.9% (vs. 2.5%).

Hyoscyamine

Hyoscyamine is a pharmacologically active levorotary isomer of atropine that is reported to have similar actions and side effects [2]. Few clinical studies are available to evaluate efficacy in the treatment of OAB [43]. A sublingual formulation of hyoscyamine sulfate is available.

Imidafenacin

Imidafenacin is a muscarinic antagonist with greater affinity for the M3 and M1 receptors than the M2 receptor [44]. The oral administration of imidafenacin in rats showed longer lasting and more selective binding to muscarinic receptors in the bladder than other tissues, with little binding in the brain [45]. Demonstration of this effect in human tissues is yet to be confirmed. The drug is primarily metabolized in the liver by cytochrome P450 enzyme CYP3A4 [46]. The drug is also excreted in the urine; however, the pharmacologic importance of this has not yet been elucidated. Clinical studies have primarily been performed in Japan, and the drug is not available in Western countries.

A double-blind phase II dose-finding RCT (n = 401) showed a dose-dependent reduction in urinary frequency, urgency, urgency incontinence episodes as well as an increase in voided volume that was significant over placebo. The 0.1 mg twice daily dose of imidafenacin was selected as the appropriate balance between efficacy and side effects [47]. In a larger study, the same authors performed a placebo and propiverine-controlled trial (n = 781) that demonstrated non-inferiority of imidafenacin 0.1 mg twice daily to propiverine 20 mg per day for the reduction of urgency incontinence episodes at 12 weeks (non-inferiority margin 14.5%, P = 0.0014) [48]. The incidence of adverse events was significantly lower with imidafenacin than propiverine (P = 0.0101) with dry mouth being the most commonly reported side effect. A long-term 52-week study by the same authors (n = 376) demonstrated a persistent improvement in voiding symptoms at the 0.1 mg twice daily dose in Japanese patients with the most common adverse event being dry mouth in 40.2% [49]. Compared to short-term treatment, long-term treatment did not increase the frequency of adverse effects. Imidafenacin has not been found to prolong QT/QTc, alter laboratory values, or increase post-void residual measures.

The effect of imidafenacin on nocturia was studied in two small open-label studies as well as a post hoc analysis of a large multicenter RCT and suggested benefit [50–52]. In stratified analysis of the large RCT, imidafenacin significantly reduced nighttime micturition (from approximately three to two times per night, P = 0.0292) as well as nocturnal percentage of 24-h urine production (from approximately 50% to 40%, P = 0.0053) and increased the interval to first nighttime void (from approximately 150 to 200 min, P < 0.0001) [52].

In a non-inferiority phase IV trial in Korea, imidafenacin was compared to fesoterodine 4 mg daily. No significant differences were detected in efficacy and dry mouth rates were similar [53].

Propantheline Bromide

The classic oral agent for antimuscarinic effects on the LUT was propantheline bromide, a nonselective quaternary ammonium compound that is poorly absorbed after oral administration [2]. It has a short plasma half-life of <2 h and varying biologic availability requiring individual titration. It is initially prescribed at 15–30 mg four times daily, but larger doses are often required [54]. Despite having antimuscarinic binding potential quite similar to atropine, there is a lack of convincing data on the effectiveness for the treatment of OAB. Contradictory studies are available that show complete response in 25/26 patients [55] and no difference from placebo in 154 and 23 patients, respectively [56, 57]. By today's standards, the effect of propantheline on OAB has not been well documented in RCTs; however, with its long history of use, it can be considered effective and may, in individually titrated doses, be clinically useful.

Scopolamine

Scopolamine, a belladonna alkaloid, has greater penetration through the blood-brain barrier than atropine and as a result produces more prominent central depressive effects even at low doses [2]. Transdermal scopolamine has been used for treating OAB at a continuous dose of 0.5 mg for 3 days [58]. A double-blind RCT was performed in 20 patients with DO. After 14 days, patients in the treatment group showed significant improvements in urinary frequency, nocturia, urgency, and UUI over the placebo group. Side effects included dizziness, ataxia, blurred vision, dry mouth, and skin irritation at patch site. No patients discontinued use during the study period [43].

Solifenacin

Solifenacin is a tertiary amine muscarinic antagonist with modest selectivity for the M3 receptor over the M2 and marginal selectivity over the M1 receptors [4, 59]. Solifenacin is metabolized in the liver utilizing the cytochrome P450 enzyme system (CYP3A4), but a modest percentage undergoes renal excretion without additional metabolism again raising the possibility that it could also work from the luminal side of the bladder. Whether this contributes to clinical efficacy remains unknown at this time.

Studies have demonstrated that solifenacin increases maximum bladder capacity and is under the bladder volume sensation curve [60, 61]. It is a once-daily antimuscarinic that is being marketed at the 5 mg and 10 mg doses allowing for titration. There have been several large trials examining the effects of solifenacin. A large phase II multinational RCT was performed comparing solifenacin 2.5, 5, 10, and 20 mg daily to TOLT immediate release (IR) 2 mg twice daily and placebo [62]. A total of 225 patients with urodynamically confirmed DO were enrolled, treated for 4 weeks, and followed for 2 additional weeks. There was a significant decrease in urinary frequency, incontinence episodes, and urgency episodes and an increase in volume voided in the 5, 10, and 20 mg solifenacin groups compared to placebo. The mean effects with TOLT were generally smaller than with solifenacin. The 5 and 10 mg doses of solifenacin had a lower dry mouth rate (14%) than TOLT (24%) but higher than placebo (2.6%). Discontinuation rates were highest for solifenacin 20 mg. Cardozo et al. performed a multinational RCT comparing solifenacin 5 and 10 mg once daily to placebo in 857 patients [63]. Both doses significantly improved urinary frequency, urgency, volume voided, and incontinence episodes compared to placebo as determined by 3-day voiding diaries. Of patients who reported any incontinence at baseline, 50% achieved continence with solifenacin treatment compared to 27.9% with placebo. Dry mouth was reported in 7.7% of patients taking solifenacin 5 mg, 23.1% in solifenacin 10 mg, and 2.3% in the placebo arm. Only a small percentage of patients (2–4%) did not complete the study due to adverse events, and this was comparable in all groups.

The STAR (Solifenacin and Tolterodine as an Active comparator in a Randomized) trial was a prospective double-blind, parallel group 12-week study comparing solifenacin 5 and 10 mg once daily to TOLT ER 4 mg once daily [64] in patients with OAB. After 4 weeks of treatment, patients were given the option to increase medication dosage. However, only those on solifenacin actually received the dose increase. The results showed non-inferiority of solifenacin's flexible dosing regimen compared to TOLT ER for voiding frequency (−2.45 vs. −2.24 void per day, $P = 0.004$). Solifenacin showed increased efficacy in decreasing urgency episodes, incontinence, and pad usage compared with TOLT ER (all $P < 0.05$). Additionally, more solifenacin patients achieved dryness, as documented by 3-day voiding diary, by the end of the study (59% vs. 49%, $P = 0.006$). However, these symptomatic improvements were accompanied by an increase in adverse events with dry mouth and constipation occurring in 30% and 6.4% of the solifenacin group, respectively, versus 23% and 2.5% in the TOLT group. The discontinuation rate was comparably low in both groups (3.5% in solifenacin group vs. 3.0%in the TOLT group).

A systematic review and meta-analysis of nine RCTs concluded that solifenacin provides significant improvement in urinary symptoms compared to placebo or TOLT [65]. Solifenacin 10 mg was statistically better than 5 mg in reducing urinary frequency (−0.29 episodes per day, $P < 0.001$) but similar in reducing urgency, urgency incontinence, and nocturia. Higher rates of dry mouth were reported with the 10 mg dose compared to the 5 mg dose ($P = 0.003$) but similar rates of constipation, blurred vision and overall number of adverse events. Solifenacin was statistically better than TOLT at reducing urgency episodes per day (−0.37, $P < 0.0001$), voids per day (−0.06, $P = 0.02$), and incontinence episodes per day (−0.48, $P < 0.0001$). Constipation (OR 2.91, $P < 0.0001$) and blurred vision (OR 3.19, $P = 0.03$) were greater with solifenacin than TOLT, but dry mouth was similar. Efficacy in mixed urinary incontinence [66], the elderly [67], and in multiple sclerosis patients [68] has been shown, as has an improvement in HRQoL [69]. An open-label study including 72 children of which 27 had neurogenic bladder demonstrated improved urodynamic capacity and improved continence [70]. Solifenacin has shown QT interval prolongation and torsade de pointes in an 81-year-old female [71]. In a large open-label post-marketing study (n=4,450) including patients with cardiovascular comorbidities and co-medication, solifenacin did not demonstrate any clinically relevant alteration in blood pressure or heart rate [72].

The efficacy and tolerability of solifenacin in patients with multiple sclerosis and spinal cord injury was assessed more recently in the SONIC trial, a prospective phase IIIb/IV parallel group RCT [73]. Approximately 25% of study participants were on concomitant muscle relaxers for spasticity, most patients with multiple sclerosis were female and most with spinal cord injury were male. Patients used a placebo run-in and were then randomized to solifenacin 5 mg, solifenacin 10 mg, oxybutynin 5 mg three times daily and placebo for 4 weeks. Solifenacin 10 mg significantly improved maximum cystometric capacity (134 ml vs. 5 ml in placebo) and quality of life scores. Improvement in bladder volume at first contraction and first leak and detrusor pressure at first leak were also seen with solifenacin 10 mg. Dry mouth rates were 2.3% for placebo, 4.2% for solifenacin 5 mg, 7.8% for solifenacin 10 mg, and 17% for oxybutynin 5 mg three times daily.

Treatment of children with solifenacin was studied in an open-label study of solifenacin in boys and girls [74]. Mean age was 9.2 years at start of treatment (n = 175). Significant improvements in number of incontinence episodes, completely dry rates, and urodynamics parameters were seen with greater improvements noted for idiopathic OAB than neurogenic OAB.

Tolterodine

TOLT is a tertiary amine with a major active metabolite, 5-HMT, which significantly contributes to the therapeutic effect of the drug [75]. Both TOLT and its metabolite have plasma half-lives of 2–3 h, but their effects on the bladder seem to be more long lasting. Whether this could be the result of urinary excretion of the drug with direct bladder mucosal effects remains unknown. TOLT does not have muscarinic subtype selectivity, but there is evidence in some experimental models that it has functional selectivity for the bladder over the salivary glands [76]. This has been shown in the guinea pig where the binding affinity of TOLT and oxybutynin (OXY) to muscarinic receptors in the bladder was very similar, but the affinity of TOLT for muscarinic receptors in the parotid gland was eight times lower than that of OXY [77]. TOLT is available in two formulations: an IR form prescribed as 2 mg twice daily and an ER form prescribed as 2 or 4 mg once daily. The ER formulation offers more stable blood levels of the drug and metabolite which appears to improve both efficacy and tolerability [78]. There appears to be a very low incidence of cognitive side effects with TOLT, which is likely due to the low lipophilicity of the drug and its metabolite, minimizing penetration into the CNS [79]. A notable subset of patients, up to 10% of whites and up to 19% of blacks, lacks the specific CYP enzyme, 2D6, which metabolizes TOLT to 5-HMT [80]. In these patients, a higher side effect profile, specifically including sleep disturbance, is seen [81]. Metabolism that does not utilize the CYP2D6 mechanism has the potential for less pharmacokinetic variability.

Several double-blind RCTs have documented the efficacy of TOLT in patients with OAB. The OBJECT (Overactive Bladder: Judging Effective Control and Treatment) trial compared TOLT IR 2 mg twice daily to OXY ER 10 mg daily [82]. This was a double-blind, parallel group RCT (n = 378) in patients with OAB treated for 12 weeks. The study showed OXY ER to be significantly more effective than TOLT in reducing urinary frequency, UUI episodes, and total incontinence episodes. The most common adverse event, dry mouth, was reported in 28% of those taking OXY ER and 33% of those taking TOLT IR. Rates of other adverse events including CNS effects were generally low and comparable between the groups. The OPERA (Overactive Bladder: Performance of Extended Release Agents) trial compared TOLT ER 4 mg once daily to OXY ER 10 mg once daily in 790 women with OAB symptoms [83]. This was a double-blind RCT with duration of 12 weeks. Improvements in UUI episodes were similar between the two groups but cure of UUI was greater in the OXY ER group (23.0% vs. 16.8%, $P = 0.03$). OXY ER was also more effective in reducing micturition frequency ($P = 0.003$) at the price of increased rates of dry mouth ($P = 0.02$). Adverse events were mild and occurred at low rates, with both groups having similar rates of discontinuation of treatment.

The ACET (Antimuscarinic Clinical Effectiveness Trial) was an open-label study of 1289 patients with OAB comparing TOLT ER 2 or 4 mg daily to OXY 5 or 10 mg daily [84]. After 8 weeks, 70% of patients taking TOLT ER 4 mg perceived an improved bladder condition compared to 60% in the TOLT ER 2 mg group, 59% in the OXY ER 5 mg group, and 60% in the OXY ER 10 mg group ($P < 0.01$). Dry mouth was dose dependent with both drugs; however, patients treated with TOLT ER 4 mg reported a significantly lower severity of dry mouth compared with OXY ER 10 mg. Fewer patients withdrew from the TOLT ER 4 mg group (12%) than either the OXY ER 5 mg group (19%) or the OXY ER 10 mg group (21%). Although the findings suggest that TOLT ER 4 mg may have improved clinical efficacy and tolerability to OXY ER 10 mg, the open-label design of this study makes for a less convincing conclusion.

In the IMPACT (Improvement in Patients: Assessing Symptomatic Control with TOLT ER) study, the efficacy of TOLT in improving patients' most bothersome symptoms was assessed [85]. It found significant reduction in patients' most bothersome symptom, which was either incontinence episodes, urgency episodes, or micturition frequency. Dry mouth occurred in 10% of patients and constipation in 4%. Conflicting data exists on the concomitant use of TOLT and pelvic floor muscle training. In a prospective, open study of 139 women with OAB who were randomized to TOLT, bladder training, or both, combination therapy was found to be most effective [86]. Similarly, a multicenter, single-blind study of 505 patients comparing TOLT alone to TOLT plus bladder training concluded that the effectiveness of TOLT could be augmented with the addition of a bladder training regimen [87]. However, a similar multinational RCT including 480 patients concluded that no additional benefit was seen with the addition of pelvic floor muscle exercises to TOLT [88].

TOLT ER has shown a significant increase heart rate in a proportion of subjects; however, this effect was not seen with darifenacin or placebo [29]. In a study of solifenacin versus TOLT ER, similar therapeutic and urodynamic effects were noted, but TOLT had a greater effect on increasing heart rate [89].

A new formulation of TOLT 2 mg IR with delayed release pilocarpine 9 mg administered twice daily (added to mitigate the adverse side effects of tolterodine on the salivary glands) was compared to TOLT 2 mg IR alone and placebo [90]. A total of 138 participants underwent double-blind randomized to 1 of the 3 treatment arms. Both treatment arms showed similar reductions in incontinence episodes and daily micturitions. The TOLT/pilocarpine combination had consistently lower scores for all dry mouth parameters compared to TOLT alone.

Trospium

Trospium is a hydrophilic, quaternary amine with limited ability to cross the blood-brain barrier. This should result in minimal cognitive related dysfunction [91], and it has demonstrated undetectable levels in the cerebral spinal fluid on day 10 of use [92]. Trospium does not have muscarinic subtype selectivity and, unlike the previous antimuscarinics mentioned, is not metabolized hepatically by the CYP enzyme system. It is mainly eliminated unchanged in the urine by renal tubular secretion and, as a result, may affect the urothelial mucosal signaling system as has been shown in the rat [93]. Whether this contributes to clinical efficacy in humans remains unknown at this time.

In a multicenter, double-blind RCT, the effect of trospium on urodynamic parameters was studied in patients with neurogenic DO secondary to SCI [94]. A 20 mg dose was given twice daily for 3 weeks. An increase in maximum cystometric capacity and bladder compliance and a decrease in maximal detrusor pressure were seen in the treatment group. A similar study compared the use of trospium and OXY in the treatment of neurogenic DO; both medications appeared to have equal efficacy, but the patients on trospium experienced fewer side effects [95].

The effectiveness of trospium in the treatment of non-neurogenic OAB has also been well documented. Allousi et al. performed a double-blind RCT comparing trospium 20 mg twice daily to placebo in 309 patients [96]. At 3 weeks, urodynamic studies revealed an increase in maximum cystometric capacity and volume at first involuntary bladder contraction in the trospium group. In a study comparing the efficacy of trospium 20 mg twice daily with TOLT IR 2 mg twice daily and placebo in patients with OAB ($n = 232$), trospium was found to be significantly more effective in decreasing the frequency of micturition than either TOLT or placebo [97]. Additionally, trospium caused a greater reduction in incontinence episodes with a similar rate of dry mouth as TOLT. A long-term tolerability and efficacy study comparing trospium 20 mg twice daily and OXY 5 mg twice daily in patients with OAB ($n = 358$) undergoing treatment for 52 weeks was performed [98]. Urodynamics and patient-recorded voiding diaries were performed at baseline, 26 weeks, and 52 weeks. Mean maximum cystometric capacity increased in the trospium group by 92 ml at 26 weeks and by 115 ml at 52 weeks. No other significant urodynamic differences were seen between the groups. The micturition diaries indicated a reduction in urinary frequency, incontinence frequency, and a reduction in urgency episodes in both treatment groups. At least one adverse event occurred in the majority of patients: 64.8% in the trospium group and 76.6% in the OXY group. The most common side effect in both groups was dry mouth. Overall, both drugs were comparable in the efficacy in improving urinary symptoms, but trospium had a better benefit-risk ratio than OXY due to better tolerability.

An ER formulation of trospium, 60 mg once daily, has been shown in RCTs to have similar efficacy and side effects as the twice-daily preparation [99]. An analysis of patients 75 years of age and older ($n = 143$) showed improvement in all voiding diary parameters and quality of life in patients on trospium ER compared to controls [100]. No central nervous system adverse effects were reported during the 12-week study; however, during the 9-month open-label follow-up, one patient reported dizziness and one reported vertigo thought to be possibly related to trospium ER.

Intravesical installation of trospium was studied with a single center, single-blind RCT with 84 patients [101]. Since intravesical trospium does not seem to be absorbed, an opportunity exists for treatment with minimal systemic antimuscarinic effects [102]. Compared to placebo, intravesical trospium produced a significant increase in maximum bladder capacity and a decrease in detrusor pressure. No improvement in uninhibited bladder contractions was seen. No adverse events were reported but an increase in residual urine was noted.

Trospium has not been reported to result in cognitive dysfunction.

Dual Musculotropic Relaxants-Antimuscarinic Agents

Some pharmacologic agents for the treatment of OAB have dual mechanisms of action. They have antimuscarinic activity as well as direct musculotropic relaxant effects on the bladder smooth muscle at a site metabolically distal to the antimuscarinic receptor. It is felt that the clinical effects of these drugs are primarily explained by antimuscarinic action.

Flavoxate

Flavoxate has direct inhibitory action on smooth muscle along with very weak anticholinergic properties [103]. The drug has also been found to possess moderate calcium antagonistic activity, exhibit local anesthetic properties, and have the ability to inhibit phosphodiesterase (PDE) [104]. In rats and in cats, there is some evidence that flavoxate may also have central effects on the inhibition of the micturition reflex [105, 106].

Clinical studies addressing the efficacy of flavoxate in the treatment of OAB have shown mixed results. In a double-blind crossover study comparing flavoxate 1200 mg daily with OXY 15 mg daily in 41 women with idiopathic OAB, the drugs had similar efficacy with flavoxate having fewer and milder side effects [107]. A very small study in the elderly population with non-neurogenic DO showed flavoxate had essentially no effect on maximum cystometric capacity and incontinence episodes [108]. Chapple et al. also suggest no beneficial effect of flavoxate in the treatment of idiopathic OAB [109]. In general, few side effects were reported during treatment. No recent RCTs addressing the efficacy of this drug have been performed.

Oxybutynin

OXY is a moderately potent antimuscarinic agent that has strong independent musculotropic relaxant activity as well as local anesthetic activity (that is likely only important during intravesical administration). It is a tertiary amine that is metabolized primarily by the CYP system into its primary metabolite, N-desethyl-oxybutynin (DEO) [110]. The recommended oral adult dose for the IR formulation is 5 mg three or four times daily. An ER once-daily oral formulation, as well as a transdermal delivery system (TDS) with twice-weekly dosing, and a transdermal gel with once-daily dosing are available. Side effects are secondary to nonspecific muscarinic receptor binding.

Initial reports documented success in depressing neurogenic DO [111], and subsequent reports documented successes in inhibiting idiopathic DO as well [112]. A meta-analysis summarizing 15 RCTs ($n = 476$) reported a 52% mean reduction in incontinence episodes, a 33% mean reduction in micturition frequency, and a mean overall improvement rate of 74%. This came at the expense of a 70% of patients experiencing an adverse event [113]. Holmes and associates compared the results of OXY and propantheline in a small group of women with OAB [57]. The experimental design was a randomized crossover trial with a patient-regulated variable dose regimen. This kind of dose titration study allows the patient to increase the drug dose to whatever is perceived to be the optimum ratio between clinical improvement and side effects. Of the 23 women in the trial, 14 reported subjective improvement with OXY as opposed to 11 with propantheline. Both drugs significantly increased the maximum cystometric capacity and reduced the maximum detrusor pressure on filling. The only significant objective difference was a greater increase in the maximum cystometric capacity with OXY. The mean total daily dose of OXY tolerated was 15 mg (range 7.5–30 mg) and that of propantheline was 90 mg (range 45–145 mg).

The therapeutic effect of OXY IR is associated with a high incidence of side effects, which are often dose limiting [114]. The ER form of OXY uses an osmotic system to release the active compound at a controlled rate over a period of 24 h. As a result there is less absorption in the proximal portion of the gastrointestinal tract and less first-pass metabolism. By decreasing the liver metabolite DEO, it was thought that fewer side effects, especially dry mouth, would occur, thus improving patient compliance [115]. Studies looking at salivary output showed markedly diminished production following administration of OXY IR or TOLT IR with gradual return to normal. In OXY ER group, salivary output was maintained at pre-dose levels throughout the day [116]. OXY IR and ER have been compared in a multicenter, double-blind RCT of 106 patients, all of whom had previously responded to IR OXY [117]. Similar efficacy and similar side effect profiles were noted for both formulations.

As noted above in the OBJECT study, OXY 10 mg ER proved superior to TOLT 2 mg IR twice daily with respect to weekly UUI episodes, total incontinence, and frequency [82]. The two drugs were equally well tolerated. The follow-up OPERA study compared OXY 10 mg ER to TOLT 4 mg ER and found no significant difference in efficacy between the two drugs [83]. The incidence of dry mouth was statistically lower in the TOLT group. One general consensus following this study was that IR formulations of one drug should not be compared to ER formulations of another drug.

Three different doses of OXY (5, 10, and 15 mg) were compared in a RCT, and a significant dose-response relationship for both UUI episodes and dry mouth was found. The greatest patient satisfaction was with the 15 mg dose [118].

Transdermal administration of OXY (OXY-TDS) alters the metabolism of the drug, further reducing the production of DEO compared to OXY ER. The 3.9 mg daily dose patch decreased both micturition frequency and incontinence episodes while increasing mean voided volume [119]. Dry mouth rate was similar to placebo. In a study comparing OXY-TDS to OXY IR, similar reductions in incontinence episodes were found, but significantly less dry mouth was seen with OXY-TDS (38% vs. 94% with OXY IR) [120]. In a third study, OXY-TDS was compared to placebo and TOLT ER [121]. Both drugs had similarly significant reduced daily incontinence episodes and increased voided volume, but TOLT ER was associated with a higher rate of adverse events. The major side effect for OXY-TDS was pruritus at the application site in 14% and erythema in 8.3%. The pharmacokinetics of OXY-TDS was studied using blood and saliva samples in a two-way crossover RCT with OXY ER [122]. The TDS route of administration resulted in greater systemic availability of drug with minimal metabolism to DEO. As a result, patients had greater salivary output and less dry mouth than when taking OXY ER. However, in a review by Cartwright and Cardozo on the published and presented data, they concluded that the good balance between efficacy and tolerability with OXY-TDS was offset by the rate of local skin reaction [123]. In a study assessing achievement of patient-selected goals of therapy, OXY-TDS demonstrated a significant improvement in daily urgency episodes with no difference in achievement of patients' own goals for therapy or health-related quality of life compared to placebo [124].

The transdermal application (3.9 md/daily) has demonstrated subjective efficacy in the pediatric population. There was a 35% skin site irritation reported and 20% of participants discontinued use [125].

In Japan, a new transdermal oxybutynin patch was developed with 73.5 mg of oxybutynin delivered daily and a new softer gentler adhesive. Daily dosing allows for utilization of a different skin site daily which can further decrease the skin site irritation [126]. A total of 1,530 patients were randomized to oxybutynin patch, propiverine, or placebo. The study showed superiority of the patch over placebo and non-inferiority with propiverine. Application site dermatitis was reported in 31.8% but generally considered mild. Dry mouth and constipation were much less frequent with the patch than with propiverine.

Intravesical administration of OXY is a conceptually attractive form of drug delivery, especially for patients who already perform intermittent catheterization. A specific intravesical formulation of the drug is not available, and currently the oral formulation, either liquid or crushed tablet in solution, is delivered by periodic insertion through a catheter. Several nonrandomized, unblinded, and non-placebo controlled studies have demonstrated efficacy of this therapy in a variety of patients with neurogenic bladders showing significant improvements in cystometric capacity, volume at first IVC, bladder compliance, and overall continence [127, 128]. In a study looking at the pharmacokinetics of intravesical OXY versus oral, it was found that plasma OXY levels following oral administration rose to 7.3 mg/ml within 2 h then precipitously dropped to <2 mg/ml at 4 h [129]. In the intravesical group, plasma levels rose gradually to a peak of 6.2 mg/ml at 3.5 h and remained between 3 and 4 mg/ml at 9 h. From these data it is unclear whether the intravesically applied drug acted locally or systemically. In a double-blind RCT in 52 women with DO, patients received once-daily intravesical OXY (20 mg in 40 ml sterile water) or placebo for 12 days [130]. The results revealed significant differences in first desire to void (from 95 ml pretreatment to 150 ml post treatment), cystometric capacity (205–310 ml), maximum pressure during filling (16–9 cmH20), daytime frequency (7.5–4), and nocturia (5.1–1.8). Side effects were similar in the treated and placebo groups. For unexplained reasons, 19/23 patients in the treated group continued to have symptomatic relief after termination of the study.

OXY topical gel is a transdermal formulation, which is applied once daily to the abdomen, thigh, shoulder, or upper arm area [131]. The 1-gram application dose delivers approximately 4 mg of drug to the circulation with stable plasma concentrations. In a multicenter RCT, 789 patients (89% women) with urge predominant urinary incontinence were assigned to OXY gel or placebo once daily for 12 weeks. Mean number of UUI episodes, as recorded on 3-day voiding diary, was reduced by 3.0 episodes/day versus 2.5 in the placebo arm ($P < 0.0001$). Urinary frequency was decreased by 2.7 episodes/day and voided volume increased by 21 ml (vs. 2.0 episodes, $P = 0.0017$ and 3.8 ml, $P = 0.0018$ in the placebo group, respectively). Dry mouth was reported in 6.9% of the treatment group versus 2.8% of the placebo group. Skin reaction at the application site was reported in 5.4% of the treatment group versus 1.0% in the placebo arm. It is felt that improved skin tolerability of the gel over the OXY TDS delivery system is secondary to lack of adhesive and skin occlusion. The gel dries rapidly upon application and leaves no residue; person-to-person transference via skin contact is largely eliminated if clothing is worn over the application site. In a phase III study of 704 patients with urgency predominant urinary incontinence, OXY topical gel resulted in improvement in daily incontinence episodes, frequency of micturition, voided volume, and health-related quality of life [132]. Dry mouth occurred in 7.4% vs. 2.8% of the placebo group ($P = 0.006$).

OXY 3% topical gel utilizes a metered dose pump dispenser and propylene glycol to assist with skin permeation. Two doses of the gel (84 mg/day and 56 mg/day) were compared to placebo in a phase III RCT ($n = 626$). The 84 mg/day dose was statistically better than placebo in improving weekly UI episodes as well as frequency and volume voided [133]. The lower dose was not statistically better than placebo. Dry mouth was seen in 12.1% (vs. 5% in placebo arm) and application site erythema was noted in 3.3% (vs. 0.5% in placebo arm).

Propiverine

Propiverine is a musculotropic smooth muscle relaxant with nonselective antimuscarinic activity. Calcium antagonistic properties have also been found, but the importance of this component for the drug's clinical effects has not been established [134]. This drug is not currently available in the United States.

In an analysis of 9 RCTs using propiverine in a total of 230 patients, a 17% reduction in micturition frequency was seen. Additionally, there was a 64 ml mean increase in bladder capacity and a 77% subjective improvement rate. Side effects were found in 14% [113]. In a study on patients with neurogenic DO, propiverine was found to increase bladder capacity and decrease maximum detrusor contractions compared to placebo [135]. Several comparative studies have confirmed the efficacy of propiverine and suggested that the drug may be equally efficacious in increasing bladder capacity and lowering bladder pressure with fewer side effects than OXY [136, 137]. A study comparing propiverine 15 mg twice daily to TOLT IR 2 mg twice daily showed comparable efficacy, tolerability, and improvement in HRQoL [138]. In 2006, Abrams and colleagues presented data that refuted these prior studies [139]. In a double-blind, placebo-controlled crossover study comparing propiverine 20 mg daily, propiverine 15 mg three times daily, OXY 5 mg three times daily, and placebo, propiverine 20 mg daily was inferior to OXY in reducing IVCs. Additionally, propiverine had a more pronounced effect on gastrointestinal, cardiovascular, and visual function. A large Japanese study of 1584 patients randomized patients to solifenacin 5 or 10 mg, propiverine 20 mg, or placebo [140]. All active treatments showed superiority to placebo in reducing voiding frequency, increasing voided volume, and improving HRQL. Solifenacin 10 mg showed greater reduction in nocturia episodes and urgency episodes, and increased volume voided compared to propiverine 20 mg. Side effects were also greater for the solifenacin 10 mg group with more dry mouth and constipation.

A recent study found the ER formulation of propiverine to be non-inferior to TOLT ER [141]. A greater reduction in bladder symptoms was seen for propiverine ER and discontinuation rates because adverse events were less (3.1% vs. 7.4% for TOLT ER).

Considerations

Three specific areas of concern with antimuscarinic medication deserve special mention: urinary retention, cognitive impairment, and glaucoma. In the past there was universal concern regarding the risk of urinary retention when prescribing antimuscarinic drugs. However, as Andersson and Wein [11] and Andersson et al. [2] propose, these drugs are usually competitive antagonists, which imply that when there is massive release of ACh during voiding, the effect of the drug should be diminished. If this did not occur, urinary retention would result from inability of the bladder to contract. And in fact, at high doses urinary retention can occur, but this is uncommon at doses typically prescribed for OAB [11]. Our current understanding is such that the dose range used for beneficial effects in OAB (the "therapeutic window") is lower than that needed to produce a significant reduction in the voiding contraction. Monitoring PVRs in patients with prostatic enlargement or incomplete bladder emptying is still recommended; however, these diagnoses should not be considered as absolute contraindications to the use of antimuscarinics.

More recently concern over the association of anticholinergics and cognitive impairment has prompted several studies evaluating reaction time, memory, confusion, and other cognitive decrements. In a longitudinal cohort study involving 372 adults age > 60 years without dementia at recruitment, the effects of continuous anticholinergic drug use on cognition was assessed [142]. Eighty percent of anticholinergic users were classified as having mild cognitive impairment compared with only 35% of nonusers. There was no difference between users and nonusers in the risk of developing dementia after 8 years of follow-up. Other studies in continent elderly volunteers have shown no significant effects on cognition [26]. A recent study looked at cumulative anticholinergic use and found that to be associated with an increased risk of dementia [143]. OXY, due to its small molecular size and increased propensity to cross the blood-brain barrier, has demonstrated the greatest potential to elicit cognitive impairment [144]. Studies with solifenacin, trospium chloride ER, and darifenacin demonstrate significantly lower risk of cognitive effect than OXY [26, 145] with little or no cognitive risk to otherwise healthy older adults with OAB. There are few data available on the cognitive consequences of anticholinergics in patients with dementia. However, cholinesterase inhibitors, which are often used to improve cognition in Alzheimer's disease, have been shown to precipitate urinary incontinence [146]. A study on 26 cognitively impaired older adults examined the addition of propiverine 20 mg daily to donepezil and found improved rates of continence with no significant effect on cognition [147]. A large observational study ($n = 3{,}563$) of long-term care residents with dementia failed to identify cognitive decline with the concomitant use of cholinesterase inhibitors and anticholinergics (OXY or TOLT) compared to cholinesterase inhibitors alone [148]. However, in the subset of higher-functioning participants on dual therapy, there was a 50% faster rate of physical function decline suggesting concomitant use may affect a subset of the older population with dementia.

Patients with OAB and glaucoma present another therapeutic dilemma for urologists. Both conditions increase in prevalence with age, and it has been estimated that the conditions coexist in approximately 11.6% of female patients (in Japan) [149]. The distinction between open-angle and narrow-angle glaucoma is an important one, and when the answer is unknown, referral to an ophthalmologist is imperative. A Japanese study reported that in approximately 75% of patients with glaucoma and OAB, the glaucoma is open angle, and this was felt to confer no additional risk to therapeutic intervention with anticholinergic medication. In the remaining 25% with narrow angle glaucoma, risk was felt to be elevated only if iridotomy has not been performed or has not successfully controlled the disease, reducing the true contraindication rate to approximately 8.3% of patients with OAB. Interestingly, the same study found that 33% of patients did not report glaucoma on their medical intake form. Underestimating the risk of glaucoma can result in blindness, albeit rarely, while overestimating (which often occurs out of fear) can result in denial of the most effective oral agents for the treatment of OAB. Complaints of eye pain, headache, or visual loss following initiation of anticholinergic therapy should be taken seriously, and prompt medical advice should be sought [150].

Conclusion

Antimuscarinic drugs are proven efficacious and safe in most adults and are the mainstay of treatment for OAB [13]. The continuous evolution and development of newer agents stems from the fact that the ideal agent has yet to be found—one that is LUT selective, easily administered, and relatively inexpensive. This search continues, and therapies with different mechanisms of action are currently being studied with great promise. Until then, the lessons we have learned from comprehensive systematic review of the literature include:

1. Older drugs such as OXY have high withdrawal rates due to side effects, while newer agents have consistently favorable tolerability
2. Newer agents such as darifenacin, solifenacin, and fesoterodine provide dose flexibility to allow individual titration for maximal efficacy versus tolerability
3. Extended-release once-a-day dosing appears to be better tolerated and potentially more efficacious in improving symptoms and HRQoL than immediate release dosing
4. Newer agents appear to pose less risk of cognitive decline in the elderly than OXY.

However, head-to-head studies comparing all of these agents are limited.

References

1. Abrams P, Cardozo L, Fall M, Griffiths D, Rosier P, Ulmsten U; Standardisation Sub-committee of the International Continence Society, et al. The standardisation of terminology of lower urinary tract function: report from the Standardisation Sub-committee of the International Continence Society. Neurourol Urodyn. 2002;21(2):167–78.
2. Andersson K-E, Cardozo L, Cruz F, Lee K-S, Sahai A, Wein AJ. Pharmacological treatment of urinary incontinence. In: Abrams P, Cardozo L, Wagg A, Wein AJ, editors. Incontinence. 6th ed. Bristol: ICI-ICS. International Continence Society; 2017. pp. 805–958.
3. Andersson KE. Pharmacology of lower urinary tract smooth muscles and penile erectile tissues. Pharmacol Rev. 1993;45(3):253–308.
4. Abrams P, Andersson KE. Muscarinic receptor antagonists for overactive bladder. BJU Int. 2007;100(5):987–1006.
5. Wein AJ, Levin RM, Barrett DM. Voiding function: relevant anatomy, physiology, and pharmacology. In: Duckett JW, Howards ST, Grayhack JT, Gillenwater JY, editors. Adult and pediatric urology. St. Louis: Mosby; 1991. p. 933–99.
6. Andersson KE, Wein AJ. Pharmacology of the lower urinary tract: basis for current and future treatments of urinary incontinence. Pharmacol Rev. 2004;56(4):581–631.

7. Jensen D Jr. Pharmacological studies of the uninhibited neurogenic bladder. II. The influence of cholinergic excitatory and inhibitory drugs on the cystometrogram of neurological patients with normal and uninhibited neurogenic bladder. Acta Neurol Scand. 1981;64(3):175–95.
8. Andersson KE, Yoshida M. Antimuscarinics and the overactive detrusor-which is the main mechanism of action? Eur Urol. 2003;43(1):1–5.
9. Chess-Williams R. Muscarinic receptors of the urinary bladder: detrusor, urothelial and prejunctional. Auton Autacoid Pharmacol. 2002;22(3):133–45.
10. Yoshida M, Miyamae K, Iwashita H, Otani M, Inadome A. Management of detrusor dysfunction in the elderly: changes in acetylcholine and adenosine triphosphate release during aging. Urology. 2004;63(3 Suppl 1):17–23.
11. Andersson KE, Wein AJ. Pharmacologic management of storage and emptying failure. In: Wein AJ, Kavoussi LR, Novick AC, Partin AW, Peters CA, editors. Campbell-Walsh Urology. 9th ed. Philadelphia: Saunders; 2007. p. 2091–123.
12. Guay DR. Clinical pharmacokinetics of drugs used to treat urge incontinence. Clin Pharmacokinet. 2003;42(14):1243–85.
13. Chapple CR, Khullar V, Gabriel Z, Muston D, Bitoun CE, Weinstein D. The effects of antimuscarinic treatments in overactive bladder: an update of a systematic review and meta-analysis. Eur Urol. 2008;54(3):543–62.
14. Witte LP, Mulder WM, de la Rosette JJ, Michel MC. Muscarinic receptor antagonists for overactive bladder treatment: does one fit all? Curr Opin Urol. 2009;19(1):13–9.
15. Food and Drug Administration (FDA). Detrol tolterodine tartrate tablets. 2012. https://www.accessdata.fda.gov/drugsatfda_docs/label/2012/020771s028lbl.pdf. LAB-0329-6.1. Reference ID: 3168088. Revised Aug 2012. Accessed 7 Mar 2018.
16. Food and Drug Administration (FDA). VESIcare (solifenacin succinate) tablets. 2008. https://www.accessdata.fda.gov/drugsatfda_docs/label/2008/021518s007lbl.pdf. 01232008VES. Revised Nov 2008. Accessed 7 Mar 2018.
17. Food and Drug Administration (FDA). Enablex (darifenacin) extended-release tablets. 2008. http://www.fda.gov/cder/foi/label/2008/021513s004lbl.pdf https://www.accessdata.fda.gov/drugsatfda_docs/label/2008/021513s005lbl.pdf. T2008-40. Revised April 2008. Accessed 7 Mar 2018.
18. European Medicines Agency (EMEA). Toviaz (fesoterodine). EPAR summary for the public. 2012. EMA/84670/2012. www.ema.europa.eu/docs/en_GB/document_library/.../WC500040179.pdf. Accessed 8 Mar 2018.
19. Andersson KE. Antimuscarinics for treatment of overactive bladder. Lancet Neurol. 2004;3(1):46–53.
20. Fader M, Glickman S, Haggar V, Barton R, Brooks R, Malone-Lee J. Intravesical atropine compared to oral oxybutynin for neurogenic detrusor overactivity: a double-blind, randomized crossover trial. J Urol. 2007;177(1):208–13.
21. Andersson KE. Potential benefits of muscarinic M3 receptor selectivity. Eur Urol. 2002;1(4):23.
22. Haab F, Stewart L, Dwyer P. Darifenacin, an M3 selective receptor antagonist, is an effective and well tolerated once daily treatment for overactive bladder. Eur Urol. 2004;45(4):420–9; discussion 429.
23. Chapple C, Steers W, Norton P, Millard R, Kralidis G, Glavind K, Abrams P. A pooled analysis of three phase III studies to investigate the efficacy, tolerability and safety of darifenacin, a muscarinic M3 selective receptor antagonist, in the treatment of overactive bladder. BJU Int. 2005;95(7):993–1001.
24. Cardozo L, Dixon A. Increased warning time with darifenacin: a new concept in the management of urinary urgency. J Urol. 2005;173(4):1214–8.
25. Dwyer P, Kelleher C, Young J, Haab F, Lheritier K, Ariely R, Ebinger U. Long-term benefits of darifenacin treatment for patient quality of life: results from a 2-year extension study. Neurourol Urodyn. 2008;27(6):540–7.

26. Lipton RB, Kolodner K, Wesnes K. Assessment of cognitive function of the elderly population: effects of darifenacin. J Urol. 2005;173(2):493–8.
27. Chancellor MB, Staskin DR, Kay GG, Sandage BW, Oefelein MG, Tsao JW. Blood-brain barrier permeation and efflux exclusion of anticholinergics used in the treatment of overactive bladder. Drugs Aging. 2012;29(4):259–73.
28. Serra DB, Affrime MB, Bedigian MP, Greig G, Milosavljev S, Skerjanec A, Wang Y. QT and QTc interval with standard and supratherapeutic doses of darifenacin, a muscarinic M3 selective receptor antagonist for the treatment of overactive bladder. J Clin Pharmacol. 2005;45(9):1038–47.
29. Olshansky B, Ebinger U, Brum J, Egermark M, Viegas A, Rekeda L. Differential pharmacological effects of antimuscarinic drugs on heart rate: a randomized, placebo-controlled, double-blind, crossover study with tolterodine and darifenacin in healthy participants > or = 50 years. J Cardiovasc Pharmacol Ther. 2008;13(4):241–51.
30. Ney P, Pandita RK, Newgreen DT, Breidenbach A, Stöhr T, Andersson KE. Pharmacological characterization of a novel investigational antimuscarinic drug, fesoterodine, in vitro and in vivo. BJU Int. 2008;101(8):1036–42.
31. Chapple CR, Yamaguchi O, Ridder A, Liehne J, Carl S, Mattiasson A, et al. Clinical proof of concept study (blossom) shows novel beta 3 andrenoceptor agonist YM178 is effective and well tolerated in the treatment of symptoms of overactive bladder (abstract 674). Eur Urol Suppl. 2008;7(3):239.
32. Michel MC. Fesoterodine: a novel muscarinic receptor antagonist for the treatment of overactive bladder syndrome. Expert Opin Pharmacother. 2008;9(10):1787–96.
33. Malhotra B, Gandelman K, Sachse R, Wood N, Michel MC. The design and development of fesoterodine as a prodrug of 5-hydroxymethyl tolterodine (5-HMT), the active metabolite of tolterodine. Curr Med Chem. 2009;16(33):4481–9.
34. de Mey C, Mateva L, Krastev Z, Sachse R, Wood N, Malhotra B. Effects of hepatic dysfunction on the single-dose pharmacokinetics of fesoterodine. J Clin Pharmacol. 2011;51(3):397–405.
35. Khullar V, Rovner ES, Dmochowski R, Nitti V, Wang J, Guan Z. Fesoterodine dose response in subjects with overactive bladder syndrome. Urology. 2008;71(5):839–43.
36. Kelleher CJ, Tubaro A, Wang JT, Kopp Z. Impact of fesoterodine on quality of life: pooled data from two randomized trials. BJU Int. 2008;102(1):56–61.
37. Herschorn S, Swift S, Guan Z, Carlsson M, Morrow JD, Brodsky M, Gong J. Comparison of fesoterodine and tolterodine extended release for the treatment of overactive bladder: a head-to-head placebo-controlled trial. BJU Int. 2010;105(1):58–66.
38. Kaplan SA, Schneider T, Foote JE, Guan Z, Carlsson M, Gong J. Superior efficacy of fesoterodine over tolterodine extended release with rapid onset: a prospective, head-to-head, placebo-controlled trial. BJU Int. 2011;107(9):1432–40.
39. Malhotra B, Wood N, Sachse R, Gandelman K. Thorough QT study of the effect of fesoterodine on cardiac repolarization. Int J Clin Pharmacol Ther. 2010;48(5):309–18.
40. Sand PK, Heesakkers J, Kraus SR, Carlsson M, Guan Z, Berriman S. Long-term safety, tolerability and efficacy of fesoterodine in subjects with overactive bladder symptoms stratified by age: pooled analysis of two open-label extension studies. Drugs Aging. 2012;29(1):119–31.
41. Kelleher CJ, Dmochowski RR, Berriman S, Kopp ZS, Carlsson M. Sustained improvement in patient-reported outcomes during long-term fesoterodine treatment for overactive bladder symptoms: pooled analysis of two open-label extension studies. BJU Int. 2012;110(3):392–400.
42. Wagg A, Khullar V, Marschall-Kehrel D, Michel MC, Oelke M, Darekar A, Bitoun CE, Weinstein D, Osterloh I. Flexible-dose fesoterodine in elderly adults with overactive bladder: results of the randomized, double-blind, placebo-controlled study of fesoterodine in an aging population trial. J Am Geriatr Soc. 2013;61(2):185–93.
43. Muskat Y, Bukovsky I, Schneider D, Langer R. The use of scopolamine in the treatment of detrusor instability. J Urol. 1996;156:1989–90.

44. Kobayashi F, Yageta Y, Yamazaki T, Wakabayashi E, Inoue M, Segawa M, Matsuzawa S. Pharmacological effects of imidafenacin (KRP-197/ONO-8025), a new bladder selective anti-cholinergic agent, in rats. Comparison of effects on urinary bladder capacity and contraction, salivary secretion and performance in the Morris water maze task. Arzneimittelforschung. 2007;57(3):147–54.
45. Yamada S, Seki M, Ogoda M, Fukata A, Nakamura M, Ito Y. Selective binding of bladder muscarinic receptors in relation to the pharmacokinetics of a novel antimuscarinic agent, imidafenacin, to treat overactive bladder. J Pharmacol Exp Ther. 2011;336(2):365–71.
46. Kanayama N, Kanari C, Masuda Y, Ohmori S, Ooie T. Drug-drug interactions in the metabolism of imidafenacin: role of the human cytochrome P450 enzymes and UDP-glucuronic acid transferases, and potential of imidafenacin to inhibit human cytochrome P450 enzymes. Xenobiotica. 2007;37(2):139–54.
47. Homma Y, Yamaguchi T, Yamaguchi O. A randomized, double-blind, placebo-controlled phase II dose-finding study of the novel anti-muscarinic agent imidafenacin in Japanese patients with overactive bladder. Int J Urol. 2008;15(9):809–15.
48. Homma Y, Yamaguchi O. A randomized, double-blind, placebo- and propiverine-controlled trial of the novel antimuscarinic agent imidafenacin in Japanese patients with overactive bladder. Int J Urol. 2009;16(5):499–506.
49. Homma Y, Yamaguchi O. Long-term safety, tolerability, and efficacy of the novel anti-muscarinic agent imidafenacin in Japanese patients with overactive bladder. Int J Urol. 2008;15(11):986–91.
50. Kadekawa K, Onaga T, Shimabukuro S, Shimabukuro H, Sakumoto M, Ashitomi K, et al. Effect of imidafenacin before sleeping on nocturia. LUTS. 2012;4(3):130–5.
51. Wada N, Watanabe M, Kita M, Matsumoto S, Osanai H, Yamaguchi S, et al. Effect of imidafenacin on nocturia and sleep disorder in patients with overactive bladder. Urol Int. 2012;89(2):215–21.
52. Yokoyama O, Homma Y, Yamaguchi O. Imidafenacin, an antimuscarinic agent, improves nocturia and reduces nocturnal urine volume. Urology. 2013;82(3):515–20.
53. Lee KS, Park B, Kim JH, Kim HG, Seo JT, Lee JG, Jang Y, Choo MS. A randomised, double-blind, parallel design, multi-institutional, non-inferiority phase IV trial of imidafenacin versus fesoterodine for overactive bladder. Int J Clin Pract. 2013;67(12):1317–26.
54. Beermann B, Hellstrom K, Rosen A. On the metabolism of propantheline in man. Clin Pharmacol Ther. 1972;13:212–20.
55. Blaivas JG, Labib KB, Michalik J, Zayed AA. Cystometric response to propantheline in detrusor hyperreflexia: therapeutic implications. J Urol. 1980;124:259–62.
56. Thüroff JW, Bunke B, Ebner A, Faber P, de Geeter P, Hannappel J, et al. Randomized, double-blind, multicenter trial on treatment of frequency, urgency and incontinence related to detrusor hyperactivity: oxybutynin versus propantheline versus placebo. J Urol. 1991;16(Suppl 1):48–61.
57. Holmes DMMF, Stanton SL. Oxybutynin versus propantheline in the management of detrusor instability. A patient-regulated variable dose trial. Br J Obstet Gynaecol. 1989;96:607–12.
58. Wiener LB, Baum NH, Suarez GM. New method for management of detrusor instability: transdermal scopolamine. Urology. 1986;28:208–10.
59. Ikeda K, Kobayashi S, Suzuki M, Miyata K, Takeuchi M, Yamada T, Honda K. M(3) receptor antagonism by the novel antimuscarinic agent solifenacin in the urinary bladder and salivary gland. Naunyn Schmiedeberg's Arch Pharmacol. 2002;366(2):97–103.
60. Tanaka Y, Masumori N, Tsukamoto T. Urodynamic effects of solifenacin in untreated female patients with symptomatic overactive bladder. Int J Urol. 2010;17(9):796–800.
61. Lowenstein L, Kenton K, Mueller ER, Brubaker L, Sabo E, Durazo-Arivzu RA, Fitzgerald MP. Solifenacin objectively decreases urinary sensation in women with overactive bladder syndrome. Int Urol Nephrol. 2012;44(2):425–9.
62. Chapple CR, Araño P, Bosch JL, De Ridder D, Kramer AE, Ridder AM. Solifenacin appears effective and well tolerated in patients with symptomatic idiopathic detrusor overactivity in a placebo- and tolterodine-controlled phase 2 dose-finding study. BJU Int. 2004;93(1):71–7.

63. Cardozo L, Lisec M, Millard R, van Vierssen TO, Kuzmin I, Drogendijk TE, et al. Randomized, double-blind placebo controlled trial of the once daily antimuscarinic agent solifenacin succinate in patients with overactive bladder. J Urol. 2004;172(5 Pt 1):1919–24.
64. Chapple CR, Martinez-Garcia R, Selvaggi L, Toozs-Hobson P, Warnack W, Drogendijk T, et al. STAR study group. A comparison of the efficacy and tolerability of solifenacin succinate and extended release tolterodine at treating overactive bladder syndrome: results of the STAR trial. Eur Urol. 2005;48(3):464–70.
65. Luo D, Liu L, Han P, Wei Q, Shen H. Solifenacin for overactive bladder: a systematic review and meta-analysis. Int Urogynecol J. 2012;23(8):983–91.
66. Kelleher C, Cardozo L, Kobashi K, Lucente V, et al. Solifenacin: as effective in mixed urinary incontinence as in urge urinary incontinence. Int Urogynecol J Pelvic Floor Dysfunct. 2006;17(4):382.
67. Wagg A, Wyndaele JJ, Siever P. Efficacy and tolerability of solifenacin in elderly subjects with overactive bladder syndrome: a pooled analysis. Am J Geriatr Pharmacother. 2006;4(1):14.
68. van Rey F, Heesakkers J. Solifenacin in multiple sclerosis patients with overactive bladder: a prospective study. Adv Urol. 2011;2011:834753.
69. Garely AD, Kaufman JM, Sand PK, Smith N, Andoh M. Symptom bother and health-related quality of life outcomes following solifenacin treatment for overactive bladder: the VESIcare Open-Label Trial (VOLT). Clin Ther. 2006;28(11):1935–46.
70. Bolduc S, Moore K, Nadeau G, Lebel S, Lamontagne P, Hamel M. Prospective open label study of solifenacin for overactive bladder in children. J Urol. 2010;184(4 Suppl):1668–73.
71. Asajima H, Sekiguchi Y, Matsushima S, Saito N, Saito T. QT prolongation and torsade de pointes associated with solifenacin in an 81-year-old woman. Br J Clin Pharmacol. 2008;66(6):896–7.
72. Michel MC, Wetterauer U, Vogel M, de la Rosette JJ. Cardiovascular safety and overall tolerability of solifenacin in routine clinical use: a 12-week, open-label, post-marketing surveillance study. Drug Saf. 2008;31(6):505–14.
73. Amarenco G, Sutory M, Zachoval R, Agarwal M, Del Popolo G, Tretter R, et al. Solifenacin is effective and well tolerated in patients with neurogenic detrusor overactivity: results from the double-blind, randomized, active- and placebo-controlled SONIC urodynamic study. Neurourol Urodyn. 2017;36(2):313–21.
74. Nadeau G, Schröder A, Moore K, Genois L, Lamontagne P, Hamel M, et al. Long-term use of solifenacin in pediatric patients with overactive bladder: extension of a prospective open-label study. Can Urol Assoc J. 2014;8(3–4):118–23.
75. Brynne N, Stahl MM, Hallén B, Edlund PO, Palmér L, Höglund P, Gabrielsson J. Pharmacokinetics and pharmacodynamics of tolterodine in man: a new drug for the treatment of urinary bladder overactivity. Int J Clin Pharmacol Ther. 1997;35(7):287–95.
76. Nilvebrant L, Sundquist S, Gillberg PG. Tolterodine is not subtype (m1-m5) selective but exhibits functional bladder selectivity in vivo (abstract). Abstracts from the 26th Annual Meeting of the International Continence Society. Neurourol Urodyn. 1996;15(4):310–1.
77. Nilvebrant L, Hallén B, Larsson G. Tolterodine—a new bladder selective muscarinic receptor antagonist: preclinical pharmacological and clinical data. Life Sci. 1997;60(13–14):1129–36.
78. Van Kerrebroeck P, Kreder K, Jonas U, Zinner N, Wein A; Tolterodine Study Group. Tolterodine once daily: superior efficacy and tolerability in the treatment of overactive bladder. Urology. 2001;57(3):414–21.
79. Hills CJ, Winter SA, Balfour JA. Tolterodine Drugs. 1998;55(6):813–20; discussion 821–2.
80. Xie HG, Kim RB, Wood AJ, Stein CM. Molecular basis of ethnic differences in drug disposition and response. Annu Rev Pharmacol Toxicol. 2001;41:815–50.
81. Diefenbach K, Jaeger K, Wollny A, Penzel T, Fietze I, Roots I. Effect of tolterodine on sleep structure modulated by CYP2D6 genotype. Sleep Med. 2008;9(5):579–82.
82. Appell RA, Sand P, Dmochowski R, Anderson R, Zinner N, Lama D; Overactive Bladder: Judging Effective Control and Treatment Study Group, et al. Prospective randomized controlled trial of extended release oxybutynin chloride and tolterodine tartrate in the treatment of overactive bladder: Results of the OBJECT study. Mayo Clin Proc. 2001;76(4):358–63.

83. Diokno AC, Appell RA, Sand PK, Dmochowski RR, Gburek BM, Klimberg IW, Kell SH; OPERA Study Group. Prospective, randomized, double-blind study of the efficacy and tolerability of the extended-release formulations of oxybutynin and tolterodine for overactive bladder: results of the OPERA trial. Mayo Clin Proc. 2003;78(6):687–695.
84. Sussman D, Garely A. Treatment of overactive bladder with once-daily extended-release tolterodine or oxybutynin: the antimuscarinic clinical effectiveness trial (ACET). Curr Med Res Opin. 2002;18(4):177–84.
85. Elinoff V, Bavendam T, Glasser DB, Carlsson M, Eyland N, Roberts R. Symptom-specific efficacy of tolterodine extended release in patients with overactive bladder: the IMPACT trial. Int J Clin Pract. 2006;60(6):745–51.
86. Song C, Park JT, Heo KO, Lee KS, Choo MS. Effects of bladder training and/or tolterodine in female patients with overactive bladder syndrome: a prospective, randomized study. J Korean Med Sci. 2006;21(6):1060–3.
87. Mattiasson A, Blaakaer J, Høye K, Wein AJ; Tolterodine Scandinavian Study Group. Simplified bladder training augments the effectiveness of tolterodine in patients with an overactive bladder. BJU Int. 2003;91(1):54–60.
88. Millard RJ; Asia Pacific Tolterodine Study Group. Clinical efficacy of tolterodine with or without a simplified pelvic floor exercise regimen. Neurourol Urodyn. 2004;23(1):48–53.
89. Hsiao SM, Chang TC, Wu WY, Chen CH, Yu HJ, Lin HH. Comparisons of urodynamic effects, therapeutic efficacy and safety of solifenacin versus tolterodine for female overactive bladder syndrome. J Obstet Gynaecol Res. 2011;37(8):1084–91.
90. Dmochowski RR, Staskin DR, Duchin K, Paborji M, Tremblay TM. Clinical safety, tolerability and efficacy of combination tolterodine/pilocarpine in patients with overactive bladder. Int J Clin Pract. 2014;68(8):986–94.
91. Todorova A, Vonderheid-Guth B, Dimpfel W. Effects of tolterodine, trospium chloride , and oxybutynin on the central nervous system. J Clin Pharmacol. 2001;41(6):636–44.
92. Staskin D, Kay G, Tannenbaum C, Goldman HB, Bhashi K, Ling J, Oefelein MG. Trospium chloride is undetectable in the older human central nervous system. J Am Geriatr Soc. 2010;58(8):1618–9.
93. Kim Y, Yoshimura N, Masuda H, De Miguel F, Chancellor MB. Intravesical instillation of human urine after oral administration of trospium, tolterodine, and oxybutynin in a rat model of detrusor overactivity. BJU Int. 2006;97(2):400–3.
94. Stöhrer M, Bauer P, Giannetti BM, Richter R, Burgdörfer H, Mürtz G. Effect of trospium chloride on urodynamic parameters in patients with detrusor hyperreflexia due to spinal cord injuries: a multicenter placebo-controlled double-blind trial. Urol Int. 1991;47(3):138–43.
95. Madersbacher H, Stöhrer M, Richter R, Burgdörfer H, Hachen HJ, Mürtz G. Trospium chloride versus oxybutynin: a randomized double blind, multicenter trial in the treatment of detrusor hyperreflexia. Br J Urol. 1995;75(4):452–6.
96. Allousi S, Laval KU, Eckert R. Trospium chloride (Spasmo-lyt) in patients with motor urge syndrome (detrusor instability): a double-blind, randomised, multicentre, placebo-controlled study. J Clin Res. 1998;1:439–51.
97. Jünemann KP, Al-Shukri S. Efficacy and tolerability of trospium chloride and tolterodine in 234 patients with urge-syndrome: a double-blind, placebo-controlled multicenter clinical trial. Neurourol Urodyn. 2000;19:488–9.
98. Halaska M, Ralph G, Wiedemann A, Primus G, Ballering-Brühl B, Höfner K, Jonas U. Controlled, double-blind, multicenter clinical trial to investigate long-term tolerability and efficacy of trospium chloride in patients with detrusor instability. World J Urol. 2003;20(6):392–9.
99. Dmochowski RR, Sand PK, Zinner NR, Staskin DR. Trospium 60 mg once daily (QD) for overactive bladder syndrome: results from a placebo-controlled interventional study. Urology. 2008;71(3):449–54.
100. Sand PK, Johnson Ii TM, Rovner ES, Ellsworth PI, Oefelein MG, Staskin DR. Trospium chloride once-daily extended release is efficacious and tolerated in elderly subjects (aged >/= 75 years) with overactive bladder syndrome. BJU Int. 2011;107(4):612–20.

101. Fröhlich G, Burmeister S, Wiedemann A, Bulitta M. Intravesical instillation of trospium chloride, oxybutynin and verapamil for relaxation of the bladder detrusor muscle. A placebo controlled, randomized clinical test. Arzneimittelforschung. 1998;48(5):486–91. *[Article in German].*
102. Walter P, Grosse J, Bihr AM, Kramer G, Schulz HU, Schwantes U, Stöhrer M. Bioavailability of trospium chloride after intravesical instillation in patients with neurogenic lower urinary tract dysfunction: a pilot study. Neurourol Urodyn. 1999;18(5):447–53.
103. Ruffmann R. A review of flavoxate hydrochloride in the treatment of urge incontinence. J Int Med Res. 1988;16(5):317–30.
104. Guarneri L, Robinston E, Testa R. A review of flavoxate: pharmacology and mechanism of action. Drugs Today. 1994;30:91–9.
105. Oka M, Kimura Y, Itoh Y, Sasaki Y, Taniguchi N, Ukai Y, et al. Brain pertussis toxin-sensitive G proteins are involved in the flavoxate hydrochloride-induced suppression of the micturition reflex in rats. Brain Res. 1996;727(1–2):91–8.
106. Kimura Y, Sasaki Y, Hamada K, Fukui H, Ukai Y, Yoshikuni Y, et al. Mechanisms of suppression of the bladder activity by flavoxate. Int J Urol. 1996;3(3):218–27.
107. Milani R, Scalambrino S, Milia R, Sambruni D, Riva L, Pulici F, et al. Double-blind crossover comparison of flavoxate and oxybutynin in women affected by urinary urge syndrome. Int Urogynecol J. 1993;4(1):3–8.
108. Briggs RS, Castleden CM, Asher MJ. The effect of flavoxate on uninhibited detrusor contractions and urinary incontinence in the elderly. J Urol. 1980;123(5):665–6.
109. Chapple CR, Parkhouse H, Gardener C, Milroy EJ. Double-blind, placebo-controlled, cross-over study of flavoxate in the treatment of idiopathic detrusor instability. Br J Urol. 1990;66(5):491–4.
110. Waldeck K, Larsson B, Andersson KE. Comparison of oxybutynin and its active metabolite, N-desethyl-oxybutynin, in the human detrusor and parotid gland. J Urol. 1997;157(3):1093–7.
111. Thompson I, Lauvetz R. Oxybutynin in bladder spasm, neurogenic bladder and enuresis. Urology. 1976;8(5):452–4.
112. Andersson KE. Current concepts in the treatment of disorders of micturition. Drugs. 1988;35(4):477–94.
113. Thüroff JW, Chartier-Kastler E, Corcus J, Humke J, Jonas U, Palmtag H, Tanagho EA. Medical treatment and medical side effects in urinary incontinence in the elderly. World J Urol. 1998;16(Suppl 1):S48–61.
114. Baigrie RJ, Kelleher JP, Fawcett DP, Pengelly AW. Oxybutynin: is it safe? Br J Urol. 1988;62(4):319–22.
115. Gupta SK, Sathyan G. Pharmacokinetics of an oral once-a-day controlled-release oxybutynin formulation compared with immediate-release oxybutynin. J Clin Pharmacol. 1999;39:289–96.
116. Chancellor MB, Appell RA, Sathyan G, Gupta SK. A comparison of the effects on saliva output of oxybutynin chloride and tolterodine tartate. Clin Ther. 2001;23(5):753–60.
117. Anderson RU, Mobley D, Blank B, Saltzstein D, Susset J, Brown JS. Once daily controlled versus immediate release oxybutynin chloride for urge urinary incontinence. OROS Oxybutynin Study Group. J Urol. 1999;161(6):1809–12.
118. Corcos J, Casey R, Patrick A, Andreou C, Miceli PC, Reiz JL; Uromax Study Group, et al. A double-blind randomized dose-response study comparing daily doses of 5, 10 and 15 mg controlled-release oxybutynin: balancing efficacy with severity of dry mouth. BJU Int. 2006;97(3):520–527.
119. Dmochowski RR, Davila GW, Zinner NR, Gittelman MC, Saltzstein DR, Lyttle S, Sanders SW; Transdermal Oxybutynin Study Group. Efficacy and safely of transdermal oxybutynin in patients with urge and mixed urinary incontinence. J Urol. 2002;168(2):580–586.
120. Davila GW, Daugherty CA, Sanders SW; Transdermal Oxybutynin Study Group. A short-term, multicenter, randomized double-blind dose titration study of the efficacy and anticholinergic side effects of transdermal compared to immediate release oral oxybutynin treatment of patients with urge urinary incontinence. J Urol. 2001;166(1):150–1.

121. Dmochowski RR, Sand PK, Zinner NR, Gittelman MC, Davila GW, Sanders SW; Transdermal Oxybutynin Study Group. Comparative efficacy and safety of transdermal oxybutynin and oral tolterodine versus placebo in previously treated patients with urge and mixed urinary incontinence. Urology. 2003;62(2):237–242.
122. Appell RA. Efficacy and safety of transdermal oxybutynin in patients with urge and mixed urinary incontinence. Curr Urol Rep. 2003;4(5):343.
123. Cartwright R, Cardozo L. Transdermal oxybutynin: sticking to the facts. Eur Urol. 2007;51(4):907–14.
124. Cartwright R, Srikrishna S, Cardozo L, Robinson D. Patient-selected goals in overactive bladder: a placebo controlled randomized double-blind trial of transdermal oxybutynin for the treatment of urgency and urge incontinence. BJU Int. 2011;107(1):70–6.
125. Gleason JM, Daniels C, Williams K, Varghese A, Koyle MA, Bägli DJ, et al. Single center experience with oxybutynin transdermal system (patch) for management of symptoms related to non-neuropathic overactive bladder in children: an attractive, well tolerated alternative form of administration. J Pediatr Urol. 2014;10(4):753–7.
126. Yamaguchi O, Uchida E, Higo N, Minami H, Kobayashi S, Sato H; Oxybutynin Patch Study Group. Efficacy and safety of once-daily oxybutynin patch versus placebo and propiverine in Japanese patients with overactive bladder: a randomized double-blind trial. Int J Urol. 2014;21(6):586–593.
127. Connor JP, Betrus G, Fleming P, Perlmutter AD, Reitelman C. Early cystometrograms can predict the response to intravesical instillation of oxybutynin chloride in myelomeningocele patients. J Urol. 1994;151(4):1045–7.
128. Szollar SM, Lee SM. Intravesical oxybutynin for spinal cord injury patients. Spinal Cord. 1996;34(5):284–7.
129. Madersbacher H, Jilg G. Control of detrusor hyperreflexia by the intravesical instillation of oxybutynin hydrochloride. Paraplegia. 1991;29(2):84–90.
130. Enzelsberger H, Helmer H, Kurz C. Intravesical instillation of oxybutynin in women with idiopathic detrusor instability: a randomized trial. Br J Obstet Gynaecol. 1995;102(11):929–39.
131. Staskin DR, Dmochowski RR, Sand PK, Macdiarmid SA, Caramelli KE, Thomas H, Hoel G. Efficacy and safety of oxybutynin chloride topical gel for overactive bladder: a randomized, double-blind, placebo controlled, multicenter study. J Urol. 2009;181(4):1764–72.
132. Sand PK, Davila GW, Lucente VR, Thomas H, Caramelli KE, Hoel G. Efficacy and safety of oxybutynin chloride topical gel for women with overactive bladder syndrome. Am J Obstet Gynecol. 2012;206(2):168.e161–6.
133. Goldfischer ER, Sand PK, Thomas H, Peters-Gee J. Efficacy and safety of oxybutynin topical gel 3% in patients with urgency and/or mixed urinary incontinence: a randomized, double-blind, placebo-controlled study. Neurourol Urodyn. 2015;34(1):37–43.
134. Haruno A. Inhibitory effects of propiverine hydrochloride on the agonist-induced or spontaneous contractions of various isolated muscle preparations. Arzneimittelforschung. 1992;42(6):815–7.
135. Stöhrer M, Madersbacher H, Richter R, Wehnert J, Dreikorn K. Efficacy and safety of propiverine in SCI patients suffering from detrusor hyperreflexia—a double-blind, placebo-controlled clinical trial. Spinal Cord. 1999;37(3):196–200.
136. Stöhrer M, Mürtz G, Kramer G, Schnabel F, Arnold EP, Wyndaele JJ; Propiverine Investigator Group. Propiverine compared to oxybutynin in neurogenic detrusor overactivity- results of a randomized, double-blind, multicenter clinical study. Eur Urol. 2007;51(1):235–242.
137. Madersbacher H, Halaska M, Voigt R, Alloussi S, Höfner K. A placebo-controlled, multicentre study comparing the tolerability and efficacy of propiverine and oxybutynin in patients with urgency and urge incontinence. BJU Int. 1999;84(6):646–51.
138. Jünemann KP, Halaska M, Rittstein T, Mürtz G, Schnabel F, Brünjes R, Nurkiewicz W. Propiverine versus tolterodine: efficacy and tolerability in patients with overactive bladder. Eur Urol. 2005;48(3):478–82.
139. Abrams P, Cardozo L, Chapple C. Comparison of the efficacy, safety, and tolerability of propiverine and oxybutynin for the treatment of overactive bladder syndrome. Int J Urol. 2006;13(6):692–8.

140. Yamaguchi O, Marui E, Kakizaki H, Itoh N, Yokota T, Okada H; Japanese Solifenacin Study Group, et al. Randomized, double-blind, placebo- and propiverine-controlled trial of the once-daily antimuscarinic agent solifenacin in Japanese patients with overactive bladder. BJU Int. 2007;100(3):579–587.
141. Leng J, Liao L, Wan B, Du C, Li W, Xie K, et al. Results of a randomized, double-blind, active-controlled clinical trial with propiverine extended release 30 mg in patients with overactive bladder. BJU Int. 2017;119(1):148–57.
142. Ancelin ML, Artero S, Portet F, Dupuy AM, Touchon J, Ritchie K. Non-degenerative mild cognitive impairment in elderly people and use of anticholinergic drugs: longitudinal cohort study. BMJ. 2006;332(7539):455–9.
143. Gray SL, Anderson ML, Dublin S, Hanlon JT, Hubbard R, Walker R, et al. Cumulative use of strong anticholinergics and incident dementia: a prospective cohort study. JAMA Intern Med. 2015;175(3):401–7.
144. Kay GG, Ebinger U. Preserving cognitive function for patients with overactive bladder: evidence for a differential effect with darifenacin. Int J Clin Pract. 2008;62(11):1792–800.
145. Staskin D, Kay G, Tannenbaum C, Goldman HB, Bhashi K, Ling J, Oefelein MG. Trospium chloride has no effect on memory testing and is assay undetectable in the central nervous system of older patients with overactive bladder. Int J Clin Pract. 2010;64(9):1294–300.
146. Hashimoto M, Imamura T, Tanimukai S, Kazui H, Mori E. Urinary incontinence: an unrecognised adverse effect with donepezil. Lancet. 2000;356(9229):568.
147. Sakakibara R, Ogata T, Uchiyama T, Kishi M, Ogawa E, Isaka S, et al. How to manage overactive bladder in elderly individuals with dementia? A combined use of donepezil, a central acetylcholinesterase inhibitor, and propiverine, a peripheral muscarine receptor antagonist. J Am Geriatr Soc. 2009;57(8):1515–7.
148. Sink KM, Thomas J 3rd, Xu H, Craig B, Kritchevsky S, Sands LP. Dual use of bladder anticholinergics and cholinesterase inhibitors: long-term functional and cognitive outcomes. J Am Geriatr Soc. 2008;56(5):847–53.
149. Kato K, Furuhashi K, Suzuki K, Murase T, Sato E, Gotoh M. Overactive bladder and glaucoma: a survey at outpatient clinics in Japan. Int J Urol. 2007;14(7):595–7.
150. Fink AM, Aylward GW. Buscopan and glaucoma: a survey of current practice. Clin Radiol. 1995;50(3):160–4.

Chapter 7
β3-Agonists for Overactive Bladder

Sophia Delpe Goodridge and Roger R. Dmochowski

Abbreviations

AE	Adverse effects
BID	Twice daily
BIM	Budget income model
BMI	Body mass index
BOO	Bladder outlet obstruction
BPM	Beats per minute
DBP	Diastolic blood pressure
HR	Heart rate
HRQOL	Health-related quality of life
HTN	Hypertension
LUTS	Lower urinary tract symptoms
NDO	Neurogenic detrusor overactivity
OAB	Overactive bladder
OAB-qSS	Overactive bladder questionnaire symptom score
PPBC	Patient perception of bladder control
PVR	Post-void residual
Qmax	Maximum flow
Qmaxpdet	Detrusor pressure at maximum flow
SBP	Systemic blood pressure
TEAE	Treatment emergent adverse effect
TS-VAS	Treatment satisfaction-visual analog scale
UDS	Urodynamics
UI	Urinary incontinence
UTI	Urinary tract infection

S. D. Goodridge · R. R. Dmochowski (✉)
Vanderbilt University, Department of Urologic Surgery, Nashille, TN, USA
e-mail: roger.dmochowski@vanderbilt.edu

L. Cox, E. S. Rovner (eds.), *Contemporary Pharmacotherapy of Overactive Bladder*, https://doi.org/10.1007/978-3-319-97265-7_7

Introduction

Overactive bladder (OAB), while not a life-threatening disease, is a debilitating condition impacting 10.7% of the population with an anticipated impact on 546 million people by 2018 worldwide [1]. It is reported that Europe has the highest prevalence followed by North America, South America, Asia, and Africa [1]. As specified by the American Urological Association and Society of Urodynamics, Female Pelvic Medicine, and Urogenital Construction, the first step in management of OAB is behavioral modification followed by a trial of medications [2]. Traditionally, anticholinergics are the first-line drug of choice; however, this class of medications may have significant side effects including dry mouth, constipation, and potential for cognitive and other central nervous system adverse events (AE). These side effects may lead to non-compliance and a poor quality of life. It has been reported that persistence with anticholinergic medication use is only 13% at 1 year [3]. Given these findings, researchers and clinicians have searched for alternative oral agent treatment options with similar efficacy and a more favorable side effect profile. Mirabegron, a β3-agonist, is the first medication in this class approved for use in the United States, Canada (Myrbetriq®, Astellas Pharma US, Northbrook IL, USA), Europe (Betmiga®, Astellas Pharma BV, Brussels, Belgium), and Japan (Betanis®, Astellas Pharma Inc., Tokyo, Japan) for the treatment of OAB.

This chapter will review the pathophysiology of micturition to understand the pharmacologic effects of β-agonists on the lower urinary tract. The pharmacokinetics of mirabegron will also be discussed followed by a review of studies demonstrating the clinical efficacy of mirabegron compared to placebo and to anticholinergic medications. Adverse effects and contraindications will also be reviewed.

Pathophysiology of Micturition

Bladder innervation is controlled by the sympathetic and parasympathetic nervous systems. Under normal circumstances, excitation of the parasympathetic system results in effective bladder wall contraction and complete bladder emptying. Conversely, excitation of the sympathetic system enables bladder wall relaxation and subsequent storage of urine via activation of β-adrenoceptors. Three such β-adrenoceptors exist: β1, β2, and β3. Specifically, β3-adrenergic receptors are expressed on nerve fibers in the mucosa and muscular layers of the bladder. Of the three subtypes, β3 is predominant in the human detrusor muscle, accounting for 97% of its β-adrenoceptor agonists and is activated by adrenergic stimulation resulting in detrusor relaxation [4, 5].

Recognition of the role of β-adrenoceptors in bladder storage led to the development of a selective β3-adrenoceptor agonist targeted at facilitating bladder wall relaxation and improvement of storage. In the 1980s and 1990s, research for a potent β3 agonist gained momentum owing to the development of mirabegron which has been shown to have a high intrinsic affinity for the β3-adrenoceptor agonist and very low intrinsic activity at β1 and β2 adrenoceptors [6, 7].

Pharmacokinetics of Mirabegron

Mirabegron is rapidly absorbed in plasma in the unchanged form. In humans it is then metabolized in the liver by cytochrome P450 (CYP) 3A4 as well as CYP2D6. Once orally ingested, it is excreted via urine (55%) and feces (34%) as metabolites and unchanged drug form. The metabolites, phase II glucuronides, are not pharmacologically active toward β3-adrenoceptors. Given its method of metabolism, mirabegron may be subject to drug-drug interactions, particularly with other medications interacting with cytochrome P450 [8–12].

Pharmacokinetic testing has been done on healthy subjects, specifically nonobese Japanese, Chinese, and Taiwanese men and women with ages ranging from 20 to 54. The subjects were tested under fasting conditions, low-fat diets, and high-fat diets with administered doses of mirabegron ranging from 25 mg to 100 mg [13]. Samples of blood and urine assessing the concentration of mirabegron were done at varying time periods. Overall, this study showed a decrease in absorption of the drug with ingestion of food. Independent of dose, a decrease in mirabegron plasma concentration was noted in patients exposed to food. A greater reduction was noted in patients following a low-fat meal compared to high-fat meals. Despite these findings, interindividual variability in the maximum concentration of drug was similar in the fasted and fed states. This suggests that dose adjustment is not necessary in the clinical setting regardless of patients' dietary intake [13, 14].

Similar studies were conducted in Europe, Australia, and North America in healthy, adult subjects between ages 18 and 55 with body mass indices (BMI) ranging between 20 and 32, with similar results [15]. Again, drug concentration was higher when medication was administered under fasting conditions in both the 50 mg and 100 mg dosages. Though there is a reduction in drug concentration in fed patients, this appears to be clinically insignificant with patients reaching therapeutic drug concentration regardless of diet and BMI. Adverse effects of reported with mirabegron use included increased blood pressure, increased heart rate, nausea, and headache. This will be discussed in further detail later in the chapter. These studies demonstrated similar findings in drug bioavailability and concentration in a diverse group of patients [13–15].

Clinical Efficacy of Mirabegron

To date, several clinical trials have been done assessing the efficacy of mirabegron [16, 17]. Chapple and associates published a review article assessing phase III clinical trials of mirabegron with similar study designs. Varying doses of mirabegron were used, and some studies compared efficacy with both placebo and tolterodine [18]. Mirabegron daily doses ranging from 25 to 100 mg demonstrated significant efficacy in urgency incontinence (UI), urgency, and micturition frequency.

In a pooled analysis of three clinical trials, Chapple et al. [18] reported on the primary endpoints assessed, including mean micturition episodes per 24 h and mean incontinence episodes per 24 h. Compared to 59.6% of patients in the placebo group, 69.5% of patients in the 50 mg group and 70.5% of patients in the 100 mg group reported ≥50% reduction in incontinence from baseline ($p \leq 0.001$). The percentage of patients with <8 micturitions/24 h at their final visit was 31.6% in the 50 mg group and 34% in the 100 mg group, compared to 24.6% of patients in the placebo group ($p \leq 0.001$). Secondary endpoints assessed were mean voided volume, level of urgency, urgency episodes, and nocturia episodes from baseline to final visit. For both mirabegron 50 mg and 100 mg groups, all secondary endpoints were improved compared to placebo in a statistically significant way ($p \leq 0.05$). In a pooled data analysis of patients ≥65, mirabegron 50 mg and 100 mg were effective in reducing the mean number of incontinence episodes per 24 h from baseline to final visit by 1.6. From baseline to final visit, the mean number of micturitions was decreased by 1.7 in the 50 mg group and 1.8 in the 100 mg group [18].

In the four trials using the overactive bladder questionnaire (OAB-q), the minimally important difference was exceeded in all domains in the mirabegron group versus placebo with the exception of the social interaction domain in three of the studies. The patient perception of bladder control (PPBC), which was evaluated for responsiveness to treatment by Coyne et al. [19], also demonstrated subjective measures of improvement in patients taking mirabegron. Significant changes were defined as major improvement (≥2 category decrease), minor improvement (≥1 category decrease), no change, or deterioration (≥1 category increase). Minor and major improvements on PPBC at the final visit compared to baseline were appreciated in mirabegron 100 mg vs placebo in two of the studies reviewed ($p \leq 0.001$). Treatment satisfaction-visual analog scale (TS-VAS) showed statistically significant improvements in both the mirabegron 50 mg and 100 mg groups versus placebo ($p \leq 0.001$) [18]. Overall, a parallel improvement was found in both subjective and objective measures in the mirabegron groups.

Nitti and colleagues conducted a multicenter, randomized, double-blind, placebo-controlled trial assessing safety and efficacy in a diverse group of subjects [20]. The subjects were men and women of varying racial backgrounds, age ≥ 18 with a diagnosis of OAB for at least 3 months in the absence of infection, chronic inflammation, severe hypertension, bladder stones, previous pelvic radiation, pelvic tumor/mass, continued use of anticholinergic medication, clinically significant stress incontinence, or stress-predominant mixed incontinence. These patients had to report a baseline daily voiding frequency of at least eight episodes in addition to three or more urgency episodes during a 3-day period.

Patients were equally divided into three groups: placebo ($n = 454$), 50 mg daily group ($n = 442$), and 100 mg daily group ($n = 433$). Demographics and baseline characteristics were similar between the three groups.

Both mirabegron groups, when compared to placebo, had decreases in micturition episodes per 24-hour period, mean level of urgency, as well as mean number of incontinence episodes ($p \leq 0.05$). Both treatment groups also had an increase in their mean voided volume of urine per void ($p \leq 0.05$). Subjectively, the mirabegron groups were noted to have significant improvements in healthcare-related quality of life (HRQOL) as assessed by the OAB-q [20].

In the United States, mirabegron is approved for usage at doses of 25 mg and 50 mg. The Food and Drug Administration, after reviewing several double-blind, placebo-controlled, multicenter randomized trials, found that efficacy in treatment with reduced number of voids per day and episodes of urgency incontinence in a 24-h period [21]. There are studies which suggest that supratherapeutic doses of mirabegron (100–200 mg) may result in increased tachycardia and hypertension [16] (Chapple phase II dose ranging).

Comparison of Mirabegron to Anticholinergic Drugs

Given the standard pharmacologic treatment for overactive bladder has been anticholinergics, a head-to-head comparison between the standard of care and mirabegron is important for clinical decision-making. Kosilov et al. conducted a randomized controlled trial evaluating the effectiveness and safety of mirabegron compared to solifenacin in patients over the age of 65 with OAB [22]. Subjects (143 women and 95 men) were split into four groups with approximately 50 people per group: (1) mirabegron 50 mg, (2) solifenacin 10 mg, (3) combination of mirabegron 50 mg and solifenacin 10 mg, and (4) placebo. Response to treatment was measured by urodynamic evaluation pre- and post-treatment, OAB questionnaires, as well as bladder diaries. Both the mirabegron only and solifenacin only groups had similar improvement in the number of incontinence episodes and voids per day. In the mirabegron only group, bladder capacity and detrusor compliance were improved ($p \leq 0.05$), but the maximum bladder capacity did not change significantly ($p \geq 0.05$), while in the solifenacin only group, all UDS parameters improved ($p \leq 0.05$). No statistically significant improvements were seen in patients receiving placebo ($p \geq 0.05$). In all groups, post-void residual (PVR) increased by no more than 15 cc [22]. Additionally, 21 patients out of 63 (33%) reported side effects in the mirabegron only group versus 11/52 (21%) in the solifenacin only group and 59 (24%) in the placebo group. The most common side effects reported were dry mouth, high blood pressure, increased heart rate, dizziness, and pain in the heart. The number of patients who refused to continue therapy due to side effects was clinically insignificant [22]. This study nicely depicts efficacy for both mirabegron and solifenacin.

Sebastianelli and colleagues completed a systematic review and meta-analysis comparing the efficacy of mirabegron 50 and 100 mg in the treatment of OAB to tolterodine 4 mg and placebo [23]. Eight randomized studies were included in this meta-analysis evaluating 10,248 patients. Both doses of mirabegron and tolterodine were significantly associated with improvement in voided volume, mean number of micturitions per 24 h, incontinence episodes per 24 h, and urgency episodes per 24 h compared to placebo. While tolterodine did not lead to a decrease in nocturia episodes in comparison to placebo ($p = 0.36$), both mirabegron doses lead to a decrease in nocturia ($p \leq 0.05$). No increase in treatment-emergent adverse events (TEAEs) was found in mirabegron compared with placebo. Tolterodine, however, was associated with a significantly greater risk overall of TEAEs compared to placebo ($p < 0.0001$). The discontinuation rate as a result of AE was not significantly changed between treatment groups and placebo.

Anticholinergics and mirabegron appear to have similar efficacy in the treatment and management of OAB. Though not indicated for nocturia, there is a response and improvement in nocturia with the use of mirabegron when compared to tolterodine or placebo. Overall, there is a higher reporting of AEs in the anticholinergic groups. AEs do not result in discontinuation of either drug class in a clinically or statistically significant way.

Combination Therapy

SYNERGY was a multicenter, randomized, double-blind, phase III trial assessing the efficacy of mirabegron monotherapy vs combination therapy with solifenacin [24]. Patients selected for this study were ≥ 18 years of age with OAB symptoms for ≥3 months. Subjects were randomized to mirabegron 25 mg, mirabegron 50 mg, solifenacin 5 mg, mirabegron 25 + solifenacin 5 mg, mirabegron 50 mg + solifenacin 5 mg, or placebo. Key questionnaires used for assessing improvement were OAB-qSS and TS-VAS. All treatment groups had a statistically significant improvement in OAB symptom bother score compared to placebo ($p \leq 0.001$); however the greatest difference was noted in the combination groups ($p \leq 0.001$). HRQOL scores were also observed to be greater in combination groups vs monotherapy groups ($p \leq 0.002$). Both combination groups showed greater improvement in TS-VAS compared to monotherapy groups [24].

Kosilov et al., when comparing effectiveness between mirabegron 50 mg/day and solifenacin 10 mg/day, assessed the efficacy of combination therapy (simultaneous administration of mirabegron 50 mg/day and solifenacin 10 mg/day). When comparing the combination group to the mirabegron only and solifenacin only groups, the combination group had the greatest improvements from baseline. In the combination group, 19/65 (29%) of subjects reported side effects [22].

Collectively, these studies nicely depict that while monotherapy is efficacious in patients with OAB, combination therapy provides increased improvement. Side effects are appreciated in all groups with no greater side effects noted in the combination group compared to mirabegron alone.

Use in Special Populations

Obesity

It is well documented that obesity and metabolic syndrome contribute to OAB and are independent risk factors for the development of urgency/urgency urinary incontinence [25]. Improvements in urinary symptoms have been noted in patients following weight loss [26]. Given this association, Krhut et al. sought to identify the impact of BMI on the efficacy of mirabegron in women with OAB [15]. A total of 169 women were studied and broken down into three groups, stratified by BMI. The three groups were as follows: BMI 18.5–24.9, BMI 25–29.9, and BMI >30. Each group had patients with dry and wet OAB with a predominance of OAB wet patients. There was no statistical difference among the three groups in previous anticholinergic use or baseline symptom severity. All patients were prescribed mirabegron 50 mg daily for a total of 3 months. Nearly all (165/169, 97.6%) patients completed the 3-month treatment course. Within all study groups, there was a statistically significant improvement ($p = <0.05$) in all parameters except for severe urgency episodes within a 24-h period. There were no statistically significant differences in efficacy among the three groups. A sub-analysis of patients who failed prior anticholinergic therapy revealed that there was a significant improvement in all parameters except patients in the group with the highest BMI (average BMI of 34) who were found to have a lower response in regard to the number of micturition episodes per 24 h. Ultimately it was noted that mirabegron is efficacious regardless of BMI and should be considered in both treatment-naïve patients and anticholinergic non-responders.

Bladder Outlet Obstruction

Many men who suffer from bladder outlet obstruction (BOO) concomitantly report lower urinary tract symptoms (LUTS) including OAB symptomatology. Though the reported risk of urinary retention in male patients treated with anticholinergics is less than 3%, there is hesitancy in prescribing these medications to men with BOO [27, 28].

A randomized, double-blind, placebo-controlled multicenter phase II study was done in North America investigating the impact of mirabegron on pressure flow studies in patients with BOO and LUTS [29]. Patients were randomized to mirabegron 50 mg, 100 mg, or placebo for 12 weeks. Urodynamic (UDS) evaluation was performed at week 1 and week 12, specifically assessing maximum flow (Qmax) and pressure at maximum flow (PdetQmax). The Qmax and PdetQmax at treatment end and adjusted average change in Qmax and PdetQmax from baseline to treatment end were similar among the three groups. A dose-dependent increase in PVR was noted at the 12-week visit in patients treated with mirabegron. The PVR from baseline to treatment end in the placebo group was increased by 0.55 ± 10.702 cc compared to 17.9 ± 10.2 cc in the mirabegron 50 mg group and 30.8 ± 10.6 cc in the 100 mg group. While this was a statistically significant change in the 100 mg group ($p = 0.046$), this was not considered clinically significant. The overall incidence of AEs was similar for the placebo and mirabegron group. In particular, urinary retention was noted in one patient in the placebo group and one patient in the mirabegron 100 mg group.

Neurogenic Detrusor Overactivity

Few data have been published on the use of mirabegron in patients with neurogenic detrusor overactivity (NDO). A retrospective review [30] of 15 patients with spinal cord injury and NDO who were treated with mirabegron 25 mg for 2 weeks and then 50 mg for at least 4 more weeks found improvements in the number of incontinence episodes per 24 h. Additionally, on urodynamic evaluation, there were increases in bladder capacity and compliance, as well as detrusor pressure during filling. Further study is warranted in this patient population to better understand the efficacy and tolerability of mirabegron for NDO.

Elderly

The side effect profile of anticholinergics makes them unfavorable drugs for use in elderly populations due to their association with delirium, cognitive impairment, and falls [31] Mirabegron may be an alternative in this vulnerable patient population. In a prospective observational study [32], patients over the age of 65 who were initiating medical treatment for OAB participated in phone surveys over a 3-month period. Patients were either treated with mirabegron or anticholinergics. There was a significant improvement in OAB symptoms for patients in each group throughout the study period. There were no significant differences in improvement found between the two groups. The results of this study suggest that mirabegron is efficacious in an elderly population and has similar efficacy to anticholinergics in this population. However, side effect data was not collected in this study.

Renal and Hepatic Failure Patients

As mentioned above, mirabegron is metabolized via the kidneys and liver. The potential influence of hepatic and renal impairment on the pharmacokinetics of mirabegron was evaluated by Dickinson et al. Male and female subjects in this study were categorized by baseline renal function as determined by estimated glomerular filtration rate or hepatic function as determined by Child-Pugh classification. Subjects in this study received 100 mg of mirabegron. The plasma concentration of mirabegron in mild, moderate, and severe renal impairment was increased by 31, 66, and 118%, respectively, in comparison to healthy subjects. Similarly, patients with mild to moderate hepatic dysfunction had increased plasma concentrations compared to matched healthy subjects by 19 and 65%, respectively. Renal and hepatic insufficiency were also associated with higher maximum concentrations of mirabegron [33, 34].

Plasma concentration and maximum concentration increased significantly in patients with severe renal insufficiency and moderate hepatic insufficiency. Changes seen in patients with mild to moderate renal insufficiency and mild hepatic insufficiency are of a smaller magnitude with less clinical significance. Dosing adjustments should be considered in patients with severe renal insufficiency and moderate hepatic insufficiency [33, 34]. Per the FDA, for patients with an eGFR of 15–29 mL/min/1.73m^2 and moderate hepatic insufficiency, mirabegron dosage should not exceed 25 mg. Treatment is not recommended in patients with end-stage renal disease or severe hepatic impairment (Child-Pugh class C) [21].

Adverse Events

Several studies have reported on the adverse events associated with mirabegron treatment; however the reported rate of serious events is low. In healthy, non-OAB patients, the incidence of serious adverse effects (AEs) with the use of mirabegron was reported as low and similar across dose groups in the fed and fasted condition. Fifty-five percent of the 50 mg group and 60.5% of the 100 mg group experienced minor and self- limited treatment-related adverse events. AEs reported include nausea, headache, mild hypertension, second-degree AV block, and increased pulse rate of >10 beats/min regardless of dose or food condition [13].

The DRAGON investigator group found that the incidence of treatment-related adverse events in patients receiving mirabegron doses ranging from 25 to 100 mg was comparable to placebo [16]. They found an increased incidence of dry mouth in subjects receiving tolterodine 4 mg compared to mirabegron. Serious AEs were reported in <2% of patients across all treatment groups. HR was found to increase in a dose-dependent fashion and only in patients receiving mirabegron doses 100 mg or higher.

Similarly, the BLOSSOM investigator group, which studied mirabegron use at higher doses, found that the incidence of treatment-related adverse events was comparable for the mirabegron and placebo groups [17]. They reported a low rate of discontinuation due to AEs: 1.5% (placebo), 4.6% (mirabegron 100 mg twice daily [BID]), 7.7% (mirabegron 150 mg BID), and 3.1% (tolterodine ER 4 mg daily). Serious adverse effects noted in these groups did not appear to be treatment related. They found that while mirabegron 150 mg BID caused a 5 beats per minute (bpm) increase in heart rate (HR) from baseline, the effects of mirabegron 100 mg BID on

HR were not clinically relevant. No clinically relevant effects on blood pressure were appreciated. Additionally, there were no clinically relevant effects on electrocardiogram, laboratory parameters, or PVR.

Nitti et al. [20] also evaluated AEs and reported them to be similar between the treatment and placebo arms. Urinary retention was not found in any study group, and constipation and dry mouth were reported at low rates (<2%) in both the treatment and placebo arms. Non-culture documented urinary tract infections (UTI) were found in greater proportions in the treatment arms (2.7% in the 50 mg arm and 3.7% in the 100 mg arm) when compared to placebo (1.8%). Two deaths were reported (one in the placebo arm and one in the 100 mg treatment arm), but neither death was deemed study related. Hypertension (HTN) was defined as new-onset hypertension or an increase in systolic blood pressure (SBP) by ≥20 mmHg or diastolic blood pressure (DBP) by ≥10 mmHg on two separate events. Both placebo and treatment groups had similar rates of HTN reported. There was a slight dose-dependent increase in heart rate (HR) in the 50 mg group versus the 100 mg group with a maximal increase in HR of <3 beats per minute. No tachyarrhythmias or QT prolongations were noted in any patient.

Cardiovascular Risks

As mentioned prior, three subtypes of β-adrenoceptors are found in the bladder with subtype 3 contributing to 97% of total β-adrenoceptors. All three of these subtypes are also expressed in the heart. β1 activation results in an increased HR and forced cardiac contractility. β3 activation may have a compounding effect in regard to HR and cardiac contractility with a positive inotropic effect on the atrial tissue and negative inotropic effect on the ventricular tissue. β2 receptors, however, are located in the smooth muscle walls of vascular tissue and activation results in vasodilation [35]. Given the potential effects of mirabegron on cardiac tissue and vasculature, a meta-analysis [36] was done evaluating the effects of β3-agonists on the cardiovascular system. Although these studies included other β3-agonists such as solabegron, ritobegron, TAK677, and BRL35135, the primary focus of the meta-analysis was mirabegron, which was compared to tolterodine 4 mg ER and placebo. Sixteen of these trials were randomized controlled studies focused on mirabegron. Three 12-week trials and one 1-year phase III trial done prospectively analyzed the cardiovascular safety of mirabegron. Doses of mirabegron used in these studies were 25 mg, 50 mg, 100 mg, and 200 mg. Men and women with OAB symptoms ≥18 years old were studied, of which 0.5–1.9% had pre-existing cardiovascular disease.

Cardiac arrhythmias, QT prolongation, and hypertension were the cardiac-related events of interest assessed. For normotensive patients, HTN was defined as average SBP ≥140 or average DBP ≥90 after two consecutive visits. For patients with baseline were consdiered sugnificant HTN, an increase in SBP ≥20 or DBP ≥10 on two consecutive visits or an initiation or increase in antihypertensive medications. Tachycardia was reported if morning and evening resting pulse were greater than 100 beats per minute on 3 separate days [36].

Hypertension was the most common adverse event noted and occurred in approximately 8.7% of the mirabegron 50 mg population and 8.5% of the placebo population, but was not reported to be statistically significant. The mean increase in SBP and DBP was 1 mmHg and was reversible with discontinuation of the medication. Interestingly, the incidence of HTN decreased as the dose of mirabegron increased from 50 mg to 100 mg. A subgroup analysis taking age into account showed similar mean changes in SBP and DBP. Cardiac death, nonfatal myocardial infarction, and nonfatal strokes were not increased in the mirabegron group versus placebo [36].

One randomized placebo, active-controlled trial corrected for HR and assessed QT prolongation. This study looked at 176 healthy men and 176 healthy women and found that at normal dose ranges of mirabegron 25–100 mg, there was no increase in QT intervals. However, in supratherapeutic doses of 200 mg, QT prolongation was noted in the female cohort. In the pooled, 12-week population, the frequency of QT prolongation was low (≤0.4%) and similar between all treatment groups: placebo, mirabegron, and tolterodine [18].

In the 12-week population studies, HR was evaluated, and the treatment group was found to have an increased HR from baseline vs placebo. This increase, however, was 1 beat per minute (BPM) from baseline and was comparable to tolterodine 4 mg ER. Heart rate was actually lower for subjects receiving mirabegron 50 mg in evening measures compared to subjects on tolterodine 4 mg ER. The 1-year study showed an adjusted mean increase from baseline in the mirabegron 100 mg group and tolterodine group, with less of a change in the mirabegron 50 mg group. Again, the adjusted changes from baseline were minimal at <3 BPM. These changes do not appear to be clinically significant [36].

In the pooled 12-week population, the overall incidence of tachycardia was <5% and similar among mirabegron, placebo, and tolterodine groups. Similarly, in the 1-year population, 1.2% of mirabegron 50 mg vs 3.2% of tolterodine ER 4 mg patients reported tachycardia. One patient on mirabegron 50 mg experienced a third-degree atrioventricular block though it is unclear if this was a TEAE [36]. Additionally, the incidence of clinically significant atrial fibrillation was higher in the tolterodine group (1%) than the mirabegron (0.4% in 50 and 100 mg groups) and placebo (0.2%) groups.

Included in this meta-analysis was a study evaluating the efficacy of mirabegron with concurrent use of β-blockers, which is important to note given their opposing physiologic impacts. Seventeen percent of the pooled 12-week population and 19% of the 1-year population reported concomitant β-blocker use, with 11–18% being nonselective β-blockers. Overall, there were reduced mean incontinence episodes and micturition episodes per 24 h from baseline to final visit regardless of the use of β-blockade. In this patient population, mirabegron continued to have good tolerability. No data was available directly comparing adverse effects in β-blocker users with concomitant use of mirabegron versus placebo [36].

Additionally, no clinically relevant cardiac adverse events have been noted in patients using combined therapy of mirabegron/tamsulosin [18].

In summary, patients with overactive bladder and concomitant cardiovascular disease should have an informed discussion with their clinicians before starting treatment for OAB. While most side effects of mirabegron on the cardiovascular system appear to be clinically insignificant, when prescribed, patients should be advised of the risks of hypertension, precipitation of arrhythmia, tachycardia, and QT prolongation. In particular, providers should be cautious in patients with uncontrolled hypertension.

Tolerability

While it is important to know that a specific drug has its intended clinical effect, it is equally as important to consider tolerability and its impact on patient quality of life and compliance.

Studies have suggested that the compliance rate for anticholinergic medications for OAB is low, with discontinuation rates ranging from 4% to 31% at the 12-week mark. This is in part due to lack of efficacy and poor tolerance [37]. In a 2002 survey administered to women in the United States querying patient satisfaction with treatment of OAB, 31% of patients reported discontinuation of OAB treatment due to poor tolerance [38]. Comparatively, Martan and associates sought to evaluate the level of medication adherence of mirabegron at 1 year in patients with OAB. A retrospective, multicenter study [39] was conducted on patients taking mirabegron 50 mg. The study included adult patients with OAB for a minimum of 3 months or patients who had failed prior anticholinergic therapy. At 6 months of follow-up, 181 of 206 (87.9%) patients remained on mirabegron 50 mg, while 7 patients had an increase in dosage to 100 mg and 18 patients had an addition of an anticholinergic (trospium or solifenacin). At 12 months, a total of 29% of patients (43/176 [24.4%] females and 17/30 [56.7%] males) had discontinued treatment. The rate of discontinuation was statistically higher in male participants ($p < 0.001$). No correlation was found between age and rate of treatment persistence. Of the 60 patients who discontinued therapy, 40% reported insufficient efficacy and 43.3% reported reasons for discontinuation as missed follow-up and hospitalization for non-medicine-related reasons. The remaining 16.7% of the patients discontinued therapy due to side effects including tachycardia, headache, vertigo, nausea, eye irritation, lower abdominal pain, and vasculitis. There were no reports of discontinuation due to blurred vision, dry mouth, or constipation. The rate of patients who remained on the initial 50 mg dosage of mirabegron who discontinued treatment was 58/181 (32%) versus the group of patients with an increased dose of 100 mg mirabegron or combination of mirabegron and antimuscarinic who had a discontinuation rate of 2/25 (8%) ($p = 0.013$).

The 29% drop-out rate reported in this study is compared to the reported drop-out rate of 60% in several clinical trials evaluating treatment persistence for antimuscarinics [40, 41]. Overall treatment compliance appears to be higher among the mirabegron monotherapy group in comparison to patients who use anticholinergics as monotherapy. Additionally, there appears to be a decreased drop-out rate in patients who use combination therapy or higher doses of mirabegron; however, the numbers in this study are small.

To compare the tolerability of mirabegron to an anticholinergic, specifically tolterodine ER, a double-blind, prospective study was conducted by Staskin and colleagues [42] assessing the level of bother associated with six side effects: constipation, dry mouth, drowsiness, headache, nausea, and blurred vision. The secondary endpoint of this study was to assess patient preference of the medication. Each drug was administered for 8 weeks before a 2-week washout. The treatment groups were broken down into two periods as follows: mirabegron-washout-tolterodine ($n = 156$), tolterodine-washout-mirabegron ($n = 157$), mirabegron-washout-mirabegron ($n = 31$), and tolterodine-washout-tolterodine ($n = 32$). In patients receiving mirabegron, the dose was up-titrated from 25 mg to 50 mg after 4 weeks. The dose of tolterodine ER remained at 4 mg. At baseline, patients had moderate to severe symptoms of OAB with urgency episodes exceeding 4 in a 24-h period, frequency of urination more than 10 per 24 h, and approximately 2.7 incontinence episodes per day. Interestingly, mean tolerability scores were higher, indicating less bother related to medication side effects, for any mirabegron use (period 1, 85.48; period 2, 87.10) when compared to any use of tolterodine ER (period 1, 82,46; period 2, 84.33) ($p = 0.004$). Patients reported a slight preference for tolterodine ER (51.7%) over mirabegron (48.3%); however this was not statistically significant. Dry mouth was experienced by 56.5% patients during the tolterodine ER period and 44.5% of the patients during the mirabegron period. This information was elicited at each follow-up visit with the medication tolerability scale of the OAB-S questionnaire. No differences were noted between treatments in objective measurements of incontinence and urinary frequency [42].

The authors demonstrated that overall drug tolerability was better in the mirabegron group compared to the tolterodine group; however patient preferences between the two drugs were comparable. Objective improvements and treatment preferences were similar between the two groups; however the AEs were higher with tolterodine.

Cost-Effectiveness

As stated earlier in the chapter, approximately 546 million people are affected by OAB resulting with a net cost in the United States of $65.9 billion in 2007 with a projected increase to $82.6 billion in 2020 [43, 44]. The majority of these costs are due to OAB-related comorbidities including UTIs, sleep disturbances, skin rashes and infections, depression, and increased patient care visits. Additional costs are associated with the untreated patient. Perk et al. [45] described a budget income model (BIM) built to study the economic and clinical impact of use of mirabegron for the treatment of OAB in US commercial payer and Medicare Advantage patients. The cost considered in this analysis included not only prescription drug cost but also the cost associated with physician visits, OAB-related comorbidities, and cognitive effects resulting in outpatient and ED visits. Costs of non-cognitive adverse effects related to pharmacotherapy were considered negligible in this analysis.

The use of mirabegron increased total prescription cost; however, medical costs decreased due to fewer adverse events associated with non-treatment. The number of comorbidities decreased overall as a portion of the untreated population was treated with mirabegron leading to an overall reduction in the cost incurred by payers.

The authors suggested that overall, mirabegron is associated with less cost due to decreased OAB-related comorbidities in addition to the absence of cognitive impacts and its associated costs. No analysis was done on cost savings associated with non-pharmacologic treatment and the impact that may have on overall healthcare costs. In the elderly population where cognitive decline is a serious consideration, mirabegron may offer efficacy with decreased OAB-related costs due to a reduction in comorbidities and the potential impact on cognition of anticholinergics, but this has not yet been specifically studied [46].

Conclusions

In the absence of satisfactory improvement in symptoms from behavioral modification, oral agents are the next step in the management of OAB. Anticholinergics have been the mainstay of treatment until recently. Since the introduction of β3-agonists, researchers and clinicians have sought to assess efficacy and the role of mirabegron in the management of OAB. Mirabegron appears to be a cost-effective, safe, efficacious, and tolerable drug and should be considered as first-line treatment or in patients who have poor tolerance to or are refractory to anticholinergics. Combination therapy with mirabegron and anticholinergics can be considered if a clinically desired response is not achieved by monotherapy because combination therapy seems to offer an even greater improvement in symptoms. There may be a role for mirabegron in neurogenic detrusor overactivity, but further research is needed in this complex population.

References

1. Irwin DE, Kopp ZS, Agatep B, Milsom I, Abrams P. Worldwide prevalence estimates of lower urinary tract symptoms, overactive bladder, urinary incontinence and bladder outlet obstruction. BJU Int. 2011;108(7):1132–8.
2. Gormley EA, Lightner DJ, Burgio KL, Chai TC, Clemens JQ, Culkin DJ; American Urological Association; Society of Urodynamics, Female Pelvic Medicine & Urogenital Reconstruction, et al. Diagnosis and treatment of overactive bladder (non-neurogenic) in adults: AUA/SUFU guideline. 2012; amended 2014. http://www.auanet.org/guidelines/overactive-bladder-(oab)-(aua/sufu-guideline-2012-amended-2014). Accessed 27 Apr 2018.

3. D'Souza AO, Smith MJ, Miller LA, Doyle J, Ariely R. Persistence, adherence and switch rates among extended release and immediate release overactive medications in a regional managed care plan. J Manag Care Pharm. 2008;14(3):291–301.
4. Yamaguchi O, Chapple CR. Beta3-adrenoceptors in urinary bladder. Neurourok Urodyn. 2007;26(6):752–6.
5. Yamaguchi O. Beta3-adrenoceptors in human detrusor muscle. Urology. 2002;59(5 Suppl 1):25–9.
6. Takasu T, Ukai M, Sato S, Matsui T, Nagase I, Maruyama T, Sasamata M, Miyata K, Uchida H, Yamaguchi O. Effect of (R)-2-(2-aminothiazol-4-yl)-4'-{2-[(2-hydroxy-2-phenylethyl)amino] ethyl} acetanilide (YM178), a novel selective beta3-adrenoceptor agonist, on bladder function. J Pharmacol Exp Ther. 2007;321(2):642–7.
7. Sacco E, Bienstinesi R, Tienforti D, Racioppi M, Gulino G, D'Agostino D. Discovery history and clinical development of mirabegron for the treatment of overactive bladder and urinary incontinence. Expert Opin Drug Discovery. 2014;9(4):433–48.
8. Takusagawa S, van Lier JJ, Suzuki K, Nagata M, Meijer J, Krauwinkel W, et al. Absorption, metabolism and excretion of mirabegron (YM178), a potent and selective β3-adrenoceptor agonist, after oral administration to healthy male volunteers. Drug Metab Dispos. 2012;40(4):815–24.
9. Takusagawa S, Miyashita A, Iwatsubu T, Usui T. In vitro inhibition and induction of human cytrochrome P450 enzymes by mirabegron, a potent and selective β3-adrenoceptor agonist. Xenobiotica. 2012;42(12):1187–96.
10. Takusagawa S, Yajima K, Miyashita A, Uehara S, Iwatsubo T, Usui T. Identification of human cytochrome P450 isoforms and esterases involved in the metabolism of mirabegron, a potent and selective β3-adrenoceptor agonist. Xenobiotica. 2012;42(10):957–67.
11. Lee J, Moy S, Meijer J, Krauwinkel W, Sawamoto T, Kerbusch V, et al. Role of cytochrome P450 isoenzymes 3A and 2D6 in the in vivo metabolism of mirabegron, a β3 adrenoceptor agonist. Clin Drug Investig. 2013;33(6):429–40.
12. Krauwinkel W, Dickinson J, Schaddelee M, Meijer J, Tretter R, van de Wetering J, et al. The effect of mirabegron a potent and selective β3 adrenoceptor agonist, on the pharmacokinetics of CYP2D6 substrates desipramine and metoprolol. Eur J Drug Metab Pharmacokinet. 2014;39(1):43–52.
13. Iitauska H, van Gelderen M, Katashima M, Takusagawa S, Sawamoto T. Pharmacokinetics of mirabegron, a β3-adrenoceptor agonist for treatment of overactive bladder in healthy East Asian subjects. Clin Ther. 2015;37(5):1031–44.
14. Lee J, Zhang W, Moy S, Kowalski D, Kerbusch V, van Gelderen M, et al. Effects of food intake on pharmacokinetic properties of mirabegron oral controlled-absorption system: a single dose, randomized, crossover study in healthy adults. Clin Ther. 2013;35(3):333–41.
15. Krhut J, Martan A, Zachoval R, Hanus T, Svabik K, Zvara P. Impact of body mass index on treatment efficacy of mirabegron for overactive bladder in females. Eur J Obstet Gynecol Reprod Biol. 2016;196:64–8.
16. Chapple CR, Dvorak V, Radziszewski P, Van Kerrebroeck P, Wyndaele JJ, Bosman B, et al. Dragon Investigator Group. A phase II dose-ranging study of mirabegron in patients with overactive bladder. Int Urogynecol J. 2013;24(9):1447–58.
17. Chapple CR, Amarenco G, López Aramburu MA, Everaert K, Liehne J, Lucas M, Vik V, et al. BLOSSOM Investigator Group. A proof-of-concept study: mirabegron, a new therapy for overactive bladder. Neurourol Urodyn. 2013;32(8):1116–22.
18. Chapple CR, Cardozo L, Nitti VW, Siddiqui E, Michel MC. Mirabegron in overactive bladder: a review of efficacy, safety, and tolerability. Neurourol Urodyn. 2014;33(1):17–30.
19. Coyne KS, Martza LS, Kopp Z, Abrams P. The validation of the patient perception of bladder condition (PPBC). A single item global measure for patients with overactive bladder. Eur Urol. 2006;49(6):1079–86.
20. Nitti VW, Auerbach S, Martin N, Calhoun A, Lee M, Herschorn S. Results of a randomized phase III trial of mirabegron in patients with overactive bladder. J Urol. 2013;189(4):1388–95.

21. Myrbetriq™ (mirabegron) extended-release tablets, for oral use. Initial U.S. Approval: Revised June 2012. Northbrook: Astellas Pharma US, Inc. https://www.accessdata.fda.gov/drugsatfda_docs/label/2012/202611s000lbl.pdf. Accessed 4 May 2018.
22. Kosilov K, Loparev S, Ivanovskaya M, Kosilova L. A randomized, controlled trial of effectiveness and safety of management of OAB symptoms in elderly men and women with standard-dosed combination of solifenacin and mirabegron. Arch Gerontol Geriatr. 2015;61(2):212–6.
23. Sebastianelli A, Russo G, Kaplan SA, McVary KT, Moncada I, Graves S, et al. Systematic review and meta-analysis on the efficacy and tolerability of mirabegron for the treatment of storage lower urinary tract symptoms/overactive bladder: comparison with placebo and tolterodine. Int J Urol. 2018;25(3):196–205.
24. Robinson D, Kelleher C, Staskin D, Mueller ER, Falconer C, Wang J, et al. Patient-reported outcomes from SYNERGY, a randomized, double-blind, multicenter study evaluating combinations of mirabegron and solifenacin compared with monotherapy and placebo in OAB patients. Neurourol Urodyn. 2018;27(1):394–406.
25. Zacche MM, Giarenis TG, Robinson D, Cardozo L. Is there an association between aspects of the metabolic syndrome and overactive bladder? A prospective cohort study in women with lower urinary tract symptoms. Eur J Obstet Gynecol Reprod Biol. 2017;217:1–5.
26. Subak LL, Whitcomb E, Shen H, Saxton J, Vittinghoff E, Brown JS. Weight loss: a novel and effective treatment for urinary incontinence. J Urol. 2005;174(1):190–5.
27. Kaplan SA, Roehrborn CG, Abrams P, Chapple CR, Bavendam T, Guan Z. Antimuscarinics for treatment of storage lower urinary tract symptoms in men: a systematic review. Int J Clin Pract. 2011;65(4):487–507.
28. Martín-Merino E, García-Rodríguez LA, Massó-González EL, Roehrborn CG. Do oral antimuscarinic drugs carry an increased risk of acute urinary retention? J Urol. 2009;182(4):1442–8.
29. Nitti VW, Rosenberg S, Mitcheson DH, He W, Fakhoury A, Martin NE. Urodynamics and safety of the β3-adrenoceptor agonist mirabegron in males with lower urinary tract symptoms and bladder outlet obstruction. J Urol. 2013;190(4):1320–7.
30. Wöllner J, Pannek J. Initial experience with the treatment of neurogenic detrusor overactivity with a new β-3agonist (mirabegron) in patients with spinal cord injury. Spinal Cord. 2016;54(1):78–82.
31. Saraf AA, Petersen AW, Simmons SF, Schnelle JF, Bell SP, Kripalani S, et al. Medications Associated with geriatric syndromes and their prevalence in older hospitalized adults discharged to skilled nursing facilities. J Hosp Med. 2016;11(10):694–700.
32. Bunniran S, Davis C, Kristy R, Ng D, Schermer CR, Uribe C, Suehs BT. A prospective study of elderly initiating mirabegron versus antimuscarinics: patient reported outcomes from the overactive bladder satisfaction scales and other instruments. Neurourol Urodyn. 2018;37(1):177–85.
33. Dickinson J, Lewand M, Sawamoto T, Krauwinkel W, Schaddelee M. Effects of renal or hepatic impairment on the pharmacokinetics of mirabegron. Clin Drug Investig. 2013;33(1):11–23.
34. Vij M, Drake MJ. Clinical use of the β3 adrenoceptor agonist mirabegron in patients with overactive bladder syndrome. Ther Adv Urol. 2015;7(5):241–8.
35. Skeberdis VA, Gendviliene V, Zablockaite D, Treinys R, Macianskiene R, Bogdelis A, et al. beta3-adrenergic receptor activation increases human atrial tissue contractility and stimulates the L-type Ca2+ current. J Clin Invest. 2008;118(9):3219–27.
36. Rosa GM, Ferrero S, Nitti VW, Wagg A, Saleem T, Chapple CR. Cardiovascular safety of β3-adrenoceptor agonists for the treatment of patients with overactive bladder syndrome. Eur Urol. 2016;69(2):311–23.
37. Sexton CC, Notte SM, Maroulis C, Dmochowski RR, Cardozo L, Subramanian D, Coyne KS. Persistence and adherence in the treatment of overactive bladder syndrome with anticholinergic therapy: a systematic review of the literature. Int J Clin Pract. 2011;65(5):567–85.
38. Dmochowski RR, Newman DK. Impact of overactive bladder on women in the United States: results of a national survey. Curr Med Res Opin. 2007;23(1):65–76.

39. Martan A, Masata J, Krhut J, Zachoval R, Hanus T, Svabik K. Persistence in the treatment of overactive bladder syndrome (OAB) with mirabegron in a multicenter clinical study. Eur J Obstet Gynecol Reprod Biol. 2017;210:247–50.
40. Haab F, Castro-Diaz D. Persistence with antimuscarinic therapy in patiens with overactive bladder. Int J Clin Pract. 2005;59(8):931–7. Review
41. Wagg A, Compion G, Fahey A, Siddiqui E. Persistence with prescribed antimuscarinic therapy for overactive bladder: a UK experience. BJU Int. 2012;110(11):1767–74.
42. Staskin D, Herschorn S, Fialkov J, Tu LM, Walsh T, Schermer CR. A prospective, double-blind, randomized, two-period crossover, multicenter study to evaluate tolerability and patient preference between mirabegron and tolterodine in patients with overactive bladder (PREFER study). Int Urygonecol J. 2018;29(2):273–83.
43. Ganz ML, Smalarz AM, Krupski TL, Anger JT, Hu JC, Wittrup-Jensen KU, Pashos CL. Economic costs of overactive bladder in the United States. Urology. 2010;75(3):526–32, 532.e1–e18.
44. Hu TW, Wagner TH. Health-related consequences of overactive bladder: an economic perspective. BJU Int. 2005;96(Suppl 1):43–5.
45. Hu TW, Wagner TH, Bentkover JD, LeBlanc K, Piancentini A, Stewart WF, et al. Estimated economic costs of overactive bladder in the United States. Urology. 2003;61(6):1123–8.
46. Perk S, Wielage RC, Campbell NL, Klein TM, Perkins A, Posta LM, et al. Estimated budget impact of increased use of mirabegron, a novel treatment for overactive bladder. J Manag Care Spec Pharm. 2016;22(9):1072–84.

Chapter 8
Combination Pharmacotherapy for Overactive Bladder

Joon Jae Park and Christopher R. Chapple

Introduction

As seen in previous chapters of this book, pharmacotherapy for overactive bladder (OAB) whilst it has traditionally relied on antimuscarinic therapy such as oxybutynin, tolterodine and solifenacin has been augmented by the introduction of the β3-receptor agonist mirabegron. Used as a monotherapy agent, both groups of medications have similar efficacy rates but with different side effect profiles [1]. The difficulty for the treating clinician comes when patients have minimal or no benefit on either of these groups of medications [2, 3]. As later chapters of this book will also show, intradetrusor botulinum injections are effective in patients with refractory OAB symptoms (particularly urgency urinary incontinence) [4]. Unfortunately, due to its more invasive nature as well as having its own unique side effects, such factors may influence its choice by both patients and the treating clinicians alike [5]. Other alternatives currently available include sacral nerve neuromodulation [6] and percutaneous tibial nerve stimulation [7], but their popularity in mainstay clinical practice is currently limited.

Clearly then, combining both groups of oral OAB medications is an attractive option, as by using different mechanisms of action, efficacy may be optimised and the incidence of side effects reduced. There are now studies showing improved efficacy when compared to both separate monotherapy groups. From a safety point of view, combining an antimuscarinic and a be β3-agonist can provide a similar efficacy to a higher dose of antimuscarinic but with a reduced incidence of side effects by lowering their antimuscarinic dosage requirements and consequently lower their associated antimuscarinic side effects such as dry mouth and constipation. In this

J. J. Park
Department of Urology, Changi General Hospital, Singapore, Singapore

C. R. Chapple (✉)
Department of Urology, Royal Hallamshire Hospital, Sheffield Teaching Hospitals NHS Foundation Trust, Sheffield, UK
e-mail: c.r.chapple@shef.ac.uk

L. Cox, E. S. Rovner (eds.), *Contemporary Pharmacotherapy of Overactive Bladder*, https://doi.org/10.1007/978-3-319-97265-7_8

chapter, we will be examining the evidence of combination therapy in the management of OAB.

At the time of this book's publication, there were a total of five clinical trials that involved an antimuscarinic agent with a β3-agonist. All of them involved the comparison of solifenacin as the antimuscarinic agent of choice and mirabegron as the only β3-agonists currently available. Four out of five of these trials were industry sponsored by Astellas Pharma as both of these agents were developed and marketed by this company. The trials involve one large phase 2 (Symphony), one small Russian randomised study, one small post-marketing phase 4 Japanese study (MILAI) and two large phase 3 studies (BESIDE and SYNERGY) [8–12].

For this book chapter, we will briefly summarise the study design and efficacy results of all of these five clinical trials, but particular attention will be given to the three larger trials (Symphony, BESIDE and SYNERGY trials). We will also review the patient-reported outcome measure (PROM) results and safety-related outcome measures from these studies, which are always important to know for the practising clinician at the time of prescribing these combination therapies [13]. Finally, we will give some practical advice in terms of ideal starting prescriptive dosage, timing of dosage increment and follow-up regime.

Please note that this chapter will not focus on the evidence looking at combination therapy between an alpha-blocker with either an antimuscarinic or β3-agonists in male patients with concomitant OAB and bladder outlet obstruction/benign prostatic hyperplasia as this is covered in Chapter 15, 'Considerations in Male OAB'.

Symphony Study by Abrams et al.

An initial animal model study showed that combining both solifenacin and mirabegron led to additive effects in increasing bladder storage function [14]. A phase I study evaluating the pharmacokinetic interaction in healthy non-OAB individuals between these two drugs did not show any significant interaction, and it was found to be generally well tolerated [15].

This paved the way for future clinical trials leading to the phase 2 study named the Symphony trial published in February 2014 [8]. This trial was a factorial designed, multicentre, multinational, randomised, double-blind, parallel group, placebo and monotherapy controlled trial in men and women with OAB. Inclusion criteria included those patients aged ≥18 years with symptoms of OAB such as urgency, urinary frequency and/or urgency incontinence of ≥3-month duration. This study had a total of 1306 patients who entered initial randomisation, and 1239 patients went on to complete the study. As for any phase 2 study, the primary objective was to evaluate the efficacy of this new combination therapy. Secondary objectives included the evaluation of the optimal dosing regime (dose-response relationship) as well as assessing for its safety and tolerability. As the ideal combination doses were unknown, there were a total of 12 randomised groups: 1 placebo, 5 monotherapy (solifenacin 2.5, 5, or 10 mg monotherapies and mirabegron 25 or 50 mg monotherapies) and 6 combination groups (solifenacin 2.5, 5, or 10 mg plus mirabegron 25 or 50 mg). The study duration was 12 weeks in each arm.

The primary end point was the change from baseline to end of treatment in mean volume voided per micturition (MVV), which is a common end point measured in OAB trials to show drug efficacy as it is an objective parameter measured in frequency volume charts. In this trial, except for the mirabegron 25 mg monotherapy group, all other groups showed statistically significant improvement in MVV when compared to placebo. Of more interest to this particular book chapter, when one compares the combination therapy groups to solifenacin 5 mg monotherapy group, four out of six solifenacin and mirabegron combination groups achieved statistically significant adjusted change in MVV. These four groups were the solifenacin 5, or 10 mg plus mirabegron 25 mg, and solifenacin 5, or 10 mg plus mirabegron 50 mg (the combination therapy groups containing solifenacin 2.5 mg did not achieve statistically significant adjusted change). The adjusted mean difference in MVV in the aforementioned four groups were 18.0 (SE 6.2) [95% CI 5.4–30.0] ($p < 0.001$), 22.0 (SE 7.4) [95% CI 7.2–36.1] ($p < 0.001$), 18.2 (SE 6.1) [95% CI 6.2–30.2] ($p < 0.003$) and 26.3 (SE 7.3) [95% CI 12.0–41.0] ($p < 0.001$), respectively.

In terms of change from baseline to end of treatment (EOT) in the mean number of micturitions per 24 h, statistically significant differences compared to both placebo and solifenacin 5 mg monotherapy were only observed in three out of six combination groups. These groups were the solifenacin 10 mg together with mirabegron 25 mg and solifenacin 5 or 10 mg plus mirabegron 50 mg. The group with the largest change in urinary frequency was seen in the higher dose group of solifenacin 10 mg together with mirabegron 50 mg. The adjusted change (SE) from baseline to EOT in mean number of micturitions per 24 h was − 1.1 ($p < 0.005$) when compared to placebo and − 1.0 ($p < 0.005$) when compared to solifenacin 5 mg monotherapy.

All 12 groups (including placebo) showed a reduction in the number of incontinence episodes from baseline to EOT. However, none of the treatment arms in this study failed to show any statistically significant reduction in the number of incontinence episodes when compared to placebo.

The main limitation of the Symphony study is that only the MVV was powered to detect any differences; consequently, the other efficacy variables were therefore underpowered.

It is important to assess if the above improvements in MVV and urinary frequency seen in combinations groups are actually meaningful to patients. It is important to show statistically significant subjective changes, but if the patient fails to notice any subjective improvements, it is unlikely to lead to any significant improvement in quality of life. Therefore it is extremely important to evaluate the patient-reported outcomes in any OAB studies. In the case of the Symphony trial, the authors published a separate paper specifically looking at this subject matter [8]. Two validated health questionnaires were used for this trial. These were the Overactive Bladder Questionnaire (OAB-q) and Patient Perception of Bladder Condition (PPBC). The OAB-q consists [16] of an 8-item symptom bother scale (0–100; lower scores indicate better QoL) and a 25-item health-related QoL (HRQoL) scale (0–100; higher scores indicate better QoL). The PPBC [17] consists of a six-point Likert scale ranging from one ('no problems at all') to six ('many severe problems').

Only two out of the six combination therapy groups achieved a statistically significant difference of ≥10-point improvement in the OAB-q symptom bother score when compared to placebo. These were solifenacin 5 mg plus mirabegron 25 mg (OR 2.14 [95%CI1.02, 4.48, p = 0.043]) and solifenacin 5 mg plus mirabegron 50 mg (OR 2.61 [95% CI 1.22, 5.58, p = 0.013]). However, no combination group showed a statistically significant difference compared to solifenacin 5 mg monotherapy. One of this combination group, the solifenacin 5 mg plus mirabegron 50 mg group showed a ≥ 10-point improvement in total HRQoL compared to both placebo (OR 2.45 [95% CI 1.22, 4.94, p = 0.012]) and solifenacin 5 mg monotherapy (OR 2.21 [95% CI 1.19, 4.09, p = 0.012]).

Looking at the PPBC questionnaire, more than 80% of patients achieved ≥1-point improvement in PPBC, but only the solifenacin 5 mg plus mirabegron 50 mg combination at EoT showed statistically significant superiority compared to both placebo and solifenacin 5 mg monotherapy ($p < 0.05$). This was also the only group that achieved a major (≥2 point) improvement versus both placebo ($p = 0.038$) and solifenacin 5 mg monotherapy ($p = 0.012$).

The previously noted secondary objective of change in the mean number of micturitions per 24 h was further analysed by the authors to assess the odds of achieving micturition normalisation with combination therapy. This was defined as a change of >8 micturitions/24 h at baseline to <8 micturitions/24 h post EOT. Results showed that in two groups, the solifenacin 10 mg plus mirabegron 25 mg and solifenacin 5 mg plus mirabegron 50 mg, 65.4% and 61.6% of patients respectively achieved normalisation of micturition. This was statistically significant when compared to both placebo and solifenacin 5 mg ($p < 0.05$). The odds of achieving micturition frequency normalisation was approximately twofold greater with the combination groups of solifenacin 10 mg with mirabegron 25 mg (OR 2.06 [95% CI 1.11, 3.84; $p = 0.023$]) and solifenacin 5 mg with mirabegron 50 mg (OR 1.91 [95% CI 1.14, 3.21; $p = 0.015$]) compared to the solifenacin 5 mg monotherapy group.

In summary, the Symphony study showed that some combination therapy groups were superior to both placebo and monotherapy groups. The ideal combination dosage seems to be the solifenacin 5 mg plus mirabegron 50 mg as it gave rise to similar/superior efficacy to the higher dosage of solifenacin 10 mg plus mirabegron 50 mg. This was achieved with a lower side effect profile compared to the latter group and will be discussed more in detail later in this book chapter.

Randomised Study by Kosilov et al.

The following year after the publication of the Symphony trial, Kosilov et al. published a randomised, single-blinded, placebo controlled trial in September 2015 looking at the efficacy and safety of solifenacin and mirabegron combination therapy in elderly OAB patients [9]. A total of 239 elderly patients (143 female and 95 male) with a mean age of 71.2 participated in this trial. The patients were randomised to receive one of four groups consisting of placebo, solifenacin 10 mg, mirabegron 50 mg or solifenacin 10 mg plus mirabegron 50 mg for 6 weeks duration.

The results showed that all three treatment groups showed improvement in the mean number of urinary incontinence episodes per day and in the mean number of micturitions per day. The combination group of solifenacin 10 mg and mirabegron 50 mg showed the highest improvement in both of these parameters with a change in mean urinary incontinence episodes per day from 5.1 to 1.3 ($p \leq 0.01$) and a change in the mean number of micturitions per day from 9.1 to 5.1 ($p \leq 0.01$). However, only the mean urinary incontinence episodes per day was statistically superior to both solifenacin and mirabegron monotherapy groups ($p \leq 0.05$). No statistically significant changes were seen in the placebo group.

Unique to this study, all patients had filling cystometric urodynamic studies both at the beginning and at the end of the study. This showed that 64.4% of patients had detrusor overactivity related urinary incontinence, 23.4% had phasic detrusor overactivity and 12.1% had terminal detrusor overactivity. All three treatment groups showed improvement in maximum bladder capacity and detrusor compliance. Once again the largest change was seen in the combination therapy group where the mean maximum bladder capacity increased from 188.7 ml to 289.9 ml at EOT whilst the bladder detrusor compliance increased from 18.5 and 32.4 ml/cm H20 at EOT ($p < 0.001$).

Treatment-related side effects were similar across the three groups (range 21–33.3%). Six patients had to discontinue treatment due to treatment-related side effects (three patients each in the solifenacin monotherapy and in the combination groups).

Although the authors of this trial should be commended in carrying out the only nonindustry-sponsored trial to date in the use of combination therapy in OAB patients, it is difficult to make solid conclusions from it due to its limitations of relatively low number of patients recruited (between 52 and 65 patients in each arm) and short duration of the trial (6 weeks of active treatment).

MILAI Study by Yamaguchi et al.

The MILAI study was a relatively small Japanese multicentre, nonrandomised, open-label phase IV study to assess the efficacy and safety of mirabegron as an 'add-on' therapy for patients with OAB treated with solifenacin published in October 2015 [10]. Due to its open-label design, there was no placebo arm, and neither the participants nor the clinicians were blinded. There was also no monotherapy arm that the combination therapy could be compared to. The study was primarily looking at the safety profile of combination therapy in a small Japanese population ($n = 218$), and they recruited postmenopausal female OAB patients and men who did not wish to have further children. This is reflected in the mean age of the participants being 64.6 years (SD 9.97, range 38–85).

The total duration of the study was 18 weeks, comprising of a 2-week screening period and a 16-week treatment period. Patients initially received either solifenacin 2.5 or 5 mg monotherapy for 2 weeks. The initial solifenacin dosage was not randomised, and although it was not specifically mentioned by the authors, we presume that it was left to the treating physician to decide the starting dose. Subsequently, at week 2, all participants received an additional mirabegron 25 mg. At week 8, the treating clinician was free to increase the dose of mirabegron to 50 mg (whilst keeping the original solifenacin dose at 2.5 mg or 5 mg) if they thought the participant had an insufficient response, if the patient was also agreeable to the increase in dosage and so long as there were no other safety concerns. Thirty-seven of 70 (53%) patients receiving solifenacin 2.5 mg plus mirabegron 25 mg went up to increase their dose of mirabegron to 50 mg, and 93/148 (63%) patients receiving 5 mg plus mirabegron 25 mg went up to increase their dose of mirabegron to 50 mg.

The MVV significantly increased from baseline to each visit in all treatment groups with the highest change observed in the solifenacin 5 mg plus mirabegron 50 mg group (36.957 ml, $p < 0.001$, 95% CI 27.971–45.943). The mean change in the number of micturitions/24 h from baseline to EOT was similar across all four groups, ranging from −1.89 to −2.36. Overall 38.2% achieved normalisation of urinary frequency of <8 micturitions/24 h. The mean number of urgency episodes/24 h significantly decreased from baseline to EOT across all groups ranging from −1.57 to −2.59. The mean change in the overactive bladder symptom score [18] from baseline to EOT ranged from −3.4 to −4.0. The PROM was measured using the overactive bladder questionnaire short form score (OAB-q SF), and all four groups saw significant improvements ($p < 0.001$). The mean changes from baseline to EOT for the mean OAB-q SF symptom bother score ranged from −16.31 to −22.25 for the different treatment groups and for OAB-q SF total HRQL score ranged from 12.56 to 17.34. The overall incidence of treatment-related adverse event (TEAE) was 23.3% with only 4.9% being classified as serious.

As mentioned earlier, the MILAI study was a relatively small post-marketing study without a placebo arm or active monotherapy arm to which the combination groups could be compared. The main conclusion that we can draw from this study is that combination therapy seems to be safe in Japanese patients with OAB.

BESIDE Trial by Drake et al.

Having established the efficacy and safety of combination therapy in the aforementioned smaller studies, two phase III studies were published shortly one after another. The first was the BESIDE study published in February 2016 [11], which looked specifically at whether patients who were still having urgency urinary incontinence (i.e OAB 'wet') with solifenacin 5 mg would go on to do better if they increased their solifenacin dose to 10 mg versus 'adding-on' mirabegron. This is a very relevant cohort group of patients in clinical practice as urgency urinary incontinence is the most bothersome OAB symptom and affects QoL the most [19]. They are also the group of patients that are most likely to contemplate more invasive procedures such as intradetrusor botox injections [20].

The study design consisted of a randomised, double-blind, parallel-group, multicentre and multinational phase IIIB study. There was no placebo arm in this study. Inclusion criteria included patients aged ≥18 years, having OAB symptoms for ≥3 months with an average of ≥2 incontinence episodes/24 h. After a 2-week screening/washout period, 2401 patients were given solifenacin 5 mg (single blind) for 4 weeks. Subsequently, only those patients who failed to achieve 100% continence went on to proceed with randomisation. So a total of 2174 patients were randomised (double-blind) to 1 of 3 arms for 12 weeks in a 1:1:1 ratio. The groups were solifenacin 5 mg (control arm), solifenacin 10 mg or combination therapy with solifenacin 5 mg plus mirabegron (25 mg for the first 4 weeks and 50 mg for the last 8 weeks). There was no mirabegron monotherapy arm. The severity of the OAB in this group of patients is reflected in their baseline characteristics, in which the number of UI episodes/24 h was quite high at 3.16 (SD 2.73), 3.31 (SD 3.05) and 3.23 (SD 3.00), respectively. These were similar to the mean urgency UI episodes/24 h episodes showing that most UI were due to urgency rather than stress UI. About 2/3 of the participants had tried at least one or more OAB medications in the past, and the mean number of pads used was almost three a day (range 2.74–2.92).

Results showed that the adjusted change from baseline to EOT in the mean number of UI episodes per 24 h (primary end point) was greater with combination (−1.80) compared to solifenacin 5 mg (−1.53) or solifenacin 10 mg (−1.67), giving rise to a statistically significant difference vs solifenacin 5 mg and 10 mg groups of −0.26 ($p = 0.001$, 95% CI −0.47 to −0.05) and − 0.13 ($p = 0.008$, 95% CI −0.34 to 0.08), respectively.

There was also statistically significantly greater improvement in the mean number of micturitions/24 h (a key secondary end point) with combination therapy (−1.59) compared to solifenacin 5 mg (−1.14) or solifenacin 10 mg (−1.12), giving rise to a statistically significant difference between the combination group vs solifenacin 5 mg and 10 mg groups of −0.45 ($p = <0.001$, 95% CI −0.67 to −0.22) and − 0.47 ($p < 0.001$, 95% CI −0.70 to −0.25), respectively.

As mentioned earlier, in this study all the patients who were randomised were incontinent at baseline despite 4 weeks of solifenacin 5 mg. Post-randomisation, those who went on to have zero incontinence episodes at EOT were higher in the combination group (46%) than in the solifenacin 5 mg (37.9%) or in the solifenacin 10 mg (40.2%) monotherapy groups. So the odds ratio of remaining dry on combination therapy compared to solifenacin 5 mg and 10 mg was 1.47 ($p = 0.001$, CI 1.17–1.84) and 1.28 (CI 1.02–1.61), respectively. In other words, one was 47% and 28% more likely to achieve complete continence on combination therapy compared to remaining on solifenacin 5 mg or increasing the solifenacin dose to 10 mg, respectively. No clinically or statistically significant difference in nocturia episodes was seen.

Quality of life was assessed using the OAB-q, the Patient Perception of Bladder Condition (PPBC) questionnaire and the Treatment Satisfaction Visual Analog Scale (TS-VAS) [21]. The combination group demonstrated superiority over solifenacin 5 and 10 mg groups for change from baseline to EOT in the symptom bother score, the total HRQoL and the PPBC. The mean adjusted difference in the symptom bother score was −4.96 ($p < 0.001$, 95% CI −6.88 to −3.04) and −3.30 ($p = 0.001$, 95% CI −5.23 to −1.37) for the combination vs solifenacin 5 and 10 mg, respectively. The mean adjusted difference in the total HRQoL were 3.15 ($p = 0.001$, 95% CI 1.35 to 4.95) and 3.38 ($p < 0.001$, 95% CI 1.58 to 5.19) for the combination vs solifenacin 5 and 10 mg, respectively. The change from baseline to EOT in the TS-VAS was statistically significantly higher for combination compared with solifenacin 5 mg but not compared with solifenacin 10 mg with a mean adjusted difference of 0.4 ($p = 0.001$, 95% CI 0.2 to 0.6) and 0.2 ($p = 0.113$, 95% CI 0.0 to 0.4), respectively.

The BESIDE trial is an important phase III study that showed that in the subgroup of patients with urgency UI persistence despite 4 weeks of solifenacin 5 mg monotherapy, adding in mirabegron rather than increasing the dose of solifenacin to 10 mg is not only better, but as we will see later, it also led to fewer side effects.

SYNERGY Trial by Herschorn et al.

The following year, in October 2017, the other phase III trial, SYNERGY, was published [12]. This is the largest clinical trial conducted so far, looking into the efficacy and safety of combination therapy of solifenacin and mirabegron in the treatment of OAB. This trial was a randomised, double-blind, parallel-group, placebo controlled, active-controlled, multicentre and multinational phase III study.

The total study duration was 18 weeks. There was an initial 4-week single-blind placebo run-in period followed by a 12 week double-blind treatment period with a final 2-week single-blind placebo run-out period.

It is important to highlight that only patients with OAB symptoms who had episodes of urinary incontinence (UI) were eligible to enter randomisation. In those patients with mixed UI, urgency UI had to be the predominant factor to be allowed to enter randomisation. So inclusion criteria were patients aged ≥18 years having OAB symptoms for ≥3 months with an average of ≥8 micturitions/24 h, ≥1 urgency episode/24 h (grade 3 or 4 on the Patient Perception of Intensity of Urgency Scale (PPIUS)/24 h [22]) and ≥3 UI episodes over a 7-day micturition diary.

A total of 3527 patients were randomised (double-blind) to 1 of 6 arms for 12 weeks in a 1:1:1:2:2 ratio. The groups were placebo, solifenacin 5 mg, mirabegron 25 mg, mirabegron 50 mg, solifenacin 5 mg plus mirabegron 25 mg and solifenacin 5 mg plus mirabegron 50 mg.

The two co-primary end points were (1) change from baseline to EOT in the mean number of UI episodes/24 h and (2) change from baseline to EOT in the mean number of micturitions/24 h. Key secondary efficacy end points were change from baseline to EOT in the MVV/micturition and change from baseline to EOT in PROM.

Results showed that the mean adjusted change from baseline to EOT for the two co-primary end points was greater in the combination therapy groups compared to both placebo and monotherapies. However, although the combined solifenacin 5 mg plus mirabegron 50 mg showed statistical superiority to solifenacin 5 mg monotherapy for change from baseline to EOT in mean number of UI episodes/24 h with a mean adjusted difference of −0.20 ($p = 0.033$, CI −0.44 to 0.04), it failed to show a statistically significant difference when compared to mirabegron 50 mg monotherapy with a mean adjusted difference of −0.23 ($p = 0.052$, CI −0.47 to 0.01). Hence the primary objective for the combined solifenacin 5 mg plus mirabegron 50 mg therapy was not met. As the null hypothesis for this test was not rejected, the subsequent hypotheses for the change in the mean number of micturitions/24 h and the MVV/micturition could not be tested. Nonetheless, at a p value of 0.052, the study came close to reaching statistical significance, and the authors goes on to explain the possible reasons why this may be so. For example, in their analysis of their data, it was noted that there was a larger effect size in patients who had received prior OAB treatment compared to patients who never had OAB treatment prior to participating in this trial (i.e. treatment-naive patients). Specifically, the mean number of UI episodes and micturitions/24 h was better in those who had prior OAB medication in the past. So bearing this in mind, one possible explanation, the authors argued, of why this trial's co-primary end point failed to reach statistical significance may be due to the fact that there was a higher proportion of treatment-naive patients in the SYNERGY study compared to the previous phase III trial (BESIDE). The number of treatment-naive patients in the SYNERGY and BESIDE trials was 54% and 31.8%, respectively. Furthermore, in the BESIDE trial, only those who remained incontinent despite 4 weeks of solifenacin 5 mg monotherapy went on to proceed with randomisation. In contrast, this preselection of patients was not performed in the SYNERGY trial.

In secondary analyses, the adjusted change from baseline to EOT in mean numbers of micturitions/24 h for mirabegron 25 mg (−2.00), mirabegron 50 mg (−2.03), solifenacin 5 mg (−2.20), solifenacin 5 mg plus mirabegron 25 mg (−2.49) and solifenacin 5 mg plus mirabegron 50 mg (−2.59) was all greater than placebo (−1.64). The adjusted mean change from baseline to EOT in MVV/micturition for mirabegron 25 mg (13.32), mirabegron 50 mg (21.99), solifenacin 5 mg (30.99), solifenacin 5 mg plus mirabegron 25 mg (34.84) and solifenacin 5 mg plus mirabegron 50 mg (39.73) was also all greater than placebo (8.44). At EOT, 52.2% of patients in the solifenacin 5 mg plus mirabegron 50 mg went on achieve zero UI episodes/24 h (based on the last 3 diary days). This was slightly lower in the solifenacin 5 mg plus mirabegron 25 mg group at 50.7%. For the monotherapy treatment groups of solifenacin 5 mg and mirabegron 50 mg, it was 42.9% and 46.3%, respectively, giving rise to an odds ratio compared to solifenacin 5 mg plus mirabegron 50 mg of 1.40 (95% CI, 1.09 to 1.81) and 1.34 (95% CI, 1.04 to 1.73), respectively.

As regards PROM results, the mean adjusted change from baseline to EOT in OAB-q symptom bother score was greater in the combination groups compared to the monotherapy groups and placebo groups. The largest change was seen in the solifenacin 5 mg plus mirabegron 25 mg (−31.1) and solifenacin 5 mg plus mirabegron 50 mg (−32.2) groups. These were statistically significant ($p < 0.001$) when compared to placebo (−19.5), mirabegron 50 mg monotherapy (−26.1) and solifenacin 5 mg monotherapy (−26.4) groups.

The mean adjusted change from baseline to EOT in HRQoL total scores was greater in the combination groups compared to the monotherapy groups and placebo groups. The largest change was seen in the solifenacin 5 mg plus mirabegron 25 mg and solifenacin 5 mg plus mirabegron 50 mg groups with an adjusted mean (SE) change from baseline to EOT of 24 and 24.3, respectively. This was statistically significant ($p < 0.001$) when compared to placebo and solifenacin 5 mg monotherapy groups but not compared to mirabegron 50 mg ($p = 0.002$).

Meta-analysis by Xu et al.

A meta-analysis was recently published in September 2017 comparing the efficacy and safety of combination therapy to solifenacin monotherapy [23]. The doses used in this meta-analysis were solifenacin (5 or 10 mg) plus mirabegron (50 mg) and solifenacin (5 or 10 mg) monotherapy. The MILAI study was excluded in their analysis as it did not have a monotherapy arm.

Results showed that the mean difference in mean number of micturitions per 24 h was −0.45 (95% CI, −0.65 to −0.26, $P < 0.00001$), the mean difference in number of episodes of incontinence per 24 h was −0.71 (95% CI, −0.14 to −0.02, $P = 0.04$) and the mean difference in mean number of urgency episodes per 24 h was −0.56 (95% CI −0.83 to −0.30, $P < 0.0001$), all favouring combination therapy over solifenacin monotherapy.

Safety Assessments of Combination Therapy

A clear clinical concern one would have at the time of considering combination therapy is whether there could be an increased side effect risk when these two classes of medications are combined. All five trials so far mentioned had safety assessments looking into treatment-emergent adverse events (TEAEs), post-void residual volumes, laboratory parameters and cardiovascular parameters (such as heart rate, blood pressure and electrocardiogram changes). We will now look into the data from these trials so that we can better counsel and monitor our patients in whom we start combination therapy.

Antimuscarinics Side Effects

During the dose-finding phase II study, Symphony [8], it was noted that the total treatment-emergent adverse events (TEAE) were highest in the treatment arms containing solifenacin 10 mg. For example, the TEAE for solifenacin 10 mg plus mirabegron 50 mg group was 59.3%, whereas in the solifenacin 5 mg plus mirabegron

50 mg group, it was lesser at 40.8%. Most TEAE were mild to moderate in severity with dry mouth being the commonest side effect with a severity incidence of 17.3% and 13.1%, respectively. Only a few patients went on to discontinue their medication by the end of the trial, and the group with the largest number of patients who had to discontinue their medication due to TEAE was in the solifenacin 10 mg plus mirabegron 50 mg group at only 3.7%. In contrast, in the solifenacin 5 mg plus mirabegron 50 mg, only 0.7% went on to discontinue their medication due to a TEAE. For this reason, the two subsequent phase III trials did not include combination therapy groups containing solifenacin 10 mg as the trial organisers felt that the side effect to benefit ratio did not warrant its use. Conversely, we, the authors, don't recommend the use of solifenacin 10 mg combination therapies in routine clinical practice.

In the phase III BESIDE trial [11], the TEAE incidences among the three treatment arms were similar with TEAE incidences of 33.1% in the solifenacin 5 mg monotherapy group, 39.4% solifenacin 10 mg monotherapy group and 35.9% in the solifenacin 5 mg plus mirabegron 50 mg combination group. In the phase III SYNERGY study [12], the total number of TEAE was also similar across the different groups, with the highest incidence seen in the solifenacin 5 mg plus mirabegron 25 mg at 40.4% and the lowest incidence in the mirabegron 25 mg at 31.9%.

Dry mouth and constipation were the commonest antimuscarinic side effects seen in both phase III trials. In the BESIDE [11] trial, the incidence of dry mouth and constipation in the combination therapy group was 5.9% and 4.6%, respectively. This was similar to solifenacin 5 mg monotherapy at 5.6% and 3% but lesser than in the solifenacin 10 mg monotherapy at 9.5% and 4.7%. In the SYNERGY trial [12], the incidence of dry mouth and constipation for the solifenacin 5 mg plus mirabegron 50 mg was 7.2% and 3.7%, respectively, which was slightly higher than the solifenacin 5 mg monotherapy group's incidence of 5.9% and 1.4%, respectively. To put things in perspective, during a 12-month-long phase III trial comparing mirabegron 50 mg and tolterodine extended release 4 mg, the incidence of TEAE was 59.7% and 62.6%, respectively, with dry mouth incidences of 2.8% and 8.6%, respectively [24].

Urinary Tract Infections (UTI)

The incidence of UTIs in the BESIDE study [11] was similar across the three treatment groups (range 2.2–2.8%). In the SYNERGY study [12], the incidence of UTIs was highest in the combination groups, with the UTI incidences in the solifenacin 5 mg plus mirabegron 25 mg and solifenacin 5 mg plus mirabegron 50 mg being 7% and 5.2%, respectively. These were only slightly higher as compared to the other groups in this trial, with UTI incidences of 4.9%, 5%, 4.3% and 3.8% in the placebo, solifenacin 5 mg, mirabegron 25 mg and mirabegron 50 mg monotherapy groups, respectively.

Post-void Residual (PVR) and Acute Retention of Urine (ARU)

In clinical trials, patients with elevated PVRs tend to be excluded from OAB trials [25, 26]. So the mean baseline PVR volume seen in both the BESIDE and SYNERGY trials was very low at 26 ml and 22.5 ml, respectively [11, 12]. In the BESIDE trial, the mean change of PVR at EOT for the solifenacin 5 mg, solifenacin 10 mg and combination groups was 3 ml, 7.4 ml and 5.5 ml, respectively. This small mean change of PVR from baseline to EOT is mirrored in the SYNERGY trial, where the highest change in the mean PVR volume was 11 mL in the solifenacin 5 mg plus mirabegron 50 mg group.

Based on the BESIDE trial, urinary retention was an uncommon occurrence, and this was reported as a TEAE in only eight patients with one (0.1%), five (0.7%) and two (0.3%) patients reported in the solifenacin 5 mg, solifenacin 10 mg and combination groups, respectively. TEAE for urinary retention were based on spontaneous reporting using a predefined list of preferred and lower-level terms.

Two patients in the solifenacin 10 mg group discontinued their treatment due to urinary retention; however, the authors stated that these two patients did not require catheterisation. There was no case of urinary retention requiring catheterisation in any treatment group reported by the authors. On the other hand, in the SYNERGY study, it seems that rates of urinary retention were more common in the combination groups. Not a single case of urinary retention occurred in the placebo and mirabegron monotherapy groups, but in the solifenacin 5 mg monotherapy, solifenacin 5 mg plus mirabegron 25 mg and solifenacin 5 mg plus mirabegron 50 mg groups, there were three (0.7%), eight (0.9%) and ten (1.2%) patients with urinary retention. Among these, a total of four patients required catheterisation, two patients (0.2%) in the solifenacin 5 mg plus mirabegron 25 mg group and two patients (0.2%) in the solifenacin 5 mg plus mirabegron 50 mg group.

Overall urinary retention rates, at least in the short term, seem to be uncommon, and checking PVR upon follow-up seems to be prudent at present.

Cardiovascular Safety

The incidence of OAB tends to increase with age, and therefore cardiovascular comorbidities tend to be more prevalent in OAB patients [27]. Safety results from all the trials conducted so far seem to indicate that there is no clinically significant added risk of cardiovascular-related TEAE with combination therapy.

The most comprehensive results published on this topic are based on the BESIDE study where the authors went on to publish a separate paper looking at this subject matter [28]. The frequency of hypertension, tachycardia and ECG QT prolongation was low across all three treatment groups of combination (1.1%, 0.3%, 0.1%), solifenacin 5 mg (0.7%, 0.1%, 0.1%) and solifenacin 10 mg (0.8%, 0%, 0.1%) groups.

Adjusted mean change from baseline to EOT in systolic and diastolic blood pressure for solifenacin 5 mg (−0.93 mm Hg, −0.45 mm Hg), solifenacin 10 mg (−1.28 mm Hg, −0.48 mm Hg) and combination groups (0.07 mm Hg, −0.35 mm Hg) was all comparable to each other. Adjusted mean change from baseline to EOT in pulse rate for solifenacin 5 mg (0.43 bpm), solifenacin 10 mg (0.27 bpm) and combination groups (0.47 bpm) was also comparable to each other. These small changes in pulse rate and blood pressures are unlikely to be of much clinical significance.

TEAE related to hypertension for the groups of solifenacin 5 mg, solifenacin 10 mg and combination group was reported in five (0.7%), six (0.8%) and eight (1.1%) patients, respectively. Seven serious CV-related TEAEs were reported, but none of these were considered by the trial investigators to be related to the OAB treatment.

Practical Prescriptive Advice

Looking at the evidence from these trials, it seems that combination therapy is safe and effective in the non-neurogenic OAB group of patients. In any given treatment-naive patient, it seems prudent that no matter how severe the symptoms of OAB may be, the data supports the view that one should try monotherapy treatment first rather than upfront combination therapy. Antimuscarinics are the commonest first-line therapy that is used clinically worldwide, with mirabegron being the obvious alternative should there be any contraindications to the use of antimuscarinics or failure to respond to them. This is in contrast to the management of patients with non-neurogenic male LUTS due to BOO secondary to benign prostatic enlargement/benign prostatic hyperplasia where long-term studies such as MTOPS and COMBAT have clearly shown that patients who are upfront started on combination therapies with an alpha-blocker and five alpha reductase inhibitors will go on to have a better short- and long-term efficacy compared to their individual monotherapy groups [29, 30].

The best indication so far for the use of combination therapy in OAB seems to be in the 'refractory' OAB patients. The precise criteria for defining the success or failure of antimuscarinic treatment that is universally accepted is as yet to be defined [31], and one could argue, based on the BESIDE study, that patients who have persistent urgency urinary incontinence despite 4 weeks of solifenacin 5 mg are a reasonable benchmark to define failure to respond to antimuscarinic therapy. So a clear evidence-based recommendation for the use of combination therapy in OAB would be in the group of patients whom initial solifenacin 5 mg monotherapy fails to achieve satisfactory improvement in urgency urinary incontinence. In this group of patients, we recommend adding on mirabegron 25 mg or 50 mg instead of increasing the solifenacin dose further and review them again 4 weeks later. If symptom control is still not satisfactory and the patient is tolerating the regime well, then one could further increase the mirabegron 25 mg dose to 50 mg. This mirrors the BESIDE trial protocol, and it seems that patients continued to notice further improvements in their symptoms at each clinical trial visit up to the EOT visit at

12 weeks. Therefore we recommend that a further clinical assessment be made 2–3 months after the start of combination therapy prior to deciding whether the patient is indeed refractory to combination therapy or not.

The latest updated 2017 European Association of Urology (EAU) guidelines on urinary incontinence reflect these changes and states that 'patients inadequately treated with solifenacin 5 mg may benefit more from the addition of mirabegron than dose escalation of solifenacin' and was given a level of evidence of 1b [32]. Unfortunately, the American Urological Association (AUA)/Society of Urodynamics, Female Pelvic Medicine and Urogenital Reconstruction (SUFU) guidelines which were last amended in 2014 do not comment on combination therapy as of yet [33].

The duration of all the clinical trials ranged from 12 to 16 weeks, so, regrettably, we do not have any long-term efficacy data of combination therapy. This would be an interesting topic of research in the future.

We acknowledge that the cost of medication is an important consideration at the time of prescribing medications and that solifenacin is by no means the cheapest antimuscarinic currently available in many markets, as it is one of the latest to enter the market and still under patent protection law. Although one could argue that combining mirabegron with other antimuscarinics medications could make financial sense, there is, unfortunately, no data to support its efficacy and safety. The only other study comparing another antimuscarinic medication with mirabegron was a small Japanese pharmacokinetic drug interaction study between mirabegron and tolterodine in healthy Japanese postmenopausal females (i.e. non-OAB patients) [34]. Therefore we, the authors, cannot recommend that any other antimuscarinics other than solifenacin should be used in combination therapy. Again this will be a good topic for further research in the future.

Conclusion

In summary, in patients with refractory urgency urinary incontinence despite solifenacin monotherapy, combination therapy leads to superior efficacy compared to increasing the solifenacin dose with an acceptable/better side effect profile. Other clinical indications such as upfront combination therapy and the use of other antimuscarinic agents other than solifenacin are currently not supported by the data available. Long-term efficacy of combination therapy is currently lacking, and further research is warranted.

References

1. Maman K, Aballea S, Nazir J, Desroziers K, Neine ME, Siddiqui E, et al. Comparative efficacy and safety of medical treatments for the management of overactive bladder: a systematic literature review and mixed treatment comparison. Eur Urol. 2014;65(4):755–65.

2. Benner JS, Nichol MB, Rovner ES, Jumadilova Z, Alvir J, Hussein M, et al. Patient-reported reasons for discontinuing overactive bladder medication. BJU Int. 2010;105(9):1276–82.
3. Sexton CC, Notte SM, Maroulis C, Dmochowski RR, Cardozo L, Subramanian D, Coyne KS. Persistence and adherence in the treatment of overactive bladder syndrome with anticholinergic therapy: a systematic review of the literature. Int J Clin Pract. 2011;65(5):567–85.
4. Chapple C, Sievert KD, MacDiarmid S, Khullar V, Radziszewski P, Nardo C, et al. OnabotulinumtoxinA 100 U significantly improves all idiopathic overactive bladder symptoms and quality of life in patients with overactive bladder and urinary incontinence: a randomised, double-blind, placebo- controlled trial. Eur Urol. 2013;64(2):249–56.
5. BOTOX [prescribing information]. Irvine: Allergan. Revised October 2017. https://www.allergan.com/assets/pdf/botox_pi.pdf. Accessed 26 Apr 2018.
6. Siddiqui NY, Wu JM, Amundsen CL. Efficacy and adverse events of sacral nerve stimulation for overactive bladder: a systematic review. Neurourol Urodyn. 2010;29(Suppl 1):S18–23.
7. Gaziev G, Topazio L, Iacovelli V, Asimakopoulos A, Di Santo A, De Nunzio C, Finazzi-Agrò E. Percutaneous tibial nerve stimulation (PTNS) efficacy in the treatment of lower urinary tract dysfunctions: a systematic review. BMC Urol. 2013;13:61.
8. Abrams P, Kelleher C, Staskin D, Rechberger T, Kay R, Martina R, et al. Combination treatment with mirabegron and solifenacin in patients with overactive bladder: efficacy and safety results from a randomised, double-blind, dose-ranging, phase 2 study (Symphony). Eur Urol. 2015;67(3):577–88.
9. Kosilov K, Loparev S, Ivanovskaya M, Kosilova L. A randomized, controlled trial of effectiveness and safety of management of OAB symptoms in elderly men and women with standard-dosed combination of solifenacin and mirabegron. Arch Gerontol Geriatr. 2015;61(2):212–6.
10. Yamaguchi O, Kakizaki H, Homma Y, Igawa Y, Takeda M, Nishizawa O, et al. Safety and efficacy of mirabegron as 'add-on' therapy in patients with overactive bladder treated with solifenacin: a post-marketing, open-label study in Japan (MILAI study). BJU Int. 2015;116(4):612–22.
11. Drake MJ, Chapple C, Esen AA, Athanasiou S, Cambronero J, Mitcheson D; BESIDE study investigators, et al.. Efficacy and safety of mirabegron add-on therapy to solifenacin in incontinent overactive bladder patients with an inadequate response to initial 4-week solifenacin monotherapy: a randomised double-blind multicentre phase 3B study (BESIDE). Eur Urol. 2016;70(1):136–145.
12. Herschorn S, Chapple CR, Abrams P, Arlandis S, Mitcheson D, Lee KS, et al. Efficacy and safety of combinations of mirabegron and solifenacin compared with monotherapy and placebo in patients with overactive bladder (SYNERGY study). BJU Int. 2017;120(4):562–75.
13. Brubaker L, Chapple C, Coyne KS, Kopp Z. Patient-reported outcomes in overactive bladder: importance for determining clinical effectiveness of treatment. Urology. 2006;68(2 Suppl):3–8.
14. Korstanje C, Someya A, Hiroshi Y, Noguchi Y, Sasamata M. Additive effects for increased bladder storage function with the antimuscarinic drug solifenacin and the selective b3-adrenoceptor agonist mirabegron in two rat models for in vivo bladder function. Poster 81 presented at: 43rd Meeting of the International Continence Society; August 26–30, 2013; Barcelona, Spain.
15. Krauwinkel WJ, Kerbusch VM, Meijer J, Tretter R, Strabach G, van Gelderen M. Evaluation of the pharmacokinetic interaction between the b3-adrenoceptor agonist mirabegron and the muscarinic receptor antagonist solifenacin in healthy subjects. Clin Pharmacol Drug Dev. 2013;2(3):255–63.
16. Garely AD, Lucente V, Vapnek J, Smith N. Solifenacin for overactive bladder with incontinence: symptom bother and health-related quality of life outcomes. Ann Pharmacother. 2007;41(3):391–8.
17. Coyne KS, Matza LS, Kopp Z, Abrams P. The validation of the patient perception of bladder condition (PPBC): a single-item global measure for patients with overactive bladder. Eur Urol. 2006;49(6):1079–86.

18. Homma Y, Yoshida M, Seki N, Yokoyama O, Kakizaki H, Gotoh M, et al. Symptom assessment tool for overactive bladder syndrome—overactive bladder symptom score. Urology. 2006;68(2):318–23.
19. Tang DH, Colayco DC, Khalaf KM, Piercy J, Patel V, Globe D, Ginsberg D. Impact of urinary incontinence on healthcare resource utilization, health-related quality of life and productivity in patients with overactive bladder. BJU Int. 2014;113(3):484–91.
20. Cox L, Cameron AP. OnabotulinumtoxinA for the treatment of overactive bladder. Res Rep Urol. 2014;6:79–89.
21. MacDiarmid S, Al-Shukri S, Barkin J, Fianu-Jonasson A, Grise P, Herschorn S, et al. Mirabegron as add-on treatment to solifenacin in incontinent overactive bladder patients with an inadequate response to solifenacin monotherapy: responder analyses and patient-reported outcomes from the BESIDE study. J Urol. 2016;196(3):809–18.
22. Notte SM, Marshall TS, Lee M, Hakimi Z, Odeyemi I, Chen WH, Revicki DA. Content validity and test-retest reliability of Patient Perception of Intensity of Urgency Scale (PPIUS) for overactive bladder. BMC Urol. 2012;12:26.
23. Xu Y, Liu R, Liu C, Cui Y, Gao Z. Meta-analysis of the efficacy and safety of mirabegron add-on therapy to solifenacin for overactive bladder. Int Neurourol J. 2017;21(3):212–9.
24. Chapple CR, Kaplan SA, Mitcheson D, Klecka J, Cummings J, Drogendijk T, et al. Randomized double-blind, active-controlled phase 3 study to assess 12-month safety and efficacy of mirabegron, a β(3)-adrenoceptor agonist, in overactive bladder. Eur Urol. 2013;63(2):296–305.
25. Kaplan SA, Roehrborn CG, Rovner ES, Carlsson M, Bavendam T, Guan Z. Tolterodine and tamsulosin for treatment of men with lower urinary tract symptoms and overactive bladder: a randomized controlled trial. JAMA. 2006;296(19):2319–28. Erratum in: JAMA. 2007:297(11):1195. JAMA. 2007;298(16):1864.
26. Haab F, Cardozo L, Chapple C, Ridder AM, Solifenacin Study Group. Long-term open-label solifenacin treatment associated with persistence with therapy in patients with overactive bladder syndrome. Eur Urol. 2005;47(3):376–84.
27. Andersson KE, Sarawate C, Kahler KH, Stanley EL, Kulkarni AS. Cardiovascular morbidity, heart rates and use of antimuscarinics in patients with overactive bladder. BJU Int. 2010;106(2):268–74.
28. Drake MJ, MacDiarmid S, Chapple CR, Esen A, Athanasiou S, Cambronero Santos J, et al. Cardiovascular safety in refractory incontinent patients with overactive bladder receiving add-on mirabegron therapy to solifenacin (BESIDE). Int J Clin Pract. 2017;71(5):e12944.
29. Bautista OM, Kusek JW, Nyberg LM, McConnell JD, Bain RP, Miller G, et al. Study design of the Medical Therapy of Prostatic Symptoms (MTOPS) trial. Control Clin Trials. 2003;24(2):224–43.
30. Roehrborn CG, Siami P, Barkin J, Damião R, Major-Walker K, Nandy I; CombAT Study Group, et al.. The effects of combination therapy with dutasteride and tamsulosin on clinical outcomes in men with symptomatic benign prostatic hyperplasia: 4-year results from the CombAT study. Eur Urol. 2010;57(1):123–131.
31. Phé V, de Wachter S, Rouprêt M, Chartier-Kastler E. How to define a refractory idiopathic overactive bladder? Neurourol Urodyn. 2015;34(1):2–11.
32. Burkhard FC, Bosch, JLHR, Cruz F, Lemack GE, Nambiar N, Thiruchelvam A, et al. EAU guidelines on urinary incontinence in adults. 2017. Arnhem: EAU Guidelines Office. http://uroweb.org/guideline/urinary-incontinence/. Accessed 26 Apr 2018.
33. Gormley EA, Lightner DJ, Burgio KL, Chai TC, Clemens JQ, Culkin DJ; American Urological Association; Society of Urodynamics, Female Pelvic Medicine & Urogenital Reconstruction, et al. Diagnosis and treatment of overactive bladder (non-neurogenic) in adults: AUA/SUFU guideline. 2012; amended 2014. http://www.auanet.org/guidelines/overactive-bladder-(oab)-(aua/sufu-guideline-2012-amended-2014). Accessed 27 Apr 2018.
34. Nomura Y, Iitsuka H, Toyoshima J, Kuroishi K, Hatta T, Kaibara A, et al. Pharmacokinetic drug interaction study between overactive bladder drugs mirabegron and tolterodine in Japanese healthy postmenopausal females. Drug Metab Pharmacokinet. 2016;31(6):411–6.

Chapter 9
Behavioral Therapy in Combination with Pharmacotherapy

Cristiano Mendes Gomes and Marcelo Hisano

Introduction

Behavioral treatments (BT) are a group of therapies that aim to improve overactive bladder (OAB) symptoms by modifying patient behavior or his/her environment. Most BT programs include multiple components and are individualized to the needs of the patient and his/her particular living situation [1]. There are two main approaches to BT for OAB. One targets the modification of bladder function by changing voiding habits, such as with bladder training and delayed voiding. The other approach focuses on the bladder outlet and includes pelvic floor muscle training to enhance strength and control and techniques for urge suppression. Distinct components of BT can include self-monitoring [bladder diary), timed voiding, delayed voiding, pelvic floor muscle training (including pelvic floor relaxation), use of pelvic floor muscles for urethral occlusion and urge suppression (urge strategies), normal voiding techniques, biofeedback, electrical stimulation, fluid management, dietary changes, weight loss, and other lifestyle changes [1, 2].

As BT presents essentially no risks to patients, most guidelines encourage its use as first-line treatment to all patients [1–5]. BT can be combined with other therapeutic techniques, and we will discuss its use in association with pharmacological therapy for OAB in this chapter.

C. M. Gomes (✉) · M. Hisano
Hospital of the University of Sao Paulo School of Medicine, Division of Urology, Sao Paulo, Brazil

L. Cox, E. S. Rovner (eds.), *Contemporary Pharmacotherapy of Overactive Bladder*, https://doi.org/10.1007/978-3-319-97265-7_9

Behavioral Treatments for OAB

Behavioral treatments are designated as first-line treatments because they are as effective in improving symptoms as pharmacological treatment [2]. In addition, they are relatively noninvasive and, contrary to medications, are rarely associated with adverse events. Nonetheless, they do require the active participation of the patient and/or caregiver along with time and effort from the clinician.

Most studies with BT for OAB focus on the treatment of urinary incontinence, and most trials have been performed with women [5]. The literature indicates that most patients experience significant reductions in symptoms and improvements in quality of life. The medical literature provides clear support for the effectiveness of bladder training with incremental voiding schedules [6] and pelvic floor muscle training with urge suppression techniques [7]. Improvements typically range from 50% to 80% in reduction of the episodes of incontinence. Reductions in voiding frequency have also been shown in men [8] and women [6, 9].

Studies have also demonstrated improvement of OAB symptoms with reduction in fluid intake and caffeine intake [5].

No single component of behavioral therapy appears to be indispensable to efficacy, and no single type of BT appears to be superior than others [1, 5].

Behavioral Treatments Versus Pharmacotherapy

A number of studies have compared the effectiveness of BT and pharmacotherapy. In randomized trials, different types of BT were generally either equivalent to [9] or superior to [7] medications in reducing incontinence episodes, improving voiding parameters such as frequency and nocturia and ameliorating quality of life (QoL). Most studies evaluated oxybutynin, but other agents such as tolterodine, imipramine and solifenacin have also been evaluated with similar results [7–10].

According to the American Urological Association/Society of Urodynamics, Female Pelvic Medicine and Urogenital Reconstruction (AUA/SUFU) guideline panel [3, 4], these data indicate that behavioral therapies can result in symptomatic improvements similar to pharmacotherapy without exposing patients to adverse events. Evidence strength is considered Grade B because most of the randomized trials were of moderate quality, follow-up durations were short in most studies (12 weeks), and sample sizes were small. Consistent with these results, the guideline recommends behavioral therapies should be offered to all OAB patients, including those that require a caregiver, who can be instructed in BT such as prompted voiding and timed voiding. The European Association of Urology (EAU) guideline also supports this recommendation [5].

Combination of Behavioral Therapy and Pharmacotherapy

Behavioral and drug therapies are frequently used in combination in clinical practice to enhance patient symptom control and QoL. Few studies indicate that starting behavioral and pharmacological therapy simultaneously may improve outcomes, including frequency, voided volume, incontinence, and symptom distress [11–14]. In patients who are not significantly improved on behavioral or drug therapy alone, there also is evidence that continuing the initial therapy and adding the alternate therapy in a stepped approach can produce further clinical improvement [15].

According to the AUA/SUFU guideline panel [3], there are no known contraindications to combining pharmacologic management and BT. They considered the evidence strength as Grade C because it is based on relatively few trials, small sample sizes, and limited follow-up durations.

Potential limitations for the use of BT include patient ability and motivation to comply and availability of, and access to, specific treatments. Behavioral therapies do require an investment of time and effort by the patient to achieve maximum benefits and may require sustained and regular contact with the clinician to maintain regimen adherence and consequent efficacy [16]. In patients who are unwilling or unable to comply with behavioral therapy regimens and instructions, it is appropriate to move to second-line pharmacologic therapies.

Given that idiopathic OAB is a chronic syndrome without an ideal treatment and no treatment will cure the condition in most patients, clinicians should be prepared to manage the transition between treatment levels appropriately. Treatment failure occurs when the patient does not have the desired change in their symptoms or is unable to tolerate the treatment due to adverse events; lack of efficacy and the presence of intolerable adverse events reduce compliance. The interaction between efficacy, tolerability, and compliance is important to achieve the best results [17].

Most studies concerning the combination of behavioral therapy and anticholinergic agents were performed for female patients without neurological conditions. One important limitation common to most studies is that it is very difficult to blind patients and researchers regarding the assignment to behavioral treatment [10].

Burgio et al. in 1998 [7] conducted a randomized trial comparing three groups of treatment for OAB confirmed by clinical evaluation and urodynamic testing. They randomized 197 women between 55 and 92 years old for behavioral therapy with biofeedback ($n = 65$ patients), anticholinergics (oxybutynin; $n = 67$), and placebo ($n = 65$). The primary outcome measure of the study was the reduction of episodes of incontinence after 8 weeks. Significant improvement of this endpoint was observed for all groups, with superior improvement for patients in the behavioral therapy group (80.7% reduction) compared to the anticholinergic group (68.5%) and placebo (39.4%). The improvement occurred mostly during the initial 4 weeks of treatment. Another parameter measured in this study was the patient's perception of improvement, which was 81.6%, 66.4%, and 45.1%, respectively. It is interesting to note that 53% of the patients had a cystogram pre- and posttreatment. Of these, bladder capacity increased by a mean of 17.3 mL in the behavioral group ($p = 0.3$) and 70.9 mL in the anticholinergic group ($p < 0.001$) and decreased by 5.9 mL in the placebo group ($p = 0.61$).

In a follow-up study, the same group published their results in terms of urodynamic changes after treatment [9]. They showed superior increase in cystometric capacity in the oxybutynin group compared to the BT and placebo groups (69.9 mL, 17.3 mL, and 6.0 mL, respectively). The effect on other urodynamic parameters was comparable for the two active intervention groups and did not parallel symptom improvement.

The finding of subjective clinical improvement after behavioral therapy despite the lack of objective improvement (like for cystogram or urodynamic test) was also demonstrated by Elser in 1999 [18]. They evaluated 181 women with stress incontinence, OAB, or mixed incontinence in three groups of treatment (bladder training, pelvic floor muscle training (PFMT), and combined therapy) and performed urodynamic tests pre- and posttreatment. They did not find objective changes in urodynamic results, except for first sensation to void, which had increased.

In an extension of their randomized controlled trial (RCT) [7], Burgio et al. offered additional treatment to patients who were not completely dry or satisfied with the outcome [15]. Patients who received BT in the first phase of the study ($n = 8$) received the addition of oxybutynin and were evaluated after 8 weeks. Additional benefit was seen in improvement from a mean 57.5% reduction of incontinence with single therapy to a mean 88.5% reduction of incontinence with combined therapy. Twenty-seven subjects crossed from drug therapy alone to combined drug and BT. They also had additional improvement, from a mean 72.7% reduction of incontinence with single therapy to a mean 84.3% reduction of incontinence with combined therapy. The authors concluded that combining drug and BT in a stepped program can produce added benefit for patients with OAB.

The ability of behavioral therapy to enable discontinuation of drug treatment was evaluated in women with urge urinary incontinence [12]. After a first phase when patients were randomized to receive tolterodine and behavioral therapy or tolterodine only for 10 weeks, patients discontinued medication and were followed for 8 months. The tolterodine dose was 4 mg daily and could be reduced to 2 mg as necessary, while behavioral therapy included bladder training and PFMT. There were no differences between the groups for the primary endpoint, defined as not needing treatments for OAB at 8 months (28% for combined therapy group and 27% for tolterodine group). Although the addition of BT did not result in improved ability to discontinue drug therapy, the combination treatment had beneficial effects on patient satisfaction, perceived improvement, and reduction of OAB symptoms.

A prospective RCT compared the efficacy of the association of BT and pharmacotherapy to antimuscarinics alone in 64 women with urodynamically proven urgency urinary incontinence [19]. Patients received extended release oxybutynin for 8 weeks; those in the combined drug-BT group also received PFMT and bladder training. No differences in reduction of incontinence episodes were observed between the groups at 8-week (91.8% reduction in the drug only group vs 86.2% in the combination group) and also at the 6- and 12-month evaluations. Groups did not differ on secondary outcomes at any point. The authors concluded that concurrent behavioral training does not enhance outcomes of drug therapy for urgency incontinence in women when the pharmacological therapy is implemented with frequent individualized dose titration, daily bladder diaries, and careful management of side effects.

A multicenter randomized single-blind study compared the effect of drug treatment with combined drug/BT therapy in 501 patients (25% men) with clinical symptoms of OAB [14]. Patients received either tolterodine alone or tolterodine and bladder training. In both groups, a significant improvement in comparison to the baseline symptoms was observed. Superior improvements with combined therapy were observed for urinary frequency reduction and voided volume after 24 weeks. No differences were observed between groups for urgency episodes and incontinence episodes.

Another multicenter study compared the combination of tolterodine with a simple PFMT to tolterodine alone [20]. All patients received 2 mg of tolterodine, and 227 patients were randomized to the combination treatment group and also received PFMT. Of the patients, 75.4% were women and they were evaluated at 12 and 24 weeks. There was an improvement in terms of incontinence episodes, micturitions per day, urgency episodes, voided volume per micturition, and patients perception for both groups compared to baseline, but no differences were observed between groups.

Chancellor et al. randomized 395 patients (89% women) with OAB in two groups: darifenacin alone (190 patients) vs darifenacin associated with BT (bladder training and Kegel exercises; 205 patients). The darifenacin dose started at 7.5 mg daily and could be increased to 15 mg, as needed. After 12 weeks of treatment, the average reduction of urinary frequency from baseline was 2.7 for both groups. Secondary parameters such as urgency urinary incontinence, urgency episodes, and nocturia were also improved for both groups, with no between-group differences.

Another multicenter randomized study compared the effects of solifenacin treatment to solifenacin and BT for patients with OAB [13]. A total of 643 patients (85% women) were randomized for the two groups (323 vs 320, respectively); they initially received 5 mg daily of the solifenacin for 8 weeks after which they could increase the dosage for 10 mg daily, as needed. The primary endpoint at 8 weeks was the micturition frequency, which decreased in both groups but was significantly better in the combination group (2.9 decrease vs 2.2 for solifenacin only group). At week 16, the reduction of micturition frequency was still greater for the combined therapy. No differences were found between groups in terms of reduction of urgency episodes, incontinence episodes, number of pads used, and urgency incontinence episodes.

A Cochrane Review compared the efficacy of pharmacotherapy vs combined therapy with BT for non-neurogenic OAB in 2012 [10]. Three studies were included for the comparison between the combination of anticholinergic drugs and bladder training versus bladder training alone. They showed superior subjective improvement for the combination therapy, while no differences were observed in terms of improvement of the number of voids per day and urgency. For the comparison of antimuscarinics in combination with BT versus antimuscarinics alone, nine trials were identified. However, because of the different types of BT applied, a meta-analysis was not possible. Three trials compared tolterodine combined to bladder training to tolterodine alone, with improvements favoring the combination group. Three other trials compared anticholinergic agents combined to bladder training and PFMT; a meta-analysis of these studies showed no differences between the two groups regarding micturitions per day. The proportion of people experiencing adverse events was similar in the trials comparing bladder training and an anticholinergic versus anticholinergic alone. The authors concluded that because of the great disparity between studies in terms of antimuscarinic agents and dosages used and the type of behavioral therapy, it was not possible to draw a definite recommendation. In addition, they highlighted the lack of data concerning the long-term results.

It is important to note that studies comparing pharmacotherapy with specific behavioral interventions (other than PFMT/timed voiding/bladder training), including fluid and dietary modification and weight loss, are lacking.

Combination of Electrical Stimulation Therapy for OAB

Electrical stimulation (ES) applied to patients with OAB involves the use of either implanted or external electrodes to stimulate efferent fibers to the striated urethral sphincter reflexively causing detrusor relaxation or the selective activation of afferent fibers causing inhibition at spinal and supraspinal levels [21, 22]. The mechanism of action of SNS is not completely understood. The therapeutic benefits of SNS may arise from the effects of electrical stimulation on afferent and efferent nerve fibers connecting the pelvic organs and the spinal interneurons to the central nervous system [21, 22]. External electrodes are broadly classified into endocavitary and percutaneous electrodes. Endocavitary electrodes can be placed intravaginally or rectally. Percutaneous approaches include transcutaneous electrical nerve stimulation (TENS) and percutaneous tibial nerve stimulation (PTNS). When the electrodes are placed on the perineal skin surface, it is termed TENS [23]; PTNS involves minimally invasive electrical stimulation of S2 to S4 sacral nerves via a 34 gauge needle placed just above the medial malleolus of the ankle [24, 25].

According to the International Consultation on Incontinence, ES may be an alternative to improve symptoms for urgency urinary incontinence (grade of recommendation: B) [1]. However, they advise that this recommendation should be viewed with caution until the findings are supported in further trials. It is also important to bear in mind that there are virtually endless combinations of current types, waveforms, frequencies, intensities, electrode types, and placements that can be used for ES. Additional confusion is created by the rapid developments in the area of ES and a wide variety of stimulation devices and protocols that have been developed even for the same conditions. So far, it is not possible to identify one particular technique that is superior to others for OAB treatment [1].

Sacral nerve modulation (SNM) is a technique that involves implanted electrodes [26, 27]. It is a two-stage invasive procedure where an electrode is placed percutaneously alongside S3 in the sacral foramina. It is not a modality of BT and will not be discussed in this chapter.

In 2010 Sancaktar et al. published a randomized trial comparing the use of PTNS combined with tolterodine ($n = 20$) versus tolterodine alone ($n = 20$) for women with OAB [28]. Patients in the combined group received PTNS sessions once a week for 12 weeks. There was a significant decrease from baseline for both groups in terms of urinary frequency, urgency episodes, incontinence episodes, and incontinence impact questionnaire (IIQ-7). Patients in the combined therapy group had superior improvements for all the aforementioned parameters. The incontinence episodes per week decreased from a mean of 22 to 12.3 in the drug group and 6.4 in the combination group therapy ($p < 0.001$).

Another study compared the treatment of OAB with TENS vs TENS and oxybutynin vs oxybutynin alone [29]. Seventy-five women with OAB were randomized for these three groups, with 25 patients in each group; clinical evaluation was performed with the International Consultation on Incontinence-Short Form (ICIQ-SF) to assess incontinence, the International Consultation on Incontinence-OAB (ICIQ-OAB) to assess the symptoms of OAB, a QoL questionnaire, and a 3-day voiding diary. Treatments were delivered for 12 weeks and patients were evaluated. They were re-evaluated after another 12-week period, during which no treatments were delivered for any group. At completion of the treatment period, the ICIQ-SF score improved for all groups, with no significant differences (7.2 in the TENS group, 9.8 in oxybutynin group, and 7.9 in combination group). However, 12 weeks after the end of the treatment, the oxybutynin group had an increase in incontinence episodes (13.3) compared to the TENS alone group and TENS plus oxybutynin group (8.3 and 7.4, respectively; $p = 0.0006$). Similar results were seen with the ICIQ-OAB score and the QoL questionnaire. The authors concluded that TENS alone or in association present longer-lasting results for improvement of clinical symptoms of OAB and QoL.

A recent meta-analysis reviewed the combination of antimuscarinics with ES or behavioral therapies to pharmacotherapy alone [30]. A total of 10 RCTs were selected for the meta-analysis, comprising 982 women with non-neurogenic OAB. The antimuscarinic agents used were tolterodine in seven, oxybutynin in two, and solifenacin in one. The behavioral therapies were electrical stimulation in eight studies and bladder training in two. For the antimuscarinics combined with ES treatment compared with antimuscarinics alone, there were significant reductions of average frequency of urination, incontinence, and urgency, with pooled standardized mean differences of −2.38, −1.32, and −0.87, respectively. There was also a significant reduction of average frequency of urination (pooled standardized mean difference = −0.30; 95% confidence interval: −0.52 to −0.08) for the antimuscarinics combined with bladder training treatment compared with antimuscarinics alone. The authors concluded that both electrical stimulation and bladder training may improve treatment of OAB symptoms when compared with isolated drug therapy.

A recent study compared the effects of transcutaneous posterior tibial nerve stimulation (TENS) three times a week with the combination of TENS and trospium chloride (20 mg daily) for women patients who had failed first-line behavioral therapy for OAB and had detrusor overactivity at urodynamics [31]. After 8 weeks of treatment, all clinical parameters measured for both groups were improved compared to baseline. The combination group had superior improvements for the OABSS, IIQ-7, urinary frequency, and mean voided volume. In addition, they outperformed the TENS only group in urodynamic parameters such as first sensation and bladder capacity.

Behavioral Therapy in Combination with Estrogens

Estrogens have been used to treat postmenopausal women with OAB for many years, but there have been few controlled trials to confirm that it is of benefit [32, 33]. In a double-blind multicenter study with 64 postmenopausal women with "urge syndrome," Cardozo et al. found similar objective and subjective improvements in symptoms in comparison to placebo [34]. All women underwent pre-treatment urodynamic investigation to ensure that they had either sensory urgency or detrusor overactivity. They were randomized to treatment with oral estriol 3 mg daily or placebo for 3 months. Compliance with therapy was confirmed by a significant improvement in the maturation index of vaginal epithelial cells in the active but not the placebo group. In another study from the same group, investigators compared the effects of estradiol implants with placebo and were not able to show any differences in terms of clinical improvement [35]. However, a higher complication rate was noted in the estradiol-treated patients (vaginal bleeding).

Although the evidence supporting the use of estrogens in lower urinary tract dysfunction remains controversial, considerable data support their use in urogenital atrophy, and the vaginal route of administration appears to offer superior relief by improving vaginal dryness, pruritis, and dyspareunia and greater improvement in cytological findings while having no or minimal serum estradiol levels [36, 37].

A meta-analysis of intravaginal estrogen treatment in the management of urogenital atrophy was reported by the Cochrane group in 2012 [38]. They evaluated trials that used varying combinations of estrogen, dose, duration of treatment, and length of follow-up. The combined result of six trials of systemic administration (oral estrogen) resulted in worse incontinence than placebo. However, there was some evidence that locally applied estrogen used as vaginal creams, pessaries, suppositories, or rings improved incontinence. Overall there was less frequency and urgency in patients treated with local estrogen.

Since vaginally applied estrogen may be useful in the treatment of perimenopausal women with OAB symptoms by improving the urethral epithelium, vaginal vessels, and connective tissue, there could be a role for combination treatment with BT [39].

An RCT evaluated the use of estrogen in combination with pelvic floor stimulation (PFS) in perimenopausal women [40]. A total of 315 patients with OAB were divided in three treatment groups: (1) vaginal PFS, (2) vaginal estrogen cream, and (3) combined vaginal PFS and estrogen cream. Vaginal estrogen cream consisted of daily 2 g of estrogen cream 0.625 mg/g. Vaginal PFS was performed with a vaginal probe twice weekly for 6 weeks in 30-min sessions. Evaluations were performed at baseline and1 week and 3 and 6 months after completion of treatment. Significant improvements in OAB symptoms, QoL scores, and urodynamic parameters were observed for all groups after 1 week of treatment. The improvement was significantly better in the combined therapy group than in group 2 in all parameters except for detrusor overactivity. Improvement was significantly better in the combined therapy group than in the vaginal PFS alone group in all parameters except for voiding frequency, incontinence episodes, and QoL. All groups showed deterioration in all evaluable parameters within 6 months of follow-up, except for incontinence episodes in the combination therapy group. The authors concluded that estrogen may augment the effect of PFS and also prolong its duration.

Behavioral Therapy in Combination with β3-Agonists

Mirabegron is the only β3-agonist approved for the treatment of OAB, and its use is discussed in another chapter of this book. As of the writing of this chapter, there were no relevant published studies. Since the effect of mirabegron appears to be similar to most antimuscarinic agents [41], one might suppose that the benefits observed with the combined use of antimuscarinics and BT should probably be observed with the combination of mirabegron and BT. However, studies addressing the effects of these combinations are needed to support the use of such multimodal treatment.

Combination Therapy for Children

The pharmacological treatment of OAB in children is the topic of another chapter of this book. We included in this chapter only data regarding the combined use of antimuscarinics and BT.

In a prospective, randomized, single-blind study, Quintiliano F. et al. compared the use of parasacral transcutaneous electrical stimulation (PTENS) with oxybutynin treatment in children with OAB [42]. A total of 28 patients (9 boys and 17 girls; age 4–17 years old) were randomized to receive PTENS in 20-min sessions 3 times per week with oral placebo daily or oral oxybutynin with scapular electrical stimulation (sham treatment) 3 times per week. After 3 months of treatment, the improvement of symptoms was similar in the two groups. However, despite the lack of statistical significance, the rate of complete resolution was about twofold in favor of PTENS (46% vs 20% in the oxybutynin group; $p = 0.204$). The voiding volume improved for both groups, but urinary frequency improved only for the oxybutynin group, when compared to baseline. Constipation was reported by 15 (53%) patients at baseline and was improved in all 6 patients (100%) in the PTENS group and in 55% (5 patients) of the oxybutynin group. No patients in the PTENS group presented with side effects. However, in oxybutynin group dry mouth, hyperthermia, and hyperemia developed in 58%, 25%, and 50% of patients, respectively. The authors concluded that PTENS is as effective as oxybutynin to treat OAB in children but more effective to treat constipation while showing no detectable side effects.

In a recent study, Borch et al. evaluated the use of TENS and oxybutynin for the treatment of children with urge urinary incontinence [43]. They randomized 66 patients to receive (1) TENS combined with oxybutynin, (2) TENS combined with placebo oxybutynin, or (3) sham TENS combined with oxybutynin. The study took 10 weeks, and patients were evaluated before treatment, at 3 weeks, and at the end of the study. The primary endpoint of the study was the number of wet days weekly. The combined therapy achieved more dry patients than the other two groups (36% vs 0% vs 13%, respectively; $p = 0.05$). Children receiving active combination therapy had an 83% higher response rate than those in the placebo sacral TENS plus active oxybutynin group (RR 1.83, CI 1.0 to 3.5, $p = 0.06$). Active sacral TENS plus oxybutynin was significantly more effective compared to group 2 regarding improvement in number of wet days per week (mean difference − 2.28, CI −4.06 to −0.49, $p < 0.01$), severity of incontinence (mean difference − 3.11, CI −5.98 to −0.23, $p < 0.05$), and frequency (mean difference − 2.82, CI −4.48 to −1.17, $p < 0.001$). The authors concluded that TENS in combination with oxybutynin is superior to monotherapy with either treatment.

Conclusions

The pharmacological treatment of OAB with antimuscarinics or mirabegron is well established. Behavioral treatments are designated as first-line treatments because they are as effective in improving symptoms as pharmacological treatment, are relatively noninvasive, and, contrary to medications, are rarely associated with adverse events. However, they require patient ability and motivation to comply and availability of and access to specific treatments. Moreover, BT demands an ongoing investment of time and effort by the patient and the clinician to maintain regimen adherence and consequent efficacy. Although there is no data to suggest that BT may promote superior results as compared to drug treatment, the effect of BT might be expected to persist in those patients who continue the regimen, which is not observed after interrupting medical therapy.

The combination of BT and pharmacotherapy for OAB may be a useful treatment strategy. It may be introduced stepwise to improve OAB symptoms of patients that did not obtain adequate symptom control with medical or behavioral therapy alone, or it can be offered upfront to enhance clinical improvement. However, from current medical literature, it is not possible to determine what is the best treatment modality or combination to use in an index OAB patient. Larger trials with longer follow-up are needed, particularly long-term results after treatment has ended. There is also a need for studies evaluating the combination of β3-agonists with BT. Finally, additional studies looking at other forms of behavioral therapy, including dietary and fluid modification and weight loss, in combination with pharmacotherapy are desirable.

References

1. Dumoulin C, Adewuyi T, Booth J, Bradley C, Burgio K, Hagen S, Hunter K, et al. Adult conservative management. In: Abrams P, Cardozo L, Wagg A, Wein A, editors. International consultation on incontinence. 6th ed. 6th International Consultation on Incontinence, Tokyo, September 2016. pp. 1443–628. Bristol: The International Continence Society (ICS) and the International Consultation on Urological Diseases (ICUD); 2017.
2. Corcos J, Przydacz M, Campeau L, Gray G, Hickling D, Honeine C, et al. CUA guideline on adult overactive bladder. Can Urol Assoc J. 2017;11(5):E142–E73.
3. Gormley EA, Lightner DJ, Burgio KL, Chai TC, Clemens JQ, Culkin DJ; American Urological Association; Society of Urodynamics, Female Pelvic Medicine & Urogenital Reconstruction, et al. Diagnosis and treatment of overactive bladder (non-neurogenic) in adults: AUA/SUFU guideline. 2012; amended 2014. http://www.auanet.org/guidelines/overactive-bladder-(oab)-(aua/sufu-guideline-2012-amended-2014). Accessed 27 Apr 2018.
4. Gormley EA, Lightner DJ, Faraday M, Vasavada SP. Diagnosis and treatment of overactive bladder (non-neurogenic) in adults: AUA/SUFU guideline amendment. J Urol. 2015;193(5):1572–80.
5. Burkhard FC, Bosch, JLHR, Cruz F, Lemack GE, Nambiar N, Thiruchelvam A, et al. EAU guidelines on urinary incontinence in adults. Arnhem: EAU Guidelines Office; 2017. http://uroweb.org/guideline/urinary-incontinence/. Accessed 26 Apr 2018.
6. Fantl JA, Wyman JF, McClish DK, Harkins SW, Elswick RK, Taylor JR, et al. Efficacy of bladder training in older women with urinary incontinence. JAMA. 1991;265(5):609–13.
7. Burgio KL, Locher JL, Goode PS, Hardin JM, McDowell BJ, Dombrowski M, et al. Behavioral vs drug treatment for urge urinary incontinence in older women: a randomized controlled trial. JAMA. 1998;280(23):1995–2000.
8. Burgio KL, Goode PS, Johnson TM, Hammontree L, Ouslander JG, Markland AD, et al. Behavioral versus drug treatment for overactive bladder in men: the Male Overactive Bladder Treatment in Veterans (MOTIVE) trial. J Am Geriatr Soc. 2011;59(12):2209–16.
9. Goode PS, Burgio KL, Locher JL, Umlauf MG, Lloyd LK, Roth DL. Urodynamic changes associated with behavioral and drug treatment of urge incontinence in older women. J Am Geriatr Soc. 2002;50(5):808–16.
10. Rai BP, Cody JD, Alhasso A, Stewart L. Anticholinergic drugs versus non-drug active therapies for non-neurogenic overactive bladder syndrome in adults. Cochrane Database Syst Rev. 2012;12:CD003193.
11. Kaya S, Akbayrak T, Beksac S. Comparison of different treatment protocols in the treatment of idiopathic detrusor overactivity: a randomized controlled trial. Clin Rehabil. 2011;25(4):327–38.
12. Burgio KL, Kraus SR, Menefee S, Borello-France D, Corton M, Johnson HW, et al. Behavioral therapy to enable women with urge incontinence to discontinue drug treatment: a randomized trial. Ann Intern Med. 2008;149(3):161–9.

13. Mattiasson A, Masala A, Morton R, Bolodeoku J, Group SS. Efficacy of simplified bladder training in patients with overactive bladder receiving a solifenacin flexible-dose regimen: results from a randomized study. BJU Int. 2010;105(8):1126–35.
14. Mattiasson A, Blaakaer J, Hoye K, Wein AJ, Tolterodine Scandinavian Study G. Simplified bladder training augments the effectiveness of tolterodine in patients with an overactive bladder. BJU Int. 2003;91(1):54–60.
15. Burgio KL, Locher JL, Goode PS. Combined behavioral and drug therapy for urge incontinence in older women. J Am Geriatr Soc. 2000;48(4):370–4.
16. Borello-France D, Burgio KL, Goode PS, Markland AD, Kenton K, Balasubramanyam A, et al. Adherence to behavioral interventions for urge incontinence when combined with drug therapy: adherence rates, barriers, and predictors. Phys Ther. 2010;90(10):1493–505.
17. Wein AJ. Diagnosis and treatment of the overactive bladder. Urology. 2003;62(5 Suppl 2):20–7.
18. Elser DM, Wyman JF, McClish DK, Robinson D, Fantl JA, Bump RC. The effect of bladder training, pelvic floor muscle training, or combination training on urodynamic parameters in women with urinary incontinence. Continence Program for Women Research Group. Neurourol Urodyn. 1999;18(5):427–36.
19. Burgio KL, Goode PS, Richter HE, Markland AD, Johnson TM 2nd, Redden DT. Combined behavioral and individualized drug therapy versus individualized drug therapy alone for urge urinary incontinence in women. J Urol. 2010;184(2):598–603.
20. Millard RJ; Asia Pacific Tolterodine Study G. Clinical efficacy of tolterodine with or without a simplified pelvic floor exercise regimen. Neurourol Urodyn. 2004;23(1):48–53.
21. Yoshimura N, de Groat WC. Neural control of the lower urinary tract. Int J Urol. 1997;4(2):111–25.
22. Leng WW, Chancellor MB. How sacral nerve stimulation neuromodulation works. Urol Clin North Am. 2005;32(1):11–8.
23. Bristow SE, Hasan ST, Neal DE. TENS: a treatment option for bladder dysfunction. Int Urogynecol J Pelvic Floor Dysfunct. 1996;7(4):185–90.
24. Vandoninck V, van Balken MR, Finazzi AE, Petta F, Micali F, Heesakkers JP, et al. Percutaneous tibial nerve stimulation in the treatment of overactive bladder: urodynamic data. Neurourol Urodyn. 2003;22(3):227–32.
25. Burton C, Sajja A, Latthe PM. Effectiveness of percutaneous posterior tibial nerve stimulation for overactive bladder: a systematic review and meta-analysis. Neurourol Urodyn. 2012;31(8):1206–16.
26. Amend B, Matzel KE, Abrams P, de Groat WC, Sievert KD. How does neuromodulation work. Neurourol Urodyn. 2011;30(5):762–5.
27. Van Kerrebroeck PE, Marcelissen TA. Sacral neuromodulation for lower urinary tract dysfunction. World J Urol. 2012;30(4):445–50.
28. Sancaktar M, Ceyhan ST, Akyol I, Muhcu M, Alanbay I, Mutlu Ercan C, et al. The outcome of adding peripheral neuromodulation (Stoller afferent neuro-stimulation) to anti-muscarinic therapy in women with severe overactive bladder. Gynecol Endocrinol. 2010;26(10):729–32.
29. Souto SC, Reis LO, Palma T, Palma P, Denardi F. Prospective and randomized comparison of electrical stimulation of the posterior tibial nerve versus oxybutynin versus their combination for treatment of women with overactive bladder syndrome. World J Urol. 2014;32(1):179–84.
30. Cao Y, Lv J, Zhao C, Li J, Leng J. Cholinergic antagonists combined with electrical stimulation or bladder training treatments for overactive bladder in female adults: a meta-analysis of randomized controlled trials. Clin Drug Investig. 2016;36(10):801–8.
31. Abulseoud A, Moussa A, Abdelfattah G, Ibrahim I, Saba E, Hassouna M. Transcutaneous posterior tibial nerve electrostimulation with low dose trospium chloride: could it be used as a second line treatment of overactive bladder in females. Neurourol Urodyn. 2018;37(22):842–8.
32. Andersson KE, Cardozo L, Cruz F, Lee K-S, Suhai A, Wein AJ. Pharmacological treatment of urinary incontinence. In: Abrams P, Cardozo L, Wagg A, Wein A, editors. Incontinence. 6th International Consultation on Incontinence, Tokyo, September 2016, pp. 805–957. The

International Continence Society (ICS) and the International Consultation on Urological Diseases (ICUD); 2017.
33. Hextall A. Oestrogens and lower urinary tract function. Maturitas. 2000;36(2):83–92.
34. Cardozo L, Rekers H, Tapp A, Barnick C, Shepherd A, Schussler B, et al. Oestriol in the treatment of postmenopausal urgency: a multicentre study. Maturitas. 1993;18(1):47–53.
35. Rufford J, Hextall A, Cardozo L, Khullar V. A double-blind placebo-controlled trial on the effects of 25 mg estradiol implants on the urge syndrome in postmenopausal women. Int Urogynecol J Pelvic Floor Dysfunct. 2003;14(2):78–83.
36. Cardozo L, Bachmann G, McClish D, Fonda D, Birgerson L. Meta-analysis of estrogen therapy in the management of urogenital atrophy in postmenopausal women: second report of the Hormones and Urogenital Therapy Committee. Obstet Gynecol. 1998;92(4 Pt 2):722–7.
37. Krause M, Wheeler TL 2nd, Richter HE, Snyder TE. Systemic effects of vaginally administered estrogen therapy: a review. Female Pelvic Med Reconstr Surg. 2010;16(3):188–95.
38. Cody JD, Jacobs ML, Richardson K, Moehrer B, Hextall A. Oestrogen therapy for urinary incontinence in post-menopausal women. Cochrane Database Syst Rev. 2012;10:CD001405.
39. Bhatia NN, Bergman A, Karram MM. Effects of estrogen on urethral function in women with urinary incontinence. Am J Obstet Gynecol. 1989;160(1):176–81.
40. Abdelbary AM, El-Dessoukey AA, Massoud AM, Moussa AS, Zayed AS, Elsheikh MG, et al. Combined vaginal pelvic floor electrical stimulation (PFS) and local vaginal estrogen for treatment of overactive bladder (OAB) in perimenopausal females. Randomized controlled trial (RCT). Urology. 2015;86(3):482–6.
41. Maman K, Aballea S, Nazir J, Desroziers K, Neine ME, Siddiqui E, et al. Comparative efficacy and safety of medical treatments for the management of overactive bladder: a systematic literature review and mixed treatment comparison. Eur Urol. 2014;65(4):755–65.
42. Quintiliano F, Veiga ML, Moraes M, Cunha C, de Oliveira LF, Lordelo P, et al. Transcutaneous parasacral electrical stimulation vs oxybutynin for the treatment of overactive bladder in children: a randomized clinical trial. J Urol. 2015;193(5 Suppl):1749–53.
43. Borch L, Hagstroem S, Kamperis K, Siggaard CV, Rittig S. Transcutaneous electrical nerve stimulation combined with oxybutynin is superior to monotherapy in children with urge incontinence: a randomized, placebo controlled study. J Urol. 2017;198(2):430–5.

Chapter 10
Pharmacotherapy for Nocturia

Ari M. Bergman and Jeffrey P. Weiss

Introduction

Nocturia is defined by the International Continence Society (ICS) as voiding that occurs during the hours of sleep, when each void is preceded and followed by sleep [1]. Though the clinical complaint is often simple, nocturia can be caused by many different conditions. Determining the underlying etiology is essential for choosing the appropriate therapy. Medical conditions causing or contributing to nocturia should be ruled out or addressed as appropriate. Subsequent pharmacologic interventions should be guided by data derived from a frequency-volume chart (FVC), which is used to subcategorize nocturia. Initial treatments include behavioral interventions and therapy for underlying medical conditions contributing to nocturnal urine production. Pharmacological treatments include medications for overactive bladder (OAB), benign prostatic hyperplasia (BPH) with bladder outlet obstruction (BOO), and those to reduce nocturnal urine production.

Prevalence

Nocturia is common and affects patients from all demographics. The Boston Area Community Health (BACH) survey, which queried 5502 men and women from ages 30 to 79, found that 28.4% of respondents reported at least one void per night [2]. According to a review of pooled data from 43 studies, 11–35% of men aged 20–40 years

A. M. Bergman (✉)
Smith Institute for Urology, Greenlawn, NY, USA
e-mail: abergman6@northwell.edu

J. P. Weiss
Department of Urology, SUNY Downstate Medical Center, Brooklyn, NY, USA

L. Cox, E. S. Rovner (eds.), *Contemporary Pharmacotherapy of Overactive Bladder*, https://doi.org/10.1007/978-3-319-97265-7_10

reported 1 or more voids per night, while 2–17% reported 2 or more voids per night. 20–44% of women aged 20–40 years reported one or more episodes of nocturia, while 4–18% reported two episodes or more. Nocturia becomes more prevalent with age. 69–93% of men >70 years reported one or more voids per night, and 29–59% reported two or more episodes of nocturia. Similarly, 74–77% of women >70 years reported one or more nightly voids, and 28–62% reported two or more nightly voids [3].

Evaluation

Numerous and varying risk factors for nocturia have been identified. The Finnish National Nocturia and Overactive Bladder (FINNO) study, a survey study of 3744 randomly chosen men and women, identified multiple conditions and diseases associated with nocturia. These included urinary urgency, benign prostatic hyperplasia, snoring, obesity, prostate cancer, antidepressant use, diabetes, and coronary artery disease. None of these correlates were present in >50% of nocturia cases in both genders, emphasizing the multifactorial nature of nocturia [4].

A frequency-volume chart (FVC), or voiding diary (which adds subjective parameters to the FVC), should be employed to characterize and quantify the patient's nocturia symptoms. FVC is a log of a patient's timing and volume of voids for a 24 h period. The log must also include the time of retiring and arising. Total urine volume (TUV) and nocturnal urine volume (NUV) should be calculated. Importantly, the first morning void should be included in the NUV, because, though it is not followed by sleep, it is urine produced while asleep. Maximum voided volume (MVV) is the largest volume of urine passed during the 24 h period. If the NUV exceeds the MVV, then the nocturnal urine production has exceeded the bladder's storage capacity. This concept is summarized by the nocturia index (Ni), defined as NUV/MVV. If Ni > 1, then the patient must awaken to void to prevent enuresis.

Nocturnal bladder capacity index (NBCi) can be used as evidence of diminished nocturnal bladder capacity. NBCi is defined as the difference between the actual number of nightly voids (ANV) and the predicted number of nightly voids (PNV), i.e., NBCi = ANV-PNV. PNV=Ni-1. NBCi >0 indicates that the nightly voids are occurring at volumes < MVV. Nocturnal polyuria index (NPi) is the proportion of total urine volume produced during sleep time, i.e., NPi = NUV/TUV.

Nocturia can be classified into three categories with data derived from the FVC. Global polyuria is an abnormally elevated total 24 h production where TUV >40 ml/kg. Nocturnal polyuria is increased nocturnal urine production, with a relative commensurate decrease in diurnal urine output, with an overall normal 24 h urine production. Diminished bladder capacity is the inability for the bladder to effectively store a normal volume of urine before voiding is triggered. The polyuric states above are considered medical/renal in etiology, while diminished bladder capacity is a pathologic state arising in the lower urinary tract itself. Differentiating between these classes of nocturia is essential for management because they require differing therapeutic interventions.

Global Polyuria

Polyuria is defined as 24 h urine output >40 ml/kg. This results in daytime frequency and nocturia due to urine production exceeding bladder capacity. Underlying etiologies include diabetes mellitus/glycosuria, diabetes insipidus, and primary polydipsia (due in turn to either behavioral issues or abnormal thirst mechanism). In these cases, management should focus on treatment of the underlying condition rather than the nocturia itself. These disease states are outside the scope of practice of most urologists and should be referred to appropriate specialists.

Nocturnal Polyuria

The International Continence Society (ICS) standardization committee defines nocturnal polyuria as NUV/TUV >33% [5], though alternative diagnostic criteria have been proposed including nocturnal urine diuresis rate >90 ml/hr [6] and NUV >6.8 ml/kg. The prevalence of nocturnal polyuria is significant, though the exact prevalence depends upon the choice of definition. An examination of data collected from 1688 men from Krimpen, the Netherlands, found 44–51% of men aged 50–54 years and 54–65% of men aged 65–69 met criteria for nocturnal polyuria when defined as >33% of 24 h urine output (NP33). Only 14–19% of men aged 50–54 years and 23–26% of men aged 65–69 met criteria when nocturnal polyuria was defined as nocturnal urine output >90 ml/hr (NUP90) [7].

Among patients with nocturia, nocturnal polyuria is highly prevalent. 1412 subjects were screened for a phase III study investigating a pharmacologic treatment for nocturia. Of the 934 patients with an average ≥2 voids per night and complete FVC data, 819 (88%) had NP, defined as >33% of 24 h urine volume [8].

Nocturnal polyuria can be caused by congestive heart failure, diabetes mellitus, obstructive sleep apnea, peripheral edema, and excessive nighttime fluid intake. A careful history and physical exam should be conducted, followed by diagnostic workup as indicated, to identify and treat any of the conditions above before initiating further treatment directed at nocturia. Once these conditions have been ruled out, the etiology of nocturnal polyuria may be ascribed to the nocturnal polyuria syndrome, thought to be due to insufficient production of endogenous arginine vasopressin during sleep [9].

Obstructive sleep apnea (OSA), or the sudden cessation of respiration due to airway obstruction during sleep, can lead to nocturnal polyuria. The increased airway resistance causes a rise in right atrial transmural pressure; this in turn stimulates a release of atrial natriuretic peptide (ANP). ANP triggers increase in urine sodium and water excretion [10].

Diminished Bladder Capacity

Common causes of decreased bladder capacity include bladder outlet obstruction (BOO), neurogenic bladder, cystitis, genitourinary malignancy, or detrusor overactivity. Treatment options for BOO include pharmacologic intervention with alpha-blockers or 5-alpha reductase inhibitors, surgical procedures such as transurethral resection of prostate, or simple prostatectomy. OAB treatment options include anticholinergics, beta-agonists, or intradetrusor botulinum toxin injection. In the absence of NP, traditional treatments for OAB or BOO may improve nocturia. These interventions should not be expected to decrease nocturnal micturitions in the setting of NP. Additional causes include learned voiding dysfunction, anxiety disorders, urolithiasis, and medications.

Antimuscarinics

Mechanism of Action Urologists are familiar with antimuscarinics, as they are the mainstay of treatment of overactive bladder (OAB). They are therefore often employed in the treatment of nocturia; however, none of the currently approved antimuscarinics are indicated for the treatment of nocturia. Antimuscarinics block the stimulation of muscarinic receptors by acetylcholine. Traditionally, it was thought that antimuscarinics block parasympathetic signals to the detrusor muscle, thereby decreasing bladder contractility. However, more recent data suggests that antimuscarinics improve overall OAB symptoms by decreasing urgency and slightly increasing bladder capacity via an afferent effect, rather than by decreasing the bladder contraction itself [11, 12].

Antimuscarinics are numerous and diverse compounds. They can be subcategorized into tertiary and quaternary amines. The tertiary amines tend to have higher lipophilicity and charge than the quaternary amines. These compounds are therefore more readily absorbed by the gastrointestinal tract but are also more likely to cross the blood-brain barrier. The tertiary amines include atropine, darifenacin, imidafenacin, oxybutynin, propiverine, solifenacin, and tolterodine. The quaternary compounds include trospium and propantheline. Antimuscarinics are metabolized by the cytochrome P450 superfamily of hemoproteins. They are subject to drug interactions with other compounds that are broken down by this system [13].

Efficacy of Antimuscarinics Critical consideration of the pathophysiology of nocturia casts doubt on the expected efficacy of antimuscarinics for this complaint. Antimuscarinics are most effective at treating the urgency component of OAB, but do not affect polyuria. As discussed above, NP is present in a majority of patients with nocturia. When nocturnal urine production exceeds bladder capacity several times over, simply decreasing the sensation of urgency should not be expected to decrease nocturia. Antimuscarinics would only be expected to be effective in the subset of patients without significant NP, whose nocturia is associated with strong urgency [14]. For example, Brubaker and Fitzgerald pooled data from four placebo-controlled studies evaluating the effect of solifenacin on OAB patients and found reduced nocturia episodes only in those patients without nocturnal polyuria [15].

Buser and colleagues examined the overall efficacy of antimuscarinics in the treatment of nocturia. Their study pooled data of 38,682 men and women from 76 randomized controlled trials. A variety of antimuscarinics were employed across these studies. Data regarding nocturia was available for 13,247 subjects. The rates of reduction in number of nocturnal voids per 24 h period were corrected for placebo. The means for each medication's reduction in voids above placebo ranged from 0.04 to 0.24 voids per night. While all but the smallest differences were statistically significant, even the more pronounced reduction, a quarter of one void per night, is arguably not clinically significant [16]. Review of studies of individual medications support this conclusion.

The VENUS (Vesicare Efficacy and safety in patieNts with Urgency Study) examined the efficacy of solifenacin in the treatment of both continent and incontinent patients with overactive bladder; a subgroup analysis presented data on the effect of solifenacin on nocturia. 707 patients were randomized to either receive solifenacin or placebo for 12 weeks. Compared to placebo, patients receiving solifenacin experienced a decrease in urgency episodes in both continent (−3.4 vs −2.3) and incontinent (−4.2 vs −2.9) subjects. A significant decrease in nocturia episodes was not demonstrated, however. Nocturia in the incontinent treatment group decreased −0.6 compared to −0.5 in the incontinent placebo group. Nocturia episodes in the continent subjects decreased −0.7 compared to −0.4 in the placebo group [17].

Similarly, from a randomized controlled trial evaluating solifenacin 5 mg and 10 mg in the treatment of overactive bladder, a subgroup analysis of 962 patients with at least one nocturnal void was performed. After 12 weeks, hours of undisturbed sleep were increased by 59 min in the 5 mg group ($p = 0.0196$ vs placebo) and 60 min in the 10 mg group ($p = 0.0195$), compared to 33 min for placebo. However, the mean nocturnal micturitions only decreased −0.46 and − 0.42 with solifenacin 5 mg and 10 mg, respectively [18].

Nitti and colleagues examined the effect of fesoterodine on 836 subjects with OAB. Patients were randomized to receive either placebo, fesoterodine 4 mg daily, or fesoterodine 8 mg. Number of urgency urinary incontinence episodes, mean voided volume, and number of urgency episodes at 12 weeks of treatment were compared to baseline, and a statistically significant decrease was seen when compared to placebo ($p < 0.05$). However, the mean change in nocturnal micturitions in the treatment arms was −0.58, compared to 0.39 in the placebo group ($p = 0.42$). The differences were neither statistically nor clinically significant [19].

Similarly, a 12 week randomized placebo controlled trial evaluated 1590 patients with OAB. Patients received either an escalating dose of fesoterodine from 4 mg to 8 mg ($n = 636$), tolterodine ER 4 mg ($n = 641$), or placebo ($n = 313$). Patients receiving either fesoterodine or tolterodine had reductions in episodes of urge urinary incontinence ($p < 0.001$ and $p = 0.011$), total number of voids in 24 h ($p < 0.001$) and urgency episodes ($p < 0.001$) when compared with placebo. However, no change in nocturia was seen. The baseline number of nocturnal voids in both of the treatment arms was 2.2, compared to 2.3 in the placebo arm. Mean changes in number of nocturnal voids in the tolterodine arm were −0.6 ($p = 0.506$), −0.6 in the fesoterodine arm ($p = 0.327$), and − 0.5 in the placebo arm [20].

A multicenter trial conducted at institutions from across Europe was conducted to evaluate the efficacy of fesoterodine for the treatment of OAB. 1132 patients were randomized to either receive placebo, tolterodine extended release 4 mg, fesoterodine 4 mg, or fesoterodine 8 mg for 12 weeks. A decrease in the mean number of total voids in 24 h was demonstrated with tolterodine (−1.73, $p = 0.001$ vs placebo), fesoterodine 4 mg (−1.76, $p < 0.001$ vs placebo), and fesoterodine 8 mg (−1.88, $p < 0.001$ vs placebo). However, the reduction in nocturnal micturitions with tolterodine (−0.40, $p = 0.336$ vs placebo), fesoterodine 4 mg (−0.39, $p = 0.394$ vs placebo), and fesoterodine 8 mg (−0.39, $p = 0.418$ vs placebo) was neither statistically nor clinically significant [21].

In a double-blind randomized trial with dose escalation, 883 patients with overactive bladder received either fesoterodine or placebo. Number of voids, urgency episodes, and episodes of incontinence were followed with surveys. Improvements from baseline in diurnal and total 24 h number of voids and urgency episodes were seen at week 12; no improvement was seen in the number of nocturnal voids or nocturnal urgency episodes [22].

A 12-week double-blind study randomized patients with OAB and nocturia to receive tolterodine 4 mg or placebo within 4 h of bedtime. Voiding episodes were graded by subjects with an urgency rating of normal, OAB, or severe OAB. Voids were documented with a 7 day voiding diary, and nocturia was reported as total nocturnal voids per week. Tolterodine reduced urgency episodes and daytime frequency but not nocturia. Mean change in nighttime micturition frequency per week in the tolterodine group was −5.5 compared to −5.1 in the placebo group. A nuanced difference can be seen when results were analyzed by urgency grading. The nocturnal episodes rated as "OAB" in the treatment group declined by 30% compared to 22% with placebo; nocturnal episodes rated as "severe OAB" in the treatment group declined by 59% compared to 43% in the placebo group [23]. In other words, the overall number of nighttime voids did not decrease, but urgency-associated nocturnal voids decreased. This further supports the supposition that antimuscarinics are effective at treating the urgency-related nocturnal awakenings.

A 12-week randomized controlled trial examined the effect of trospium chloride in OAB patients. 523 subjects were randomized to receive either trospium chloride 20 mg twice daily or placebo. Symptoms were documented with FVC at 1, 4, and 12 weeks. At 12 weeks, mean nocturnal micturitions decreased from a baseline of 2.1–1.63 in the trospium group compared to 1.71 from 2.0 in the placebo group ($p < 0.05$) [24].

Rudy and colleagues had similar results with a similar study. 658 OAB patients at 52 clinical sites were randomized to either trospium 20 mg twice daily or placebo. After 12 weeks, FVC data showed improvement in daytime urgency and frequency as well as increased volume per void. Again, a statistically significant improvement in nocturia was demonstrated, with nocturnal micturitions in the treatment group decreasing from 2.00 to 1.43 at 12 weeks ($p = 0.0026$), compared to 1.71 from 2.0 in the placebo group [25].

To review, the data supporting the use of antimuscarinics in the treatment of nocturia is largely taken from studies in which the primary endpoints are related to OAB as a whole. Reduction in nocturia episodes are often secondary endpoints. The changes in nocturia parameters are sometimes statistically significant, but not clinically significant. Nocturia is usually not bothersome to patients if it does not exceed two awakenings per night [26]. Patients with bothersome nocturia typically report greater nocturia severity. Most of the studies in the OAB literature report mean baseline nocturnal micturitions of around two. Hence, the substrate for improvement in such studies is rather minimal to begin with. Further, reductions in nocturnal voids were not found to be greater than one void per night; clearly not an improvement that would satisfy most patients.

Alpha-Blockers

Mechanism of Action Alpha-1 adrenergic receptor antagonists are first-line agents in the treatment of LUTS in men. Alpha-1 adrenergic receptors are G protein-coupled receptors, and their activation initiates the inositol triphosphate second messenger signaling cascade. The predominant subtype in the prostate is the Alpha-1A receptor, activation of which causes smooth muscle contraction. Blockade of these receptors results in reduction of both bladder outlet tone and obstruction. Alpha adrenergic receptor antagonists with more specificity to the alpha-1A receptor have fewer effects outside the genitourinary tract, such as hypotension and vision changes [27].

Efficacy of Alpha-Blockers Similar to antimuscarinics, alpha-blockers are familiar to urologists and frequently used in the treatment of a common urologic condition, in this case for benign prostatic enlargement/obstruction. Studies have shown statistically significant reductions in the number of episodes of nocturia. However, just like the antimuscarinic trials discussed above, the studies showed reductions of <1 void per night from baselines of 2–3 voids per night and substantially less when correcting for the placebo effect; thus these findings are of questionable clinical utility.

Yoshimura et al. found tamsulosin to reduce nocturia episodes in a minority of BPH patients with nocturia. 505 patients with BPH were enrolled in the study, and 359 of these men were identified as having nocturia with survey data. Of the men with BPH and nocturia who were placed on tamsulosin 0.4 mg daily, 17.9% had a reduction in nocturia episodes. This was compared to 32.2% of men with BPH and nocturia who underwent transurethral resection of prostate. This was not a randomized study, and comparison to placebo was not performed [28].

Tamsulosin oral-controlled absorption system (OCAS) was shown to reduce the mean number of nighttime voids from 3.1 to 2, compared to 2.3 from 3 in the placebo group. Change in the time to first void was not statistically significant [29, 30]. A decrease in the first period of uninterrupted sleep has a significant detrimental impact on subjective sleep quality assessment and daytime function [31]. Therefore, increasing the interval before the first nocturnal void is an important goal of nocturia treatment.

In a secondary analysis of the Department of Veterans Affairs Cooperative Study, Johnson et al. examined the effects of BPH medications on nocturia. The study randomized 1229 men aged 45–80 years with BPH to receive either terazosin, finasteride, a combination of both medications, or placebo. Terazosin was given at an increasing dose from 1 mg on days 1–3, 2 mg on days 4–7, 5 mg on days 8–14, and 10 mg from day 15 through the end of the study. Finasteride 5 mg daily was given. At 12 months, the terazosin group reported a mean of 1.8 nocturia episodes per night, from a baseline of 2.5 episodes. This compares to a mean of 2.1 from 2.5, 2.0 from 2.4, and 2.1 from 2.4 in the finasteride, combination, and placebo groups, respectively. Of patients with two or more voids per night, a 50% reduction in nocturia episodes was found in 39%, 25%, 32%, and 22% of the terazosin, finasteride, combination, and placebo groups, respectively [32].

In a secondary analysis of the Medical Therapy of Prostatic Symptoms (MTOPS) trial, Johnson and colleagues evaluated the effects of doxazosin 8 mg daily, finasteride 5 mg daily, and combination therapy in the 2583 participants who reported 1 or more voids per night. Baseline mean number of nocturia episodes were 2.3, 2.4, 2.3, and 2.3 in the doxazosin, finasteride, combination, and placebo groups, respectively. At 1 year, mean nocturnal voids was reduced 0.54, 0.40, 0.58, and 0.35 in doxazosin, finasteride, combination, and placebo; reductions from baseline were 0.53, 0.42, 0.55, and 0.38 at 4 years. The decreases in the doxazosin and combination groups were statistically significant ($p < 0.05$) [33].

Roehrborn and colleagues performed a pooled analysis of three randomized placebo-controlled trials examining the efficacy of alfuzosin on BPH symptoms. Data from 954 men with BPH were included. At 12 weeks, men in the treatment arm averaged 2.6 voids per night from 3.4, compared to 2.5 from 3.6 in those men receiving placebo ($p = 0.04$) [34].

A randomized controlled trial compared silodosin to tamsulosin and placebo. After 12 weeks of either active drug or placebo, the reduction in mean nocturia episodes was −0.9, −0.8, and − 0.7 for silodosin, tamsulosin, and placebo, respectively. The reduction in the silodosin group was statistically significant ($p = 0.013$) compared to placebo, but this was not found for the tamsulosin group [35].

Beta-Adrenoreceptor Agonist

Mechanism of Action All three subtypes of beta-adrenoreceptors are found in the detrusor muscle [10]. Beta-3 adrenoreceptor agonists increase bladder capacity and promote bladder relaxation [36]. Mirabegron is currently the only selective beta-3 adrenoreceptor agonist commercially available in the United States. It is widely used for OAB in patients who do not respond to or cannot tolerate the side effects associated with anticholinergics.

Efficacy of Mirabegron. Nitti and colleagues conducted a randomized controlled trial to evaluate the therapeutic effects of mirabegron on OAB patients. Patients were randomized to either mirabegron 50 or 100 mg or placebo. At 12 weeks, the reductions in mean nocturnal micturitions were – 0.38 from 1.9, −0.57 from 1.9, and – 0.57 from 2.0 in the placebo, the 50 mg, and 100 mg groups, respectively [37].

Mirabegron is not currently indicated for the treatment of nocturia.

Botulinum Toxin

Mechanism of Action Botulinum toxin is a potent neurotoxin produced by the anaerobic bacteria *Clostridium botulinum*. The toxin binds to presynaptic cholinergic nerve terminals, is taken up into the cell, and ultimately results in irreversible inhibition of acetylcholine release [38]. Parasympathetic cholinergic nerves play an integral role in stimulating detrusor contraction; their blockade results in decreased contractility or even acontractile bladder. Botulinum toxin is also thought to block the transduction of bladder afferent nerve signaling, reducing sensory symptoms. There are multiple commercially available formulations of botulinum toxin, but onabotulinumtoxinA is the most studied and utilized intradetrusor injection therapy [10].

OnabotulinumtoxinA has been shown to have a statistically significant, if modest, effect on nocturia. In a study of the efficacy of onabotulinumtoxinA intradetrusor injection therapy, 557 patients with overactive bladder and urgency incontinence were randomized to either 100 U of active drug or placebo injected into the detrusor muscle. At 12 weeks, patients who received onabotulinumtoxinA experienced a decrease in nocturia episodes of −0.45 compared to a reduction of −0.24 in the placebo group ($p < 0.05$). These changes were from baselines of 2.2 and 2.0 voids per night in the treatment arm and the placebo arm, respectively [39]. Another study of nearly identical design found onabotulinumtoxinA reduced mean nocturia by 0.54 episodes from 2.2, compared to 0.25 from 2.1 [40].

Desmopressin

Mechanism of action Desmopressin is a vasopressin/antidiuretic hormone analogue, which functions as a selective V2-receptor agonist. Water permeability is increased at the renal tubule, enhancing renal water reabsorption; urine concentration is increased, and urine volume is thereby decreased. Stimulation of V2-receptors in the basolateral membrane of the renal tubular cell activates a cascade of second messenger-mediated events resulting in vesicles that contain aquaporin 2 (AQP2) fusing with the luminal plasma membrane of the collecting tubule. AQP2 allows water to enter the cell. Passive resorption of water along osmotic gradients by other water channels subsequently leads to water retention [41]. Desmopressin lacks the unwanted pressor or uterotonic activities of vasopressin which occur at V1-receptors primarily [42]. In addition, V2-receptor activation increases urea permeability in the medullary collecting duct, increasing urea deposition in the renal medulla and facilitating increased urine concentration through enhancement of the renal countercurrent mechanism [44].

Efficacy of Desmopressin Desmopressin is recommended for treatment of nocturia by the International Consultation on Incontinence and the European Association of Urology [44, 45]. Desmopressin is available in various countries around the world in one or more forms such as a tablet, melt, or intranasal formulation. It has been available in a tablet form in the USA for many years but does not carry the indication for the treatment of nocturia in this form. Recently, two new formulations of DDAVP have become available.

A large-scale double-blind randomized controlled trial investigated the role of desmopressin orally disintegrating tablet ("melt") in the treatment of nocturia. Desmopressin melt has the advantage of not requiring water ingestion with dosing; bioavailability is approximately 50% greater with melt than with oral tablet. Hence, 50 mcg of melt would provide the bioequivalence of 75 mcg desmopressin tablet. 1412 men and women were screened, at 78 sites in the USA and Canada, for 2 or more voids per night. 799 subjects were enrolled and randomized to receive placebo or desmopressin at 10, 25, 50, or 100 μg. Mean baseline number of voids was 3.27, 3.21, 3.35, 3.39, and 3.22. Statistically significant reduction from baseline in nighttime voids was seen with 50 and 100 μg, with change of −1.18 and − 1.43 ($p < 0.05$). Increase in initial period of undisturbed sleep from baseline was 51, 83, 85, and 107 min in the 10 μg, 25 μg, 50 μg, and 100 μg groups, respectively, compared to 39 min for the placebo group [46].

The Noctupus trials were a series of studies conducted to evaluate the effects of the desmopressin tablet on nocturia. Three short-term, double-blind, randomized placebo-controlled studies examined the effect of desmopressin on nocturia in men and women with ≥2 voids per night. Subjects with disorders causing polyuria which necessitate condition-specific treatments, such as polydipsia, diabetes insipidus, or multiple sclerosis, were excluded from the study. Of 1003 subjects screened for all 3 studies, 641 had NP and complete FVC data. NP was defined as nocturnal urine volume, including first morning void, exceeding 33% of 24 h urine production. At 3 weeks, 33% of men and 46% of women in the treatment arms demonstrated a reduction in mean number of nocturia episodes by >50% [47–50].

Patients in the treatment arm of the above studies were enrolled in a long-term open-label trial. Eighty-eight percent of original subjects participated. They were followed for 10 or 12 months. The men had an initial baseline mean of 3.1 voids per night, and the baseline among the women was 2.9. In subjects receiving treatment for 10 months, the nocturnal voids were reduced to 1.6 in men and 1.3 in women. In the 12 month group, nocturia was reduced to 1.3 in men and 1.2 in women. The percentage of patients experiencing >50% reduction in nighttime voids was 67% in both men and women by the end of the study [51]. Desmopressin nasal spray (Noctiva®) was approved for use in nocturia by the FDA in March 2018. The nasal spray formulation was studied in two randomized placebo controlled trials. A combined analysis of the two studies examined data from a total of 1333 men and women who were randomized to receive intranasal desmopressin at 1.66 mcg, 0.83 mcg, or placebo for 12 weeks. At the end of this period, mean number of voids per night decreased by 1.4 episodes with 0.83 mcg ($p < 0.0001$) and 1.5 with 1.66 mcg ($p < 0.0001$) compared to a decrease of 1.2 episodes with placebo. Hyponatremia, defined as serum sodium <125 mmol/L or <130 mmol/L with symptoms, was 1.1%, 0%, and 0.2% in the 1.66 mcg, 0.83 mcg, and placebo groups, respectively [52]. The FDA-approved Noctiva is for patients younger than 65 years of age who are not at increased risk for hyponatremia. It is recommended to start at 1 spray of Noctiva 0.83 mcg approximately 30 min before bed. The dose can be titrated up to 1.66 mcg at bedtime after 7 days with serum sodium monitoring.

Desmopressin promotes retention of free water to reduce urine production. This thereby risks hyponatremia in patients who take in excess water during circulation of active drug [42]. The US and Canada study found this risk was significantly higher in patients >65 years of age. In patients <65, serum sodium levels of less than 134 mmol/L were detected in 15%, 22%, and 24% in the 25 μg, 50 μg, and 100 μg groups. This is compared to the higher rates of 28%, 46%, and 51% for subjects >65. In patients <65 years, serum sodium <125 mmol/L was seen in 2.4% and 0 subjects receiving 50 μg and 100 μg, respectively. In patients >65 years, rates of 2.6% and 4.7% were seen. Serum sodium of <125 mmol/L were not seen in any patients receiving 10 μg or 25 μg [42]. The Noctupus study found similar results and the authors recommended against desmopressin tablet administration to patients >65. Other factors associated with hyponatremia were higher 24 h urine volumes, low baseline serum sodium levels, lower creatinine clearance, female gender, and smaller body size [42, 43]. Adverse events reported as related to treatment with desmopressin have included symptoms of dizziness, cardiac failure, headache, vomiting, chest pain, hypertension, vertigo, and nausea [53]. Patients receiving desmopressin should have normal baseline serum sodium and have their sodium checked at 1 week, 1 month, and 3 months after initiation or dose increment. Subsequent sodium testing should be done on an individualized basis.

Conclusion

Nocturia is a common and bothersome complaint; the underlying causes are myriad and diverse. A systematic approach must be used to identify underlying medical conditions. Nocturia should be classified with a FVC. In the absence of NP, medications for BPH or OAB may be employed. NP is highly prevalent among patients with nocturia; antidiuretic therapy should be considered when measures to address serious underlying etiologic conditions are ineffective. Hyponatremia is a concern with desmopressin, and patients >65 years are at greatest risk.

References

1. Van Kerrebroeck P, Abrams P, Chaikin D, Donovan J, Fonda D, Jackson S, et al. Standardisation Sub-committee of the International Continence Society. The standardisation of terminology in nocturia: report from the Standardisation Sub-committee of the International Continence Society. Neurourol Urodyn. 2002;21(2):179–83.
2. Fitzgerald MP, Litman HJ, Link CL, McKinlay JB, Survey Investigators BACH. The association of nocturia with cardiac disease, diabetes, body mass index, age and diuretic use: results from the BACH survey. J Urol. 2007;177(4):1385–9.
3. Bosch JL, Weiss JP. The prevalence and causes of nocturia. J Urol. 2010;184(2):440–6. Review.
4. Tikkinen KA, Auvinen A, Johnson TM, Weiss JP, Keränen T, Tiitinen A, et al. A systematic evaluation of factors associated with nocturia—the population-based FINNO study. Am J Epidemiol. 2009;170(3):361–8.
5. Kirkland JL, Lye M, Levy DW, Banerjee AK. Patterns of urine flow and electrolyte excretion in healthy elderly people. Br Med J. 1983;287(6406):1665–7.
6. Hofmeester I, Kollen BJ, Steffens MG, Bosch JL, Drake MJ, Weiss JP, et al. Impact of the International Continence Society (ICS) report on the standardisation of terminology in nocturia on the quality of reports on nocturia and nocturnal polyuria: a systematic review. BJU Int. 2015;115(4):520–36.
7. Blanker MH, Bohnen AM, Groeneveld FP, Bernsen RM, Prins A, Ruud Bosch JL. Normal voiding patterns and determinants of increased diurnal and nocturnal voiding frequency in elderly men. J Urol. 2000;164(4):1201–5.
8. Weiss JP. Prevalence of nocturnal polyuria in nocturia. J Urol. 2009;181((4):538.
9. Asplund R, Aberg H. Diurnal variation in the levels of antidiuretic hormone in the elderly. J Intern Med. 1991;229(2):131–4.
10. Yalkut D, Lee LY, Grider J, Jorgensen M, Jackson B, Ott C. Mechanism of atrial natriuretic peptide release with increased inspiratory resistance. J Lab Clin Med. 1996;128(3):322–8.
11. Abrams P, Andersson KE. Muscarinic receptor antagonists for overactive bladder. BJU Int. 2007;100(5):987–1006.
12. Andersson KE, Wein AJ. Pharmacologic management of lower urinary tract storage and emptying failure. In: Wein AJ, Kavoussi LR, Partin AW, Peters CA, editors. Campbell-Walsh urology. 11th ed. Philadelphia: Elsevier; 2016. p. 1836–74.
13. Guay DR. Clinical pharmacokinetics of drugs used to treat urge incontinence. Clin Pharmacokinet. 2003;42(14):1243.
14. Dmochowski R, Wein AJ. Lower urinary tract pharmacotherapy for nocturia. In: Weiss JP, Blaivas JG, Van Kerrebroeck P, Wein AJ, editors. Nocturia: causes, consequences and clinical approaches. New York: Springer Science+Business Media; 2012. p. 127–34.
15. Brubaker L, Fitzgerald MP. Nocturnal polyuria and nocturia relief in patients treated with solifenacin for overactive bladder symptoms. Int Urogynecol J Pelvic Floor Dysfunct. 2007;18(7):737–41.
16. Buser N, Ivic S, Kessler TM, Kessels AG, Bachmann LM. Efficacy and adverse events of antimuscarinics for treating overactive bladder: Network meta-analysis. Eur Urol. 2012;62(6):1040–60.
17. Toglia MR, Ostergard DR, Appell RA, Andoh M, Fakhoury A, Hussain IF. Solifenacin for overactive bladder: secondary analysis of data from VENUS based on baseline continence status. Int Urogynecol J. 2010;21(7):847–54.

18. Yokoyama O, Yamaguchi O, Kakizaki H, Itoh N, Yokota T, Ishizuka O, et al. Efficacy of solifenacin on nocturia in Japanese patients with overactive bladder: impact on sleep evaluated by bladder diary. J Urol. 2011;86(1):170–4.
19. Nitti VW, Dmochowski R, Sand PK, Forst HT, Haag-Molkenteller C, Massow U, et al. J Urol. 2007;178(6):2488–94.
20. Herschorn S, Swift S, Guan Z, Carlsson M, Morrow JD, Brodsky M, Gong J. BJU Int. 2010;105(1):58–66.
21. Chapple C, Van Kerrebroeck P, Tubaro A, Haag-Molkenteller C, Frost HT, Massow U, et al. Clinical efficacy, safety, and tolerability of once-daily fesoterodine in subjects with overactive bladder. Eur Urol. 2007;52(4):1204–12.
22. Dmochowski RR, Peters KM, Morrow JD, Guan Z, Gong J, Siami P, Staskin DR. Randomized, double-blind, placebo-controlled trial of flexible-dose fesoterodine in subjects with overactive bladder. Urology. 2010;75(1):62–8.
23. Rackley R, Weiss JP, Rovner ES, Wang JT, Guan Z. Nighttime dosing with tolterodine reduces overactive bladder-related nocturnal micturitions in patients with overactive bladder and nocturia. Urology. 2006;67(4):731–6.
24. Zinner N, Gittelmen M, Harris R, Susset J, Kanelos A, Auerbach S, Trospium Study Group. Trospium chloride improves overactive bladder symptoms: a multicenter phase II trial. J Urol. 2004;171(6 Pt 1):2311–5.
25. Rudy D, Cline K, Harris R, Goldberg K, Dmochowski R. Multicenter phase III trial studying trospium chloride in patients with overactive bladder. Urology. 2006;67(2):275–80.
26. Tikkinen KA, Johnson TM, Tammela TL, Sintonen H, Haukka J, Huhtala H, Auvinen A. Nocturia frequency, bother, and quality of life: how often is too often? A population-based study in Finland. Eur Urol. 2010;57(3):488–96.
27. Bylund DB. Subtypes of alpha 1- and alpha 2-adrenergic receptors. FASEB J. 1992;6(3):832–9.
28. Yoshimura K, Ohara H, Ichioka K, Terada N, Matsui Y, Terai A, Arai Y. Nocturia and benign prostatic hyperplasia. Urology. 2003;61(4):786–90.
29. Djavan B, Milani S, Davies J, Bolodeoku J. The impact of tamsulosin oral controlled absorption system (OCAS) on nocturia and the quality of sleep: preliminary results of a pilot study. Eur Urol Suppl. 2005;4(2):61–8.
30. Speakman M. Efficacy and safety of tamsulosin OCAS. BJU Int. 2006;98(Suppl 2):13–7.
31. Bliwise DL, Holm-Larsen T, Goble S, Norgaard JP. Short time to first void is associated with lower whole-night sleep quality in nocturia patients. J Clin Sleep Med. 2015;11(1):53–5.
32. Johnson TM, Jones K, Williford WO, Kutner MH, Issa MM, Lepor H. Changes in nocturia from medical treatment of benign prostatic hyperplasia: secondary analysis of the Department of Veterans Affairs Cooperative Study Trial. J Urol. 2003;170(1):145–8.
33. Johnson TM, Burrows PK, Kusek JW, Nyberg LM, Tenover JL, Lepor H, et al. The effect of doxazosin, finasteride and combination therapy on nocturia in men with benign prostatic hyperplasia. J Urol. 2007;178(5):2045–51.
34. Roehrborn CG, Van Kerrebroeck P, Nordling J. Safety and efficacy of alfuzosin 10 mg once-daily in the treatment of lower urinary tract symptoms and clinical benign prostatic hyperplasia: a pooled analysis of three double-blind, placebo-controlled studies. BJU Int. 2003;92(3):257–61.
35. Chapple CR, Montorsi F, Tammela TL, Wirth M, Koldewijn E, Fernandez Fernandez E, European Silodosin Study Group. Silodosin therapy for lower urinary tract symptoms in men with suspected benign prostatic hyperplasia: results of an international, randomized, double-blind, placebo- and active-controlled clinical trial performed in Europe. Eur Urol. 2011;59(3):342–52.
36. Hicks A, McCafferty GP, Riedel E, Aiyar N, Pullen M, Evans C, et al. GW427353 (solabegron), a novel, selective beta3-adrenergic receptor agonist, evokes bladder relaxation and increases micturition reflex threshold in the dog. J Pharmacol Exp Ther. 2007;323(1):202–9.
37. Nitti VW, Auerbach S, Martin N, Calhoun A, Lee M, Herschorn S. Results of a randomized phase III trial of mirabegron in patients with overactive bladder. J Urol. 2013;189(4):1388–95.

38. Montecucco C, Molgó J. Botulinal neurotoxins: revival of an old killer. Curr Opin Pharmacol. 2005;5(3):274–9.
39. Nitti VW, Dmochowski R, Herschorn S, Sand P, Thompson C, Nardo C, et al. OnabotulinumtoxinA for the treatment of patients with overactive bladder and urinary incontinence: results of a phase 3, randomized, placebo controlled trial. J Urol. 2013;189(6):2186–93.
40. Chapple C, Sievert KD, MacDiarmid S, Khullar V, Radziszewaki P, Nardo C, et al. OnabotulinumtoxinA 100 U significantly improves all idiopathic overactive bladder symptoms and quality of life in patients with overactive bladder and urinary incontinence: a randomised, double-blind, placebo-controlled trial. Eur Urol. 2013;64(2):249–56.
41. Hammer M, Vilhardt H. Peroral treatment of diabetes insipidus with a polypeptide hormone analogue, desmopressin. J Pharmacol Exp Ther. 1985;234(3):754–60.
42. Vilhardt H. Basic pharmacology of desmopressin. Drug Invest. 1990;2(Suppl 5):2.
43. Sands JM. Molecular mechanisms of urea transport. J Membr Biol. 2003;191(3):149–63.
44. Abrams P, Andersson KE, Birder L, Brubaker L, Cardozo L, Chapple C, et al. Fourth International Consultation on Incontinence Recommendations of the International Scientific Committee: Evaluation and treatment of urinary incontinence, pelvic organ prolapse, and fecal incontinence. Neurourol Urodyn. 2010;29(1):213–40.
45. Sakalis VI, Karavitakis M, Bedretdinova D, Bach T, Bosch JLHR, Gacci M, et al. Medical treatment of nocturia in men with lower urinary tract symptoms: systematic review by the European Association of Urology Guidelines Panel for Male Lower Urinary Tract Symptoms. Eur Urol. 2017;72(5):757–69.
46. Weiss JP, Zinner NR, Klein BM, Norgaard JP. Desmopressin orally disintegrating tablet effectively reduces nocturia: results of a randomized, double-blind, placebo-controlled trial. Neurourol Urodyn. 2012;31(4):441–7.
47. Van Kerrebroeck P. Nocturia and antidiuretic therapy. In: Weiss JP, Blaivas JG, Van Kerrebroeck P, Wein AJ, editors. Nocturia: causes, consequences and clinical approaches. New York: Springer Science+Business Media; 2012. p. 135–44.
48. Mattiasson A, Abrams P, Van Kerrebroeck P, Walter S, Weiss J. Efficacy of desmopressin in the treatment of nocturia: A double-blind placebo-controlled study in men. BJU Int. 2002;89(9):855–62.
49. Lose G, Lalos O, Freeman RM, Van Kerrebroeck P, Nocturia Study Group. Efficacy of desmopressin (Minirin) in the treatment of nocturia: A double-blind placebo-controlled study in women. Am J Obstet Gynecol. 2003;189(4):1106–13.
50. Van Kerrebroeck P, Rezapour M, Cortesse A, Thuroff J, Riis A, Norgaard JP. Desmopressin in the treatment of nocturia: A double-blind, placebo-controlled study. Eur Urol. 2007;52(1):221–9.
51. Lose G, Mattiasson A, Walter S, Lalos O, Van Kerrebroeck P, Abrams P, Freeman R. Clinical experiences with desmopressin for long-term treatment of nocturia. J Urol. 2004;172(3):1021–5.
52. Kaminetsky J, Fein S, Dmochowski R, MacDiarmid S, Abrams S, Cheng M, Wein A. Efficacy and safety of SER120 nasal spray in nocturia patients pooled analysis of 2 randomized, double-blind, placebo-controlled phase 3 trials. J Urol. 2018; https://doi.org/10.1016/j.juro.2018.04.050. Article in Press.
53. Friedman FM, Weiss JP. Desmopressin in the treatment of nocturia: clinical evidence and experience. Ther Adv Urol. 2013;5(6):310–7.

Chapter 11
Intravesical Chemodenervation and Toxins

Melissa T. Sanford and David A. Ginsberg

Abbreviations

ACh	Acetylcholine
AUA	American Urological Association
BDNF	Brain-derived neurotrophic factor
BoNT	Botulinum neurotoxin
BoNT-A	Botulinum neurotoxin type A
BoNT-B	Botulinum neurotoxin type B
CIC	Clean intermittent catheterization
DO	Detrusor overactivity
DRG	Dorsal root ganglia
MCC	Maximum cystometric capacity
MDP	Maximal detrusor voiding pressure
NDO	Neurogenic detrusor overactivity
NGF	Nerve growth factor
OAB	Overactive bladder
PVR	Post-voiding residual volume
QoL	Quality of life
RCT	Randomized controlled trial
RTX	Resiniferatoxin
SNAP-25	Synaptosomal-associated protein 25
SNARE	Soluble N-ethylmaleimide-sensitive fusion attachment protein receptor

M. T. Sanford
Department of Urology, University of Southern California, Los Angeles, CA, USA

D. A. Ginsberg (✉)
University of Southern California, Department of Urology, Los Angeles, CA, USA
e-mail: Ginsberg@med.usc.edu

L. Cox, E. S. Rovner (eds.), *Contemporary Pharmacotherapy of Overactive Bladder*, https://doi.org/10.1007/978-3-319-97265-7_11

TRPV1	Transient receptor potential vanilloid 1
U	Unit/units
UTI	Urinary tract infection
UUI	Urgency urinary incontinence

Introduction

Initial treatment options for OAB include behavioral modification and oral therapies (antimuscarinics and/or β3-agonist). Patients that continue to be symptomatic despite oral pharmacologic management, or who are unable to tolerate drug side effects, may benefit from further treatment with intravesical therapy. In contrast to oral therapies, intravesical therapy offers the ability to administer high concentrations of agents directly into bladder tissue and also utilize agents that may be inappropriate for systemic administration. There are currently two main types of injectable intravesical agents: botulinum neurotoxin (BoNT) and vanilloid compounds. Chemodenervation with BoNT is recommended as a third-line option for the treatment of OAB in refractory patients [1]. Intravesical injection of vanilloid compounds (capsaicin and resiniferatoxin [RTX]) is also an option for treatment but less readily utilized due to their lack of FDA approval for this indication and documented efficacy and safety. The aim of this chapter is to describe the clinical applications of these intravesical agents for OAB and discuss their mechanism of actions, outcomes, and safety.

Botulinum Toxin

Mechanism of Action

BoNT is a neurotoxin formed by the gram-positive, anaerobic spore-forming bacteria *Clostridium botulinum* and is responsible for human botulism. Molecularly, it is a polypeptide consisting of a heavy and light chain joined by a disulfide bond. Eight exotoxin serotypes have been described (A, B, C1, C2, D, E, F, G) with varying amino acid sequences [2]. Initially BoNT was only thought to work on efferent pathways by blocking the release of the neurotransmitter acetylcholine (ACh) at the neuromuscular junction, ultimately resulting in muscle paralysis; however, additional research in both urology and other subspecialties has found that the mechanism of action is more complex with involvement of afferent pathways as well [3].

In the classic efferent pathway, the BoNT heavy chain binds to synaptic vesicle protein 2 (SV2) on the presynaptic cholinergic neuron [4]. In humans SV2 isoforms can be found on a variety of nerves (parasympathetic, sympathetic, and sensory) throughout all layers of the bladder, with OAB patients demonstrating overexpression of these receptors in the detrusor [3, 5, 6]. After binding to the external surface of the nerve, the toxin is internalized by endocytosis, and the disulfide bond breaks. The free light chain then cleaves its molecular target, synaptosomal-associated protein 25 (SNAP-25). Normally SNAP-25 interacts with synaptobrevin and syntaxin to form the SNARE (soluble N-ethylmaleimide-sensitive fusion attachment protein receptor) complex, which is necessary for vesicular release of neurotransmitter at the nerve terminal. By cleaving SNAP-25, BoNT deactivates the SNARE complex and prevents release of neurotransmitters (including ACh) into the neuromuscular junction, thus preventing muscle contraction [3]. SNAP-25, or similar isoforms, has been located throughout the detrusor, suburothelium, and urothelium in both animal and human studies [3, 5]. While some studies have demonstrated the presence of cleaved SNAP-25 products after injection of BoNT, the finding of these proteins does not necessarily correlate with efficacy suggesting that other factors beyond modulation of the efferent pathway contribute to patient results [7, 8].

BoNT has additionally been shown to have afferent desensitization effects both at the level of the bladder and centrally. Intravesical administration of BoNT inhibits ATP release, which conveys information about filling and irritation via purinergic receptors; reduces suburothelial transient receptor potential vanilloid 1 (TRPV1), which is involved in mechanical sensation and pain; and reduces purinergic receptor subtype P2X3, which correlates with urgency [5, 9]. BoNT effects also extend centrally. After intravesical administration, BoNT can be directly isolated from the dorsal root ganglia (DRG) suggesting retrograde transport to the central nervous system. Intravesical BoNT is associated with downregulation of TRPV1 and P2X3 from the DRG via bladder nerve growth factor (NGF) and reductions in neuropeptides and neurotransmitters (such as substance P, calcitonin gene-related peptide, and nNOS) in bladder-projecting neurons in the DRG. Extending even more centrally, intravesical Botox has been associated with reductions in c-fos expressing cell counts in L6-S1 spinal cord segments and reduction in brain-derived neurotrophic factor (BDNF) [3, 10].

The toxin requires 24–72 h to take initial effect with 90% of parasympathetic and 50% of sympathetic fibers being affected at 1 week. While prior studies have found that function returns by formation of new nerve terminals in skeletal muscle, this does not appear to be the case in the bladder. It is unclear how the effect of BoNT dissipates, as the duration of effect is significantly shorter in movement disorders compared to autonomic dysfunction [2, 3, 11, 12].

Commercial Formulations and Dosing Considerations

Of the eight BoNT serotypes available, only types A (BoNT-A) and B (BoNT-B) have been used clinically. There are three commercially available formulations of BoNT-A: onabotulinumtoxinA (Botox®, Allergan, Irvine, CA, USA), abobotulinumtoxinA (Dysport®, Ipsen Limited, Paris, France), and incobotulinumtoxinA (Xeomin®, Merz Pharmaceuticals, Frankfurt, Germany). Only onaBoNT-A has been extensively studied and has FDA approval to treat OAB [13]. The dose, efficacy, and safety profiles across the three different compounds are not the same, and formal comparator studies between the different formulations have not been done. In general incoBoNT-A has a conversion of 1:1 with onaBoNT-A in other medical specialties, but there is only one study demonstrating its use in the bladder in the neurogenic detrusor overactivity (NDO) population [14, 15]. A conversion rate of 1:2 or 1:3 is recommended for onaBoNT-A to aboBoNT-A. While the efficacy between aboBoNT-A and onaBoNT-A is similar, aboBoNT-A is associated with almost double the rate of symptomatic retention requiring initiation of clean intermittent catheterization (CIC) (23% onaBoNT-A vs. 42% aboBoNT-A) [16, 17]. Of note, aboBoNT-A has been used for onaBoNT-A failure in NDO prior to proceeding with more invasive surgical measures, and this could be extrapolated for use in the OAB population. At this point it is unclear why aboBoNT-A may be efficacious in the face of onaBoNT-A failure, but proposed mechanisms include differences in diffusion patterns, immunogenicity, or dose equivalences [18]. For completeness sake, a conversion rate of 4:1 is recommended for aboBoNT-A to incoBoNT-A; however, this study was not performed in urologic patients [19].

There is one commercially available formulation of BoNT-B: rimabotulinumtoxinB (Neurobloc/Myobloc®, Solstice Neurosciences Inc., San Francisco, CA, USA) (Table 11.1). The literature on BoNT-B in the bladder is limited with most studies focusing on its use for bladder dysfunction refractory to BoNT-A [20, 21]. Only one small, randomized controlled trial (RCT) has been performed that demonstrated significant differences in voided volumes, weekly frequency, and weekly incontinence compared to placebo [22]. There are no studies directly comparing BoNT-A to BoNT-B in urology, but in other medical specialties, BoNT-B has shorter onset of effect, shorter duration of effect, and more immunogenicity and causes more pain than BoNT-A, making it a potentially less desirable drug [12, 16, 22] (see Table 11.1).

Table 11.1 Commercial formulations and dosing considerations

Trade name	Drug name	Serotype	Manufacturer	Vial dose (units)	Proposed conversion to onabotulinumtoxinA
Botox®	OnabotulinumtoxinA	A	Allergan	50 100 200	–
Dysport®	AbobotulinumtoxinA	A	Ipsen	300 500	1:2–1:3
Xeomin®	IncobotulinumtoxinA	A	Merz	50 100	1:1
Myobloc®	RimabotulinumtoxinB	B	Solstice	2500 5000 10,000	NA

Treatment for Overactive Bladder

Indications

The use of BoNT injection in the lower urinary tract was first studied by Dykstra et al. in 1988 for the treatment of detrusor external sphincter dyssynergia (DESD) in spinal cord injury (SCI) patients [23]. Following this, the number of investigations regarding urologic applications of BoNT increased dramatically. BoNT was utilized off-label in the bladder for many years prior to its FDA approval for NDO in 2011 and OAB in 2013. Given that onaBoNT-A is the only approved formulation of BoNT for intravesical use, the remainder of this chapter will focus on its outcomes and administration unless otherwise specified.

The American Urogynecologic Society and American College of Obstetricians and Gynecologists guidelines recommend BoNT-A as an alternative to oral pharmacotherapy for second-line therapy in patients refractory to behavioral management on the basis of the Anticholinergic versus OnabotulinumtoxinA Comparison (ABC) study [24, 25]. Conversely, the American Urological Association (AUA) and European Association of Urology (EAU) guidelines recommend intravesical BoNT-A as a third-line option to treat OAB in patients refractory to behavioral management and oral pharmacotherapy. Alternative third-line therapies include sacral neuromodulation or percutaneous tibial nerve stimulation. Third-line therapies can be offered to patients in any order, and patients who fail to respond to one third-line therapy may be offered alternative third-line therapies prior to proceeding with more invasive treatment [1, 26].

Outcomes

After several trials in the early 2000s demonstrated the effectiveness of onaBoNT-A in the NDO population, researchers began extrapolating these findings to the OAB population. Initial prospective cohort studies reported promising findings in regard to patient symptoms, urodynamic findings, and quality of life measures [27, 28].

Early, small randomized controlled trials (RCT) in the OAB population compared intradetrusor trigone-sparing injections of either 200 U or 300 U onaBoNT-A to placebo and also found statistically significant differences from baseline in frequency (−1.3 to −6.19 vs. −0.8 to −1.14), urgency incontinence (−3.50 to −4.5 vs. +0.7 to −0.71), urodynamic findings (maximum cystometric capacity (MCC) 82.06 vs. −29.89), symptom scores (Urinary Distress Index-6 (UDI-6) −5.63 to −18.6 vs. +0.5 to +3.1), and quality of life measures (Incontinence Impact Questionnaire-7 (IIQ-7) −10.38 to −39.5 vs. 0 to +0.61). Unfortunately these studies also found concerning enough rates of urinary tract infection (UTI) (13–44% vs. 0–28%) and the need for clean intermittent catheterization (CIC) (6.7–43% vs. 0%) in the onaBoNT-A arms that one of these trials was put on a clinical hold after only 4 weeks [29–31] (Table 11.2 [29–41]).

Table 11.2 Results of onaBoNT-A randomized controlled trials

Study	Groups (n)	Data time point	Injection site	Frequency	Urgency	Urgency incontinence	Symptom score	Patient-reported measure	Urodynamic findings	Ach medication	Post-void residual (mL)	%CIC	%UTI
Sahai (2007) [29]		12 weeks	Detrusor, trigone sparing	Δ/*d* from baseline	Δ/*d* from baseline	Δ/*d* from baseline	Δ UDI-6 from baseline	Δ IIQ-7 from baseline	Δ MCC from baseline	% Stopped using ACh	Δ from baseline at 1 month		
	200U (16)			−6.19[a]	−8.19	−3.50[a]	−5.63[a]	−10.38[a]	+82.06[a]	83%	+52.06[a]	37.5%	43.7%
	Placebo (18)			−1.14	−0.92	−0.71	+0.50	+0.61	−29.89	0%	+8.89	0%	0%
Brubaker (2008) (RUBI trial) [30]		4 weeks, stopped due to clinical hold for high CIC and UTI rates	Detrusor, trigone sparing			>75% reduction from baseline	Δ UDI-urge subscale from baseline	Δ PGI-I score from baseline		No patients taking ACh medications			
	200U (28)					72%	31[a]	2.7[a]				43%	44%
	Placebo (15)					0% reduction	52	4.0				0%	22%
Flynn (2009) [31]		6 weeks	Detrusor, trigone sparing	Δ/*d* from baseline		Δ/*d* from baseline	Δ UDI-6 from baseline	Δ IIQ-7 from baseline	Δ MCC from baseline	No patients taking ACh medications	Δ from baseline		
	200U or 300U (15)			−1.3		−4.5[a]	−18.6[a]	−39.5[a]	No difference between groups		+82	6.7%	13%
	Placebo (7)			−0.8		+0.7	+3.1	0			−3		28%

Cohen (2009) [32]		12 weeks	Detrusor, trigone sparing	Δ/*d* from baseline in OAB dry		Δ/*d* from baseline in OAB wet		Δ VAS from baseline	Δ MCC from baseline	No patients taking ACh medications	Δ from baseline at 1 month		
	100U (Dry 10, Wet 12)			−6.1 ([a]from baseline, NS between groups)		−6 ([a]from baseline, NS between groups)		−5.6 ([a]from baseline, NS between groups)	NS between groups		+37 ([a]from baseline, NS between groups)	4.5%	16% both groups
	150U (Dry 10, Wet 12)			−13.6 ([a]from baseline, NS between groups)		−6.5 ([a]from baseline, NS between groups)		−5.8 ([a]from baseline, NS between groups)				4.5%	
Dmochowski (2010) [33]/ Rovner (2011) [34] (Phase II dose-finding trial)		12 weeks	Detrusor, trigone sparing	Δ/*d* from baseline in DO/no DO		Δ/*d* from baseline			Δ MCC from baseline	No patients taking ACh medications	Δ from baseline		
	50U (57)			−18.6/−3.6		−20.7			+50.0		27.6	3.6%	33.9%
	100U (54)			−21.4/−23.4		−18.4			+71.0		49.3	9.1%	36.4%
	150U (49)			−10.1/−39.8		−23.0			+101.7		74.7	12.7%	44.0%
	200U (53)			−18.9/−22.9		−19.6			+91.5		107.6	18.2%	48.1%
	300U (56)			−20.1/−22.8		−19.4			+130.8		62.5	16.4%	34.5%
	Placebo (44)			−11.3/+5.4		−17.4			+49.5		1	0%	16.3%

(continued)

Table 11.2 (continued)

Study	Groups (n)	Data time point	Injection site	Frequency	Urgency	Urgency incontinence	Symptom score	Patient-reported measure	Urodynamic findings	Ach medication	Post-void residual (mL)	%CIC	%UTI
Dowson (2011) [35]		12 weeks	Detrusor, trigone sparing	Δ/*d* from baseline	Δ/*d* from baseline	Δ/*d* from baseline	Δ UDI-6 from baseline	Δ IIQ-7 from baseline	Δ MCC from baseline	No patients taking ACh medications	Δ from baseline		
	100U (10)			−0.7	+0.1	−0.1	−1.8	−5	106[a]		57	30%	40%
	Placebo (11)			0	+1	+0.9	+0.3	+2.3	0		7	0%	9.1%
Altaweel (2011) [36]		12 weeks	Detrusor, trigone sparing	Δ/*d* from baseline	Δ/*d* from baseline	Δ/*d* from baseline	Δ UDI-6 from baseline	Δ IIQ-7 from baseline	Δ MCC from baseline	No patients taking ACh medications	Δ from baseline		
	100U (11)			−7.8 ([a]from baseline, NS between groups)	−7.3 ([a]from baseline, NS between groups)	−0.5 ([a]from baseline, NS between groups)	Approx −30 ([a]from baseline, NS between groups)	Approx −30 ([a]from baseline, NS between groups)	+71 ([a]from baseline, NS between groups)		29	9.1%	9.1%
	200U (11)			−7.3 ([a]from baseline, NS between groups)	−6.4 ([a]from baseline, NS between groups)	+0.1 ([a]from baseline, NS between groups)	Approx −30 ([a]from baseline, NS between groups)	Approx −30 ([a]from baseline, NS between groups)	+132 ([a]from baseline, NS between groups)		50	18.2%	9.1%

Denys (2012) [37] (Phase II dose-finding trial)		12 weeks	Detrusor, trigone sparing			% Complete continence		>75% reduction in symptoms	Δ MCC from baseline	ACh medications continued, eight patients restarted during the study			
	50U (21)					15.8%		6%	38.4			9.5%	5.6%
	100U (22)					55.0%[a]		42%[a]	85.5			4.5%	4.8%
	150U (27)					50.0%[a]		42%[a]	91.3[a]			11.1%	9.1%
	Placebo (29)					10.7%		22%	22.9			0%	0%
Tincello (2012) [38] (RELAX study)		12 weeks	Detrusor, trigone sparing	Δ/*d* from baseline	Δ/*d* from baseline	Δ/*d* from baseline	Δ IUSS from baseline	Δ IQOL from baseline		Additional medication use at 6 months		At 6 months	At 6 months
	200U (122)			−2.3	−5	−5.2	−0.8	+40.37		14%		16%	31%
	Placebo (118)			−1.03	−0.7	−0.87	−0.2	+1.7		32%		4%	11%
Nitti (2013) [39] (EMBARK study)		12 weeks	Detrusor, trigone sparing	Δ/*d* from baseline	Δ/*d* from baseline	Δ/*d* from baseline	Positive response on TBS	Δ IQOL from baseline		No patients taking ACh medications	Δ from baseline at 2 weeks		
	100U (280)			−2.15[a]	−2.93[a]	−2.65[a]	60.8%[a]	+21.9			+49.5	5.4%	15.5%
	Placebo (277)			−0.91	−1.21	−0.87	29.2%	+6.8			+1.1	0.4%	5.9%

(continued)

Table 11.2 (continued)

Study	Groups (n)	Data time point	Injection site	Frequency	Urgency	Urgency incontinence	Symptom score	Patient-reported measure	Urodynamic findings	Ach medication	Post-void residual (mL)	%CIC	%UTI
Chapple (2013) [40] (Phase III)		12 weeks	Detrusor, trigone sparing	Δ/*d* from baseline	Δ/*d* from baseline	Δ/*d* from baseline	Positive response on TBS	Δ IQOL from baseline		No patients taking ACh medications			
	100U (277)			−2.56[a]	−3.67[a]	−2.80[a]	62.8%	+23.1[a]				6.9%	20.4%
	Placebo (271)			−0.83	−1.24	−0.82	26.8%	+6.3				0.7%	5.2%
Jabs (2013) [41]		24 weeks	Detrusor, trigone sparing	Δ/*d* from baseline		Δ/*d* from baseline	Δ UDI-6 from baseline	Δ IIQ-7 from baseline	Δ MCC from baseline				
	100U (11)			−2.7[a]		−4.1	−28.5	−34.7	64.1[a]	Five patients continued		0%	54.5%
	Placebo (10)			+0.5		+0.4	−11.1	−3.8	−97.5	Seven patients continued		0%	40%

U units, Δ change, *d* day, *UDI* urinary distress inventory scale, *IIQ* incontinence impact questionnaire, *IQOL* incontinence quality of life, *TBS* treatment benefit scale, *IUSS* Indevus Urgency Severity Score, *Ach* anticholinergic, *CIC* clean intermittent catheterization, *UTI* urinary tract infection

[a]Statistically significant ($p < 0.05$)

Given the adverse effect rates, the next wave of RCTs focused on dose finding. Two studies compared active doses of either 100 U vs. 150 U or 100 U vs. 200 U and again found significant differences in symptoms, patient-reported outcomes, and urodynamic findings when compared to baseline but no significant differences between groups, suggesting equivalent efficacy. One of these studies reported double the rate of CIC with a higher dose of 200 U, but rates of UTI were similar across all groups [32, 36]. Two larger Phase II dose-finding studies compared various doses of onaBoNT-A ranging from 50 U to 300 U to placebo and found a clear dose-response pattern with minimal additional clinical benefit at doses greater than 150 U, sustained clinical efficacy, improved urodynamic findings, and improved patient-reported symptoms beginning at a dose of 100 U. Post-void residual was also found to have a dose-dependent response with the highest rate and longest duration of CIC in the 200 U group [33, 34, 37].

As 100 U appeared to be the optimal dose that allowed for adequate efficacy while minimizing adverse outcomes, the last wave of RCTs focused on 100 U vs. placebo. Compared to placebo, these trials found statistically significant differences from baseline in frequency (−2.15 to −2.7 vs. +0.5 to −0.91), urinary incontinence (−2.65 to −4.1 vs. +0.4 to −0.87), urodynamic findings (MCC +64.1 mL vs. –97.5 mL), symptom scores (UDI-6 −28.5 vs. −11.1), and quality of life measures (IIQ-7 –34.7 vs. −3.8). While rates of UTI and CIC continued to be higher in treatment groups compared to placebo, they were less than in prior studies comparing 200 U to placebo (UTI, placebo 5.2–22%, 100 U 15.5–20.4%, 200 U 44%; CIC, placebo 0.4–0.7%, 100 U 5.4–6.9%, 200 U 37.5–43%) [29, 30, 39–41]. The large, Phase III, multicenter, randomized, placebo-controlled, double-blind trials by Nitti and Chapple are the basis for the FDA approval of 100 U onaBoNT-A for OAB.

A recent meta-analysis and systematic review of the literature included 11 trials consisting of 2149 patients for comparison and found that compared to placebo at 12 weeks, patients receiving 100 U onaBoNT-A injections had 0.56 less episodes of micturition, 1.26 less episodes of urgency, 0.8 less episodes of urinary incontinence, a relative risk of 11.49 of urinary retention (defined as PVR >200 mL), and a relative risk of 2.73 of UTI [42].

Long-Term Follow-Up

Although onaBoNT-A has been utilized for OAB for over 10 years, there is little published data on long-term outcomes with the majority of papers reporting follow-up between 1.1 and 3.2 years on a small numbers of patients (approximately 100 or less) receiving a range of onaBoNT-A doses (100–300 U) and a variety of repeat injections (2–10) [43].

The largest body of evidence comes from an extension of the Phase III trial that followed 829 patients for a median of 3.2 years with 52% of patients completing the 3.5-year trial [44]. Over the course of six injections, they found sustained improvements in clinical symptoms and patient-reported outcomes with mean reduction in frequency − 2.6 to −2.9, mean reduction in urgency −3.8 to −4.2, mean reduction in UI episodes per day −3.1 to −3.8, and high patient satisfaction ranging from 74% to 82.1% on a Treatment Benefit Scale (TBS). The rate of discontinuation due to lack of efficacy was 5.7%, which is low in comparison to anticholinergic trials where 13.5% of patients discontinued the drug due to persistent OAB symptoms [45]. The mean duration of effect was 7.6 months with 34.2% of patients requesting retreatment prior to 6 months, 37.2% of patients requesting retreatment from 6 to 12 months, and 28.5% of patients requesting retreatment after 12 months. The duration of effectiveness remained stable or increased over time. The rates of UTI and de novo CIC declined over the course of the injections from 17% to 14.4% and from 4% to 0.8%, respectively. Only 0.5% of patients discontinued therapy due to treatment-related adverse effects.

The longest published follow-up reported on 128 women with OAB who received 200 U onaBoNT-A was followed for at least 5 years with a mean follow-up of 8.1 years [46]. At the completion of the study, only 30% of patients were still using onaBoNT-A injections to manage their OAB symptoms. The vast majority of patients in the trial received only one injection (47%) prior to discontinuation, with 19% receiving two injections, 7% receiving three injections, 11% receiving four injections, 7% receiving five injections, and 9% receiving more than five injections. They found significantly higher discontinuation rates due to lack of efficacy (27% vs. 5.7%) or treatment-related adverse effects (43% vs. 0.5%) than the Phase III extension trial. Of note, the rates of de novo CIC were quite high, with 23% of patients performing CIC after the first injection, likely due to the higher onaBoNT-A dose and protocol requirement of CIC for any PVR >150 mL regardless of symptoms. This particular adverse effect likely contributed to the high discontinuation rate of 67% after the first injection.

Neutralizing Antibodies

One concern about repeated injections of onaBoNT-A is the development of neutralizing serum antibodies leading to treatment failure. Prior to 1998 a more antigenic version of onaBoNT-A was utilized which did result in a significant proportion of patients (9.5%) developing antibodies after undergoing treatment for cervical dystonia. The version of onaBoNT-A currently on the market has a lower protein load and is significantly less antigenic with no patients developing antibodies after injection [47]. When looking at the small amount of literature regarding serum antibodies after injection of the newer version of onaBoNT-A, positive titers developed in 6–16% of patients, and borderline-positive titers developed in 16–29% of patients. Of those with positive titers, 75–100% experience lack of efficacy, while 20–75% of those with borderline titers experienced lack of efficacy. There was no correlation with number of prior injections, total lifetime dose of onaBoNT-A injected, or interval since last injection [48, 49]. While the presence of neutralizing antibodies is one possible explanation for treatment failure, other factors must also be considered including errors in drug storage or preparation, improper injection technique, or disease evolution. If indeed formation of neutralizing antibodies seems to be the cause of treatment failure, one can consider a "drug holiday" for 6–12 months or switching to BoNT-B formulation [20, 21, 48].

Predictors of Success and Adverse Events

Several studies have attempted to determine predictors of success and adverse events for onaBoNT-A treatment (Table 11.3). On multivariate linear regression, female gender (coefficient (CE) 0.76) and presence of urgency incontinence (CE 0.79) were significantly associated with "successful onaBoNT-A treatment," which was defined as a moderately positive response on the Global Response Assessment (Hsiao 2016). Secondary analyses of the ROSETTA trial data found that women with lower baseline BMI, higher health-related QoL survey scores, and lower functional comorbidity index had greater reduction in mean daily incontinence episodes and that women less than 65 years old had a 3.3 greater odds of attaining greater than 75% reduction in incontinence episodes [50, 51]. At this point it is still unclear how the degree of OAB severity factors into success rates as both lower symptom scores and more baseline incontinence episodes have both been found to be predictors of success on multivariate analyses [50, 52]. In men, overall lower success rates (defined as continued onaBoNT-A therapy) have been reported compared to female-only populations (21% vs. 30%) with higher discontinuation rates due to lack of efficacy (44% vs. 27%). Men who suffered from post-prostate cancer therapy (prostatectomy +/− radiation) had higher success rates (29%) compared to men with idiopathic OAB (21%) or

Table 11.3 Predictors of success and adverse outcomes

Predictors of success	
Female gender Urge incontinence Lower BMI Higher health-related QoL survey Lower functional comorbidity index	
Predictors of adverse outcomes	
Elevated PVR/urinary retention Male gender Older age (>61–76 years) Frailty Vaginal parity >3 Elevated baseline PVR (>100mL) Elevated preoperative bladder capacity (>400mL) Poor baseline voiding efficiency (<86%) Low daytime frequency (<25 voids in 3 days)	*Urinary tract infection* Female gender Younger age (<60 years) Elevated baseline PVR (>100mL)

BMI body mass index, *QoL* quality of life, *PVR* post-voiding residual volume post-transurethral resection of the prostate (11%) [53], whereas, compared to women with idiopathic OAB, women with prior midurethral sling placement and de novo OAB have similar success rates after injection of onaBoNT-A (42% idiopathic vs. 39% de novo dry at 3 months) [54]. While 1 small retrospective study of 85 subjects found that patients who failed anticholinergic therapy due to intolerability rather than lack of efficacy had more successful subsequent onaBoNT-A therapy (86%vs. 60%, $p = 0.02$), another pre-specified pooled analysis of the 2 Phase III RCTs comprised on 1105 patients found that efficacy of onaBoNT-A did not depend on the reason for prior anticholinergic failure. Both of these studies found that the total number of prior anticholinergics tried did not determine the rate of onaBoNT-A success [55, 56]. Finally, as with other therapeutic options for OAB, the baseline presence or absence of detrusor overactivity (DO) on urodynamic studies (UDS) does not affect onaBoNT-A efficacy, likely because not all patients with OAB demonstrate DO on UDS and because there is a considerable sensory aspect of OAB that does not necessarily correlate with motor response [34, 57]. Interestingly, while onaBoNT-A has been shown to reduce levels of CGRP and NGF, higher levels of these compounds at baseline are associated with less reduction in patient-reported bother [58].

Given the risk of retention with onaBoNT-A, a number of studies have sought to determine either patient-related factors or urodynamic factors which correlate with elevated PVR or need to perform CIC. One study has reported male gender as a predictor of urinary retention (14% vs. 2% $P = 0.001$) but not PVR >150 mL (49% vs. 45%, $p = 0.358$), while another found that in a heterogeneous population of men, the de novo CIC rate was only 5%, which is consistent with prior reported rates [53, 59]. Age has been found by multiple studies to be associated with increased PVR +/− urinary retention with increased risk associated over the ages of 61–75 depending on the study [59, 60]. However, another study found that compared to healthy elderly (age >65 years) patients, those with frailty (defined as at least 3 of the following: unintentional weight loss, self-reported exhaustion, weakness, slow walking speed, or low physical activity) were more likely to develop both elevated PVR and urinary retention (61% vs. 40%, $p = 0.018$ and 12% vs. 6%, $p = 0.2$) as well as take longer to recover normal voiding if retention did occur (3.5 months vs. 1 month in healthy elderly and 0.5 month in patients less than 65 years) [61]. These findings suggest that frailty may be a more important predictor of adverse outcomes than actual age. While diabetes has been implicated in one study as a predictor of elevated PVR >150 mL (60% vs. 33%, $p = 0.007$), this and other comorbidities have not borne out on multivariate analysis [60, 62, 63]. Despite excluding pelvic organ prolapse greater than stage 1, 1 study of 208 women found that 3 or more vaginal deliveries (but not cesarean section) were associated with PVR >200 mL or need to CIC. The authors surmised this might be due to pelvic floor or nerve damage associated with the deliveries and subsequent voiding dysfunction [60].

Not surprisingly, elevated preoperative PVR (greater than 100 mL) was found on multivariate logistic regression to be associated with urinary retention after the first trial of onaBoNT-A (OR 1.39), and urinary retention after the first injection of onaBoNT-A was associated with urinary retention after subsequent injections (odds ratio (OR) 30.2) [52]. While elevated preoperative bladder capacity (greater than 400 mL) and low daytime frequency (less than 25 voids in 3 days) have been found to be associated with urinary retention, a more accurate description of the problem involves poor voiding efficiency (calculated as the percentage of voided volume of the total bladder capacity) which predicts PVR greater than 150 mL at 3 months after treatment (OR 0.9) [64, 65]. The sensitivity and specificity of voiding efficiency as a diagnostic test for elevated PVR post-onaBoNT-A are 63.8% and 57.1%, respectively, with an ideal value greater than 87% [52]. Finally in regard to UTI, female gender, younger age, and elevated baseline PVR are all associated with increased incidence of UTI (female 22% vs. 9% $p = 0.002$, age <60 22%, 61–75 15%, >76 10%, $p = 0.03$, PVR <100 10%, PVR >100 35%, $p = 0.03$) [63].

Comparison to Alternative Therapies

A double-blind, placebo-controlled randomized trial (ABC trial) comparing 241 women with OAB to either 100 U onaBoNT-A or anticholinergic therapy found similar reductions in urinary incontinence episodes per day (−1.6 vs. −1.7, $p = 0.81$), symptom scores, and improvements in QoL measures but higher rates of complete continence in the onaBoNT-A group (27% vs. 13%, $p = 0.003$). At 6 months 70% of onaBoNT-A subjects and 71% of anticholinergic subjects had adequate control of their symptoms based on the Patient Global Symptom Control score. As expected, subjects treated with anticholinergic therapy had higher rates of dry mouth (46% vs. 31%), while those treated with onaBoNT-A had higher rates of CIC (due to PVR >300 mL with or without symptoms or PVR >150 mL with symptoms) (5% vs. 0%) and UTI (33% vs. 13%) [25]. A recent meta-analysis utilized data from 102 trials comparing onaBoNT-A, mirabegron, and a variety of anticholinergic therapies to one another or placebo for a minimum of 12 weeks. They found that onaBoNT-A reduced frequency more than all drugs compared except solifenacin 10 mg daily and oxybutynin ER 10 mg daily, had higher odds of reducing incontinence by 50% compared to all drugs except darifenacin 15 mg daily, and had higher odds of complete continence compared to all drugs [66].

A multicenter open-label trial comparing 200 U onaBoNT-A to sacral neuromodulation (SNS) in 364 women with OAB (ROSETTA trial) found greater reductions in frequency (−3.9 vs. −3.3, $p = 0.01$), urinary incontinence episodes (−4.4 vs. −3.7), and higher rates of complete continence (20% vs. 4%) in the onaBoNT-A group at 6 months as well as greater improvements in symptom scores, and higher treatment satisfaction. Women in the onaBoNT-A group had higher rates of UTI (35% vs. 11%, $p < 0.001$) and 16% required CIC 2 weeks after injection which may be directly related to the higher dose of 200 U used. In the SNS group, 3% of women had the device revised or removed [67].

Administration and Injection Technique

Patient Selection

Patients should be formally evaluated prior to undergoing BoNT-A injection with a basic urologic work-up and demonstration of prior failed conservative therapy or failure of other third-tier OAB options. OnaBoNT-A is a category C drug in pregnancy and thus not recommended in women who are pregnant or attempting to conceive. It should be used with caution in those women who are breastfeeding [24]. Systemic events can occur due to migration of toxin beyond the detrusor muscle, leading to muscle weakness or hyposthenia in non-targeted adjacent muscles or distal ones. While this is a rare complication (2.4%), especially with the lower doses used for OAB, it should be noted that it occurs more commonly in the frail elderly undergoing injection [61]. Given this risk, onaBoNT-A should be used with caution in patients with pre-existing neuromuscular disorders (e.g., myasthenia gravis or Lambert-Eaton syndrome), dysphagia, or compromised respiratory function [68].

Pre-procedure Considerations

A urinalysis should be performed, and patients presenting with UTI should be treated appropriately prior to injection. The manufacturer recommends avoiding aminoglycoside antibiotics due to a theoretical risk of potentiation of onaBoNT-A effects. Patients who are in urinary retention or regularly have a PVR of greater than 200 mL and are not catheterizing should not undergo onaBoNT-A therapy unless they are willing and able to perform intermittent urethral catheterization. Given the risk of de novo retention, some providers recommend that patients learn CIC prior to injection to demonstrate their ability should they experience voiding difficulty post-injection. While the manufacturer recommends discontinuing anticoagulant medication at least 3 days prior to injection, we have anecdotally noted that continuation of these medications does not typically cause increased bleeding. The decision of whether to stop anticoagulants, continue them, or bridge using an alternative medication should be discussed with the patient and the provider who prescribed the anticoagulation (typically the primary care provider or cardiologist) in terms of the patient's thromboembolic risk and the risks of the procedure. Of note, should patients continue their anticoagulation, one could consider using less injection sites to reduce the risk of bleeding. When treating patients who receive onabotulinumtoxinA for other indications (i.e., muscle spasticity or migraines), the total dose needs to be monitored. It is recommended the total dose of onaBoNT-A does not exceed 400 U in a 3-month period [68, 69] (Table 11.4).

Table 11.4 Indications and contraindications for use of onabotulinumtoxinA

Indications
Diagnosis of OAB with failure of behavioral interventions and oral pharmacotherapy, with or without failure of SNM and/or PTNS
No more than 260U of onabotulinumtoxinA in the prior 12 weeks for any indication
Patient willingness and ability to catheterize if necessary post-procedure
Contraindications
Current UTI
Acute urinary retention in a patient not performing catheterization
Unwillingness or unable to catheterize post-procedure if necessary
Known hypersensitivity to onabotulinumtoxinA or any of its components
Pregnancy or women attempting to conceive

OAB overactive bladder, *SNM* sacral neuromodulation, *PTNS* percutaneous tibial nerve stimulation, *UTI* urinary tract infection

Storage and Reconstitution

OnabotulinumtoxinA vials come in 50, 100, and 200 U doses. Prior to reconstitution the vials should be stored in a refrigerator (2–8 °C) or freezer (at or below −5 °C). It should be noted that prior to reconstitution, the vials appear almost completely empty except for a tiny amount of white material at the bottom. The vial should be reconstituted with 10 mL of sterile 0.9% sodium chloride and very gently mixed by rotating the vial. Proper mixing of BoNT-A is of utmost importance to keep the toxin effective as shaking can lead to toxin denaturation. After reconstitution vials can be stored in the refrigerator and should be used within 24 h. The vial is single use only and should be discarded after use [68, 69].

Injection Technique

The procedure of BoNT-A injection can be performed using either a rigid or flexible cystoscope under general, spinal, or local anesthesia. A variety of needles for each type of scope are available. Possible needle variables to consider include cost, working length, tip length, tip sharpness, and flexibility. The optimal needle gauge should be between 22 and 27 with a tip length of 4 mm [70]. The majority of patients tolerate the procedure very well with local anesthesia and a flexible scope in the office setting [71]. To administer local anesthesia, the bladder should first be drained with a catheter, and then 30 cc of 1% lidocaine should be administered via catheter to dwell for 20 min. Prior to placement of the flexible cystoscope, 10 mL of 2% lidocaine gel should be inserted into the urethra.

During cystoscopy the bladder is filled to approximately 100–200 mL to allow for adequate visualization but to avoid overdistension. Careful cystoscopy should be performed to ensure that the patient does not have any previously undocumented bladder tumors or bladder stones. There is currently no universally accepted protocol regarding the location and number of injections. During the FDA approval trials, 20 injections of 0.5 mL were injected 2 mm into the detrusor approximately 1 cm apart throughout the bladder, avoiding the trigone [39, 40]. Historically the target layer for injection is the detrusor muscle because of the previously proposed method of action; however, studies have demonstrated no difference in patient symptoms or urodynamic outcomes when comparing intradetrusor to suburothelial injections likely because there is some element of diffusion of onaBoNT-A between layers and because of the more recently documented afferent effects that contribute to the overall outcome [7, 72, 73]. Penetration of the bladder wall and an injection into the perivesical tissues should be avoided both due to lack of efficacy and risk of complications (such as generalized muscle weakness). Injections to the trigone have traditionally been spared out of concern for producing VUR; however, this theoretical concern was disproven [74]. While an older meta-analysis of 6 studies including 258 patients found no significant difference between trigonal and extratrigonal injections in terms of efficacy or adverse events, this analysis is complicated by including studies with a variety of doses, combination of OAB and NDO patients, and lack of separation in the trigone group between trigone-only vs. trigone-inclusive injections [75]. A more recent meta-analysis of 8 studies including 419 patients found improved efficacy and no differences in adverse events when comparing trigone-inclusive injections to trigone-sparing injections but is also limited by inclusion of studies utilizing a variety of doses and a combination of NDO and OAB patients [73]. Some recent studies suggest efficacy may be maintained with fewer injections. Both Denys et al. and Liao et al. found that fewer injections (10 or 15) had similar outcomes compared to more injections (20, 30 or 40) [76, 77]. Avallone et al. reported 50% subjective improvement in lower urinary tract symptoms using a total of 1–3 injections, although unfortunately there was not a comparison to placebo or standard number of injection sites [78]. Finally, while some authors have advocated for adding methylene blue to the onaBoNT-A injection solution to aid injection technique, we find that this additional step is not necessary as providers gain experience with the procedure [79].

Post-procedure

Patients should receive a single dose of antibiotics during the time of injection for antimicrobial prophylaxis, but no additional therapy is indicated. Given the recent FDA black box warning regarding fluoroquinolone use, a different category of antibiotic is recommended [80, 81].

Patients should void prior to leaving the clinic. Significant bleeding is rarely encountered during the injection even in patients on anticoagulants, but patients should be informed that they could see blood in the urine for a day and have dysuria with voiding for up to 48 h due to urethral manipulation.

Patients should be counseled that the effects are not immediate and may take up to 2 weeks to fully manifest. Patients should follow up within 2 weeks to check a post-void residual (PVR) and ensure adequate emptying. Based on the Phase III trial recommendations of initiating catheterization for PVR >200 ml with symptoms or greater than 350 ml without symptoms, 6–7% of patients will require CIC. However, a recent study of 187 injections found that initiation of CIC by symptoms alone, without regard to the PVR, reduced the CIC rate to 1.6% with no increased risk of UTI (UTI rate in PVR >350 ml 17%, UTI rate in PVR <200 ml 36%) and no increased risk of frank retention [82]. Thus, the decision regarding the criteria for initiation of CIC is provider and patient dependent.

Future Work

Investigators continue to search for alternative ways to optimize the delivery of onaBoNT-A to the bladder that does not involve cystoscopic injection. While intravesical instillation is not presently a viable option due to the high molecular weight of injected preparations, other techniques have been tried. Krhut et al. attempted to augment the time urothelium is exposed to instilled onaBoNT-A by embedding it in a hydrogel. The technique demonstrated some promise compared to placebo but was not compared to the gold standard injection [83]. Kajbafazadeh et al. evaluated the use of electromotive administration (maximal current of 10 mA for 15 min) with 10 U/kg of onaBoNT-A in 15 children with NDO. Significant improvements were seen, but the study was limited by the small number of participants and lack of placebo comparison [84]. Chuang et al. utilized low-energy shock waves in a chemical cystitis animal model to facilitate successful delivery of onaBoNT-A into urothelial tissue, but human data is still lacking [85]. A recent double-blind, placebo-controlled RCT examined the intravesical liposomal delivery of onaBoNT-A in 57 patients and found mixed results with statistically significant decreases in frequency compared to placebo (−4.6 vs. −0.19, p <0.005) but no differences in urgency or UUI. While this study is somewhat promising, it is limited by small sample size and lack of comparison to the gold standard injection [86].

Vanilloid Compounds

Mechanism of Action

Vanilloid receptors are found throughout the lower urinary tract including sensory neurons, urothelial cells, and the detrusor muscle and regulate the frequency of reflex bladder contraction due to pain and/or inflammation. One proposed etiology of OAB is activation of the vanilloid receptors on the unmyelinated c-fiber sensory neurons resulting in urgency and uninhibited contractions via a sacral mediated reflex [87]. Capsaicin and resiniferatoxin are both vanilloid compounds that can bind to a specific vanilloid receptor, TRPV1. Capsaicin is the active ingredient in the hot pepper from the *Capsicum* genus and results in burning and irritation of the skin and mucous membranes. Resiniferatoxin is derived from a cactus-like plant, *Euphorbia resinifera*, and was used in the traditional medicine of North African populations as an analgesic [88]. Activation of TRPV1 results in massive inward Ca2+ and Na + currents that can be completely blocked by capsazepine, a capsaicin antagonist. Inward currents evoked by capsaicin are strong in amplitude with a short duration, while those evoked by RTX are weak with a longer duration [89]. Consecutive applications of TRPV1 agonists result in a progressive decrease in the amplitude of the inward currents and subsequent desensitization. This is accompanied by a decreased responsiveness of the TRPV1-expressing sensory neurons to natural stimuli. It is, therefore, desensitization, and not excitation, that offers potential for clinical application.

Commercial Formulations and Dosing Considerations

While capsaicin was the first TRPV1 agonist used intravesically, it caused such intense pain during the excitation phase despite local anesthesia that it is not routinely used [90]. RTX offers the best therapeutic profile as it induces a low intensity excitation phase and less pain to the patient but a prolonged desensitization effect.

RTX is currently available as dry powder (Sigman-Aldrich) that must be prepared on-site. A stock ethanol solution of 10 mM of RTX in pure ethanol must be created and stored in a glass container in a dark area at 4 °C [87].

Treatment for Overactive Bladder

The outcomes of RTX treatment are controversial, and the literature is limited by studies with small sample sizes and heterogeneous groups (Table 11.5 [91–94]). One placebo-controlled randomized trial of 58 women with OAB found that 50 nM of RTX had no significant difference when compared to placebo in either clinical or urodynamic parameters [94]. Two small retrospective reviews of 10 and 13 patients with OAB who underwent instillation with 50 nM of RTX found significant differences in both clinical parameters and urodynamic parameters at 30 days with decreased frequency by 1.7–2.3 voids, decreased UI by 1.6–4.3 episodes, increased MCC by 43–181 ml, and increased volume at first detrusor contraction by 27–270 ml [91, 92]. Finally another placebo-controlled randomized trial of 54 patients with either NDO or OAB found that 4 weekly instillations of 10 nM RTX had improved clinical outcomes, urodynamic outcomes, and patient satisfaction compared to placebo [93]. Only one meta-analysis has been performed which found no difference in urinary frequency and nocturia but a significant increase in MCC. Unfortunately this meta-analysis combined both NDO and OAB patients, so its applicability to OAB patients is challenging [95]. Finally, one group has found that responders to RTX, compared to nonresponders, have a trend toward higher TRPV1 expression levels, possibly indicating a subgroup of patients that may more fully benefit from RTX therapy [96]. At this point in time, the

Table 11.5 Results of resiniferatoxin (RTX) randomized controlled trials

Study	Groups (*n*)	Data time point	RTX dose	Frequency	Urgency incontinence	Patient-reported measure	Urodynamic findings	Adverse events
Silva (2002) [91]	RTX 13	4 weeks	50nM in 100ml	Δ/*d* from baseline	Δ/*d* from baseline	NA	Δ MCC from baseline	Avg discomfort on VAS during procedure: 3 (range 0–8)
				−2.3[a]	−3.4[a]		+181[a]	
Yokoyama (2004) [92]	RTX 10	4 weeks	50nM in 100ml	Δ/*d* from baseline	Δ/*d* from baseline	Δ IQoL from baseline	Δ MCC from baseline	Avg discomfort on VAS during procedure: 5.6 (range 0–10)
				−1.7[a]	−1.6[a]	+9.5[a]	+43[a]	
Kuo (2006) [93]		12 weeks	4 weekly instillations of 10nM in 30ml	NA	Δ/*d* from baseline	% Success	Δ MCC from baseline	NA
	RTX 26				−8[a]	62[a]	+38[a]	
	Placebo 28 (10% ethanol)				+1.4	21	−7	
Rios (2007) [94]		4 weeks	50nM in 100ml	Δ/*d* from baseline	Δ/*d* from baseline	%Satisfied with treatment	% Improvement MCC from Baseline	Discomfort during procedure:
	RTX 34			−0.65	−0.43	63.6%	4%	Pain: 35.2% (mild) Dysuria: 45.4% Hematuria: 3%
	Placebo 24 (10% ethanol)			−0.84	−1.26	55%	8%	Pain: 16.6% (mild) Dysuria: 30% Hematuria: 15%

Δ change, *d* day, *IQOL* incontinence quality of life, *MCC* maximum cystometric capacity
[a]Statistically significant ($p < 0.05$)

safety and efficacy of RTX have not been demonstrated in any large, multicenter trials with long-term follow-up, and for this reason its use beyond experimental procedures is not recommended.

Administration Technique

Drug Preparation

RTX is administered via instillation. Each dose must be prepared immediately before use using the stock solution previously created. Each instillation is 100 mL and consists of 0.5 ml of stock solution, 90 mL of saline, and 9.5 ml of pure ethanol [91].

Instillation

The RTX solution is administered via clean catheterization and maintained in the bladder for 30 min. In clinical trials patients did not complain of pain during the instillation, and anesthesia was not given. Average discomfort on a visual analog score was 3 (range 0–8). During the procedure patients experience urgency and itching or a warm sensation over the lower abdomen. After 30 min the bladder is drained and then irrigated with normal saline. The catheter is removed and patients must void prior to leaving the clinic [91].

Conclusion

Intravesical therapy serves as a valuable surrogate treatment for OAB patients who either are refractory or are unable to tolerate oral therapy. With the advent of BoNT-A, the practitioner has an important tool in the armamentarium of treatment for OAB. BoNT-A injection is an effective, safe, and well-tolerated option for patients and is regarded as the current mainstay of intravesical therapy. While vanilloid compounds for intravesical therapy are present, at this point in time, their efficacy and safety have not been sufficiently documented to recommend their use.

References

1. Gormley EA, Lightner DJ, Faraday M, Vasavada SP. American Urological Association; Society of Urodynamics, Female Pelvic Medicine. Diagnosis and treatment of overactive bladder (non-neurogenic) in adults: AUA/SUFU guideline amendment. J Urol. 2015;193(5):1572–80.

2. Nigam PK, Nigam A. Botulinum toxin. Indian J Dermatol. 2010;55(1):8–14.
3. Apostolidis A. Rahnama'i MS, Fry C, Dmochowski R, Sahai A. Do we understand how botulinum toxin works and have we optimized the way it is administered to the bladder? ICI-RS 2014. NeurourolUrodyn. 2016;35(2):293–8.
4. Dong M, Yeh F, Tepp WH, Dean C, Johnson EA, Janz R, Chapman ER. SV2 is the protein receptor for botulinum neurotoxin A. Science. 2006;312(5773):592–6.
5. Hanna-Mitchell AT, Wolf-Johnston AS, Barrick SR, Kanai AJ, Chancellor MB, de Groat WC, Birder LA. Effect of botulinum toxin A on urothelial-release of ATP and expression of SNARE targets within the urothelium. NeurourolUrodyn. 2015;34(1):79–84.
6. Yiangou Y, Anand U, Otto WR, Sinisi M, Fox M, Birch R, et al. Increased levels of SV2A botulinum neurotoxin receptor in clinical sensory disorders and functional effects of botulinum toxins A and E in cultured human sensory neurons. J Pain Res. 2011;4:347–55.
7. Coelho A, Cruz F, Cruz CD, Avelino A. Spread of onabotulinumtoxinA after bladder injection. Experimental study using the distribution of cleaved SNAP-25 as the marker of the toxin action. Eur Urol. 2012;61(6):1178–84.
8. Liu HT, Chen SH, Chancellor MB, Kuo HC. Presence of cleaved synaptosomal-associated protein-25 and decrease of purinergic receptors P2X3 in the bladder urothelium influence efficacy of botulinum toxin treatment for overactive bladder syndrome. PLoS One. 2015;10(8):e0134803.
9. Apostolidis A, Popat R, Yiangou Y, Cockayne D, Ford AP, Davis JB, et al. Decreased sensory receptors P2X3 and TRPV1 in suburothelial nerve fibers following intradetrusor injections of botulinum toxin for human detrusor overactivity. J Urol. 2005;174(3):977–82. discussion 982–3.
10. Collins VM, Daly DM, Liaskos M, McKay NG, Sellers D, Chapple C, Grundy D. OnabotulinumtoxinA significantly attenuates bladder afferent nerve firing and inhibits ATP release from the urothelium. BJU Int. 2013;112:1018–26.
11. Haferkamp A, Schurch B, Reitz A, Krengel U, Grosse J, Kramer G, et al. Lack of ultrastructural detrusor changes following endoscopic injection of botulinum toxin type a in overactive neurogenic bladder. Eur Urol. 2004;46(6):784–91.
12. Naumann M. Clinical comparison of botulinum toxin in motor and autonomic disorders. Similarities and differences. Toxicon. 2015;107(Pt A):68–71.
13. Chancellor MB, Elovic E, Esquenazi A, Naumann M, Segal KR, Schiavo G, et al. Evidence-based review and assessment of botulinum neurotoxin for the treatment of urologic conditions. Toxicon. 2013;67:129–40.
14. Scaglione F. Conversion ratio between Botox®, Dysport®, and Xeomin® in clinical practice. Toxins (Basel). 2016;8(3):65.
15. Conte A, Giannantoni A, Gubbiotti M, Pontecorvo S, Millefiorini E, Francia A, et al. Intradetrusorial botulinum toxin in patients with multiple sclerosis: a neurophysiological study. Toxins (Basel). 2015;7:3424–35.
16. Weckx F, Tutolo M, De Ridder D, Van der Aa F. The role of botulinum toxin A in treating neurogenic bladder. Transl Androl Urol. 2016;5(1):63–71.
17. Ravindra P, Jackson BL, Parkinson RJ. Botulinum toxin type A for the treatment of non-neurogenic overactive bladder: does using onabotulinumtoxinA (Botox®) or abobotulinumtoxinA (Dysport®) make a difference? BJU Int. 2013;112(1):94–9.
18. Bottet F, Peyronnet B, Boissier R, Reiss B, Previnaire JG, Manunta A, et al. Groupe d'Etude de Neuro-Urologie de Langue Française (GENULF) and the committee of NeuroUrology of the French Association of Urology (AFU).Switch to Abobotulinum toxin A may be useful in the treatment of neurogenic detrusor overactivity when intradetrusor injections of Onabotulinum toxin A failed. NeurourolUrodyn. 2018;37(1):291–7.
19. Grosset DG, Tyrrell EG, Grosset KA. Switch from abobotulinumtoxinA (Dysport®) to incobotulinumtoxinA (Xeomin®) botulinum toxin formulation: a review of 257 cases. J Rehabil Med. 2015;47:183–6.
20. Pistolesi D, Selli C, Rossi B, Stampacchia G. Botulinum toxin type B for type A resistant bladder spasticity. J Urol. 2004;171(2 Pt 1):802–3.

21. Reitz A, Schurch B. Botulinum toxin type B injection for management of type A resistant neurogenic detrusor overactivity. J Urol. 2004;171(3Pt 1):804. discussion 804–5.
22. Ghei M, Maraj BH, Miller R, Nathan S, O'Sullivan C, Fowler CJ, et al. Effects of botulinum toxin B on refractory detrusor overactivity: a randomized, double-blind, placebo controlled, crossover trial. J Urol. 2005;174(5):1873–7. discussion 1877.
23. Dykstra DD, Sidi AA, Scott AB, Pagel JM, Goldish GD. Effects of botulinum A toxin on detrusor-sphincter dyssynergia in spinal cord injury patients. J Urol. 1988;139(5):919–22.
24. American Urogynecologic Society and American College of Obstetricians and Gynecologists. Committee opinion: onabotulinumtoxinA and the bladder. Female Pelvic Med Reconstr Surg. 2014;20(5):245–7.
25. Visco AG, Brubaker L, Richter HE, Nygaard I, Paraiso MF, Menefee SA, et al. Pelvic Floor Disorders Network. therapy vs. onabotulinumtoxina for urgency urinary incontinence. N Engl J Med. 2012;367(19):1803–13.
26. Lucas MG, Bosch RJ, Burkhard FC, Cruz F, Madden TB, Nambiar AK, et al. European Association of Urology. EAU guidelines on surgical treatment of urinary incontinence. Actas Urol Esp. 2013;37(8):459–72.
27. Flynn MK, Webster GD, Amundsen CL. The effect of botulinum-A toxin on patients with severe urge urinary incontinence. J Urol. 2004;172(6 Pt 1):2316–20.
28. Schmid DM, Sauermann P, Werner M, Schuessler B, Blick N, Muentener M, et al. Experience with 100 cases treated with botulinum-A toxin injections in the detrusor muscle for idiopathic overactive bladder syndrome refractory to anticholinergics. J Urol. 2006;176(1):177–85.
29. Sahai A, Khan MS, Dasgupta P. Efficacy of botulinum toxin-A for treating idiopathic detrusor overactivity: results from a single center, randomized, double-blind, placebo controlled trial. J Urol. 2007;177(6):2231–6.
30. Brubaker L1, Richter HE, Visco A, Mahajan S, Nygaard I, Braun TM, et al. Pelvic Floor Disorders Network. Refractory idiopathic urge urinary incontinence and botulinum A injection. J Urol. 2008;180(1):217–22.
31. Flynn MK, Amundsen CL, Perevich M, Liu F, Webster GD. Outcome of a randomized, double-blind, placebo controlled trial of botulinum A toxin for refractory overactive bladder. J Urol. 2009;181(6):2608–15.
32. Cohen BL, Barboglio P, Rodriguez D, Gousse AE. Preliminary results of a dose-finding study for botulinum toxin-A in patients with idiopathic overactive bladder: 100 versus 150 units. NeurourolUrodyn. 2009;28(3):205–8.
33. Dmochowski R, Chapple C, Nitti VW, Chancellor M, Everaert K, Thompson C, et al. Efficacy and safety of onabotulinumtoxinA for idiopathic overactive bladder: a double-blind, placebo controlled, randomized, dose ranging trial. J Urol. 2010;184(6):2416–22.
34. Rovner E, Kennelly M, Schulte-Baukloh H, Zhou J, Haag-Molkenteller C, Dasgupta P. Urodynamic results and clinical outcomes with intradetrusor injections of onabotulinumtoxinA in a randomized, placebo-controlled dose-finding study in idiopathic overactive bladder. NeurourolUrodyn. 2011;30(4):556–62.
35. Dowson C, Sahai A, Watkins J, Dasgupta P, Khan MS. The safety and efficacy of botulinum toxin-A in the management of bladder oversensitivity: a randomised double-blind placebo-controlled trial. Int J Clin Pract. 2011;65(6):698–704.
36. Altaweel W, Mokhtar A, Rabah DM. Prospective randomized trial of 100u vs 200u botox in the treatment of idiopathic overactive bladder. Urol Ann. 2011;3(2):66–70.
37. Denys P, Le Normand L, Ghout I, Costa P, Chartier-Kastler E, Grise P, et al. VESITOX study group in France. Efficacy and safety of low doses of onabotulinumtoxinA for the treatment of refractory idiopathic overactive bladder: a multicentre, double-blind, randomised, placebo-controlled dose-ranging study. Eur Urol. 2012;61(3):520–9.
38. Tincello DG, Kenyon S, Abrams KR, Mayne C, Toozs-Hobson P, Taylor D, Slack M. Botulinum toxin a versus placebo for refractory detrusor overactivity in women: a randomised blinded placebo-controlled trial of 240 women (the RELAX study). Eur Urol. 2012;62(3):507–14.
39. Nitti VW, Dmochowski R, Herschorn S, Sand P, Thompson C, Nardo C, et al.; EMBARK Study Group OnabotulinumtoxinA for the treatment of patients with overactive bladder

and urinary incontinence: results of a phase 3, randomized, placebo controlled trial. J Urol. 2013;189(6):2186–93.
40. Chapple C, Sievert KD, MacDiarmid S, Khullar V, Radziszewski P, Nardo C, et al. OnabotulinumtoxinA 100 U significantly improves all idiopathic overactive bladder symptoms and quality of life in patients with overactive bladder and urinary incontinence: a randomised, double-blind, placebo-controlled trial. Eur Urol. 2013;64(2):249–56.
41. Jabs C, Carleton E. Efficacy of botulinum toxin a intradetrusor injections for non-neurogenic urinary urge incontinence: a randomized double-blind controlled trial. J Obstet Gynaecol Can. 2013;35(1):53–60.
42. López Ramos H, Torres Castellanos L, Ponce Esparza I, Jaramillo A, Rodríguez A, Moreno Bencardino C. Management of overactive bladder with onabotulinumtoxina: systematic review and meta-analysis. Urology. 2017;100:53–8.
43. Eldred-Evans D, Sahai A. Medium-to long-term outcomes of botulinum toxin A for idiopathic overactive bladder. Ther Adv Urol. 2017;9(1):3–10.
44. Nitti VW, Ginsberg D, Sievert KD, Sussman D, Radomski S, Sand P, et al. 191622-096 Investigators.Durable efficacy and safety of long-term onabotulinumtoxina treatment in patients with overactive bladder syndrome: final results of a 3.5-year study. J Urol. 2016;196(3):791–800.
45. Sand PK, Heesakkers J, Kraus SR, Carlsson M, Guan Z, Berriman S. Long-term safety, tolerability and efficacy of fesoterodine in subjects with overactive bladder symptoms stratified by age: pooled analysis of two open-label extension studies. Drugs Aging. 2012;29(2):119–31.
46. Marcelissen TA, Rahnama'i MS, Snijkers A, Schurch B, De Vries P. Long-term follow-up of intravesical botulinum toxin-A injections in women with idiopathic overactive bladder symptoms. World J Urol. 2017;35(2):307–11.
47. Jankovic J, Vuong KD, Ahsan J. Comparison of efficacy and immunogenicity of original versus current botulinum toxin in cervical dystonia. Neurology. 2003;60(7):1186–8.
48. Schulte-Baukloh H, Bigalke H, Miller K, Heine G, Pape D, Lehmann J, Knispel HH. Botulinum neurotoxin type A in urology: antibodies as a cause of therapy failure. Int J Urol. 2008;15(5):407–15. discussion 415.
49. Schulte-Baukloh H, Herholz J, Bigalke H, Miller K, Knispel HH. Results of a BoNT/A antibody study in children and adolescents after onabotulinumtoxin A (Botox®) detrusor injection. Urol Int. 2011;87(4):434–8.
50. Richter HE, Amundsen CL, Erickson SW, Jelovsek JE, Komesu Y, Chermansky C, et al. NICHD Pelvic Floor Disorders Network. Characteristics associated with treatment response and satisfaction in women undergoing onabotulinumtoxinA and sacral neuromodulation for refractory urgency urinary incontinence. J Urol. 2017;198(4):890–6.
51. Komesu YM, Amundsen CL, Richter HE, Erickson SW, Ackenbom MF, Andy UU, et al. Eunice Kennedy Shriver National Institute of Child Health and Human Development Pelvic Floor Disorders Network. Refractory urgency urinary incontinence treatment in women: impact of age on outcomes and complications. Am J Obstet Gynecol. 2018;218(1):111.e1–9.
52. Hsiao SM, Lin HH, Kuo HC. Factors associated with therapeutic efficacy of intravesical onabotulinumtoxina injection for overactive bladder syndrome. PLoS One. 2016;11(1):e0147137.
53. Rahnama'i MS, Marcelissen TA, Brierley B, Schurch B, de Vries P. Long-term compliance and results of intravesical botulinum toxin A injections in male patients. NeurourolUrodyn. 2017;36(7):1855–9.
54. Miotla P, Futyma K, Cartwright R, Bogusiewicz M, Skorupska K, Markut-Miotla E, Rechberger T. Effectiveness of botulinum toxin injection in the treatment of de novo OAB symptoms following midurethral sling surgery. Int Urogynecol J. 2016;27(3):393–8.
55. Makovey I, Davis T, Guralnick ML, O'Connor RC. Botulinum toxin outcomes for idiopathic overactive bladder stratified by indication: lack of anticholinergic efficacy versus intolerability. NeurourolUrodyn. 2011;30(8):1538–40.
56. Sievert KD1, Chapple C, Herschorn S, Joshi M, Zhou J, Nardo C, Nitti VW. OnabotulinumtoxinA 100U provides significant improvements in overactive bladder symptoms in patients with urinary incontinence regardless of the number of anticholinergic

therapies used or reason for inadequate management of overactive bladder. Int J Clin Pract. 2014;68(10):1246–56.
57. Kuo HC. Reduction of urgency severity is associated with long-term therapeutic effect after intravesical onabotulinumtoxin A injection for idiopathic detrusor overactivity. NeurourolUrodyn. 2011;30(8):1497–502.
58. Richter HE, Moalli P, Amundsen CL, Malykhina AP, Wallace D, Rogers R, Myers D. Pelvic Floor Disorders Network. Urinary biomarkers in women with refractory urgency urinary incontinence randomized to sacral neuromodulation versus onabotulinumtoxina compared to controls. J Urol. 2017;197(6):1487–95.
59. Kuo HC, Liao CH, Chung SD. Adverse events of intravesical botulinum toxin a injections for idiopathic detrusor overactivity: risk factors and influence on treatment outcome. Eur Urol. 2010;58(6):919–26.
60. Miotla P, Cartwright R, Skorupska K, Bogusiewicz M, Markut-Miotla E, Futyma K, Rechberger T. Urinary retention in female OAB after intravesical Botox injection: who is really at risk? Int Urogynecol J. 2017;28(6):845–50.
61. Liao CH, Kuo HC. Increased risk of large post-void residual urine and decreased long-term success rate after intravesical onabotulinumtoxinA injection for refractory idiopathic detrusor overactivity. J Urol. 2013;189(5):1804–10.
62. Wang CC, Liao CH, Kuo HC. Diabetes mellitus does not affect the efficacy and safety of intravesical onabotulinumtoxinA injection in patients with refractory detrusor overactivity. NeurourolUrodyn. 2014;33(8):1235–9.
63. Jiang YH, Ong HL, Kuo HC. Predictive factors of adverse events after intravesical suburothelial onabotulinumtoxina injections for overactive bladder syndrome-A real-life practice of 290 cases in a single center. NeurourolUrodyn. 2017;36(1):142–7.
64. Osborn DJ, Kaufman MR, Mock S, Guan MJ, Dmochowski RR, Reynolds WS. Urinary retention rates after intravesical onabotulinumtoxinA injection for idiopathic overactive bladder in clinical practice and predictors of this outcome. NeurourolUrodyn. 2015;34(7):675–8.
65. Hsiao SM, Lin HH, Kuo HC. Urodynamic prognostic factors for large post-void residual urine volume after intravesical injection of onabotulinumtoxinA for overactive bladder. Sci Rep. 2017;7:43753.
66. Drake MJ, Nitti VW, Ginsberg DA, Brucker BM, Hepp Z, McCool R, et al. Comparative assessment of the efficacy of onabotulinumtoxinA and oral therapies (anticholinergics and mirabegron) for overactive bladder: a systematic review and network meta-analysis. BJU Int. 2017;120(5):611–22.
67. Amundsen CL, Richter HE, Menefee SA, Komesu YM, Arya LA, Gregory WT, et al. OnabotulinumtoxinA vs sacral neuromodulation on refractory urgency urinary incontinence in women: a randomized clinical trial. JAMA. 2016;316(13):1366–74.
68. BOTOX [prescribing information]. Irvine, CA: Allergan. Revised Oct 2017. https://www.allergan.com/assets/pdf/botox_pi.pdf. Accessed 26 Apr 2018.
69. Rovner E. Chapter 6: Practical aspects of administration of onabotulinumtoxinA. NeurourolUrodyn. 2014;33(Suppl 3):S32–7.
70. Karsenty G, Baverstock R, Carlson K, Diaz DC, Cruz F, Dmochowski R, et al. Technical aspects of botulinum toxin type A injection in the bladder to treat urinary incontinence: reviewing the procedure. Int J Clin Pract. 2014;68(6):731–42.
71. Cohen BL, Rivera R, Barboglio P, Gousse A. Safety and tolerability of sedation-free flexible cystoscopy for intradetrusor botulinum toxin-A injection. J Urol. 2007;177(3):1006–10. discussion 1010.
72. Kuo HC. Comparison of effectiveness of detrusor, suburothelial and bladder base injections of botulinum toxin a for idiopathic detrusor overactivity. J Urol. 2007;178(4 Pt 1):1359–63.
73. Jo JK, Kim KN, Kim DW, Kim YT, Kim JY, Kim JY. The effect of onabotulinumtoxinA according to site of injection in patients with overactive bladder: a systematic review and meta-analysis. World J Urol. 2018;36(2):305–17.
74. Karsenty G, Elzayat E, Delapparent T, St-Denis B, Lemieux MC, Corcos J. Botulinum toxin type a injections into the trigone to treat idiopathic overactive bladder do not induce vesicoureteral reflux. J Urol. 2007;177(3):1011–4.

75. Davis NF, Burke JP, Redmond EJ, Elamin S, Brady CM, Flood HD. Trigonal versus extratrigonal botulinum toxin-A: a systematic review and meta-analysis of efficacy and adverse events. Int Urogynecol J. 2015;26:313–9.
76. Denys P, Del Popolo G, Amarenco G, Karsenty G, Le Berre P, Padrazzi B. Picaut P; Dysport Study Group. Efficacy and safety of two administration modes of an intra-detrusor injection of 750 units dysport® (abobotulinumtoxinA) in patients suffering from refractory neurogenic detrusor overactivity (NDO): A randomised placebo-controlled phase IIa study. NeurourolUrodyn. 2017;26(2):457–62.
77. Liao CH, Chen SF, Kuo HC. Different number of intravesical onabotulinumtoxinA injections for patients with refractory detrusor overactivity do not affect treatment outcome: A prospective randomized comparative study. NeurourolUrodyn. 2016;35(6):717–23.
78. Avallone MA, Sack BS, El-Arabi A, Guralnick ML, O'Connor RC. Less is more—A pilot study evaluating one to three intradetrusor sites for injection of OnabotulinumtoxinA for neurogenic and idiopathic detrusor overactivity. NeurourolUrodyn. 2017;36(4):1104–7.
79. Szczypior M, Połom W, Markuszewski M, Ciura K, Buszewska-Forajta M, Jacyna J, et al. Overactive bladder treatment: application of methylene blue to improve the injection technique of onabotulinum toxin A. Scand J Urol. 2017;51(6):474–8.
80. Wolf JS, Bennett CJ, Dmochowski RR, Hollenbeck BK, Pearle MS, Schaeffer AJ. Urologic Surgery Antimicrobial Prophylaxis Best Practice Policy Panel. Best practice policy statement on urologic surgery antimicrobial prophylaxis. J Urol. 2008;179(4):1379–90.
81. U.S. Food and Drug Administration. FDA Drug Safety Communication: FDA updates warnings for oral and injectable fluoroquinolone antibiotics due to disabling side effects. Updated 8 Mar 2018. http://www.fda.gov/Drugs/DrugSafety/ucm511530.htm. Accessed 27 Apr 2018.
82. Patel DN, Jamnagerwalla J, Houman J, Anger JT, Eilber KS.What is the true catheterization rate after intravesical onabotulinumtoxinA injection?. Int Urogynecol J. 2017. https://doi.org/10.1007/s00192-017-3440-2. [Epub ahead of print].
83. Krhut J, Navratilova M, Sykora R, Jurakova M, Gärtner M, Mika D, et al. Intravesical instillation of onabotulinum toxin A embedded in inert hydrogel in the treatment of idiopathic overactive bladder: A double-blind randomized pilot study. Scand J Urol. 2016;50(3):200–5.
84. Kajbafzadeh AM, Ahmadi H, Montaser-Kouhsari L, Sharifi-Rad L, Nejat F, Bazargan-Hejazi S. Intravesical electromotive botulinum toxin type A administration--part II: Clinical application. Urology. 2011;77(2):439–45.
85. Chuang YC, Huang TL, Tyagi P, Huang CC. Urodynamic and immunohistochemical evaluation of intravesical botulinum toxin a delivery using low energy shock waves. J Urol. 2016;196(2):599–608.
86. Chuang YC, Kaufmann JH, Chancellor DD, Chancellor MB, Kuo HC. Bladder instillation of liposome encapsulated onabotulinumtoxina improves overactive bladder symptoms: a prospective, multicenter, double-blind, randomized trial. J Urol. 2014;192(6):1743–9.
87. Avelino A, Cruz F. TRPV1 (vanilloid receptor) in the urinary tract: expression, function and clinical applications. Naunyn Schmiedebergs Arch Pharmacol. 2006;373(4):287–99.
88. Kim DY, Chancellor MB. Intravesical neuromodulatory drugs: capsaicin and resiniferatoxin to treat the overactive bladder. J Endourol. 2000;14(1):97–103.
89. Cruz F. Vanilloid receptor and detrusor instability. Urology. 2002;59(5 Suppl 1):51–60. Review.
90. Cruz F, Guimarães M, Silva C, Rio ME, Coimbra A, Reis M. Desensitization of bladder sensory fibers by intravesical capsaicin has long lasting clinical and urodynamic effects in patients with hyperactive or hypersensitive bladder dysfunction. J Urol. 1997;157(2):585–9.
91. Silva C, Ribeiro MJ, Cruz F. The effect of intravesical resiniferatoxin in patients with idiopathic detrusor instability suggests that involuntary detrusor contractions are triggered by C-fiber input. J Urol. 2002;168(2):575–9.
92. Yokoyama T, Nozaki K, Fujita O, Nose H, Inoue M, Kumon H. Role of C afferent fibers and monitoring of intravesical resiniferatoxin therapy for patients with idiopathic detrusor overactivity. J Urol. 2004;172(2):596–600.
93. Kuo HC, Liu HT, Yang WC. Therapeutic effect of multiple resiniferatoxin intravesical instillations in patients with refractory detrusor overactivity: a randomized, double-blind, placebo controlled study. J Urol. 2006;176(2):641–5.

94. Rios LAS, Panhoca R, Mattos D, Srugi M, Brruschini H. Intravesical resiniferatoxin for the treatment of women with idiopathic detrusor overactivity and urgency incontinence: A single dose, 4 weeks, double-blind, randomized, placebo controlled trial. NeurourolUrodyn. 2007;26(6):773–8.
95. Guo C, Yang B, Gu W, Peng B, Xia S, Yang F, et al. Intravesical resiniferatoxin for the treatment of storage lower urinary tract symptoms in patients with either interstitial cystitis or detrusor overactivity: a meta-analysis. PLoS One. 2013;8(12):e82591.
96. Liu HT, Kuo HC. Increased expression of transient receptor potential vanilloid subfamily 1 in the bladder predicts the response to intravesical instillations of resiniferatoxin in patients with refractory idiopathic detrusor overactivity. BJU Int. 2007;100(5):1086–90.

Chapter 12
Other Treatments for Overactive Bladder, Including Intravesical

Alison C. Levy and Lara S. MacLachlan

Oral Agents

Centrally Acting Drugs

There is a strong association between psychiatric disorders, including depression, and overactive bladder [1].Treatment of either depression or bladder symptoms may improve the other condition suggesting that the disorders may share a common pathogenesis [2]. Several relevant neurotransmitters are involved in normal and pathologic micturition pathways.

Urine storage is mediated centrally by serotonin increasing sympathetic and somatic action and suppressing parasympathetic control. Norepinephrine has dose- and receptor-dependent effects on the sympathetic and somatic systems of the lower urinary tract.

Duloxetine, an antidepressant, is a selective serotonin and norepinephrine reuptake inhibitor (SNRI) that is also approved for the treatment of stress urinary incontinence (SUI) in some countries. In phase III testing of duloxetine for SUI, patients demonstrated improvement in intervals between voiding suggesting positive effects on bladder relaxation [3]. A randomized controlled trial (RCT) in women with overactive bladder was conducted in 2007 with positive results [4]. Three hundred six women with a minimum of 3 months of urgency predominant symptoms, daytime voiding interval less than or equal to 2 h, and urodynamic confirmation of detrusor overactivity (DO) or bladder capacity less than 400 mL secondary to urgency were enrolled. Patients were randomized to receive twice daily dose of 40 mg of duloxetine for 4 weeks and then 60 mg twice daily for 8 weeks or identical-appearing placebo. The study met its primary outcome showing a reduction of mean voiding

A. C. Levy · L. S. MacLachlan (✉)
Department of Urology, Lahey Hospital and Medical Center, Burlington, MA, USA
e-mail: Lara.MacLachlan@lahey.org

L. Cox, E. S. Rovner (eds.), *Contemporary Pharmacotherapy of Overactive Bladder*, https://doi.org/10.1007/978-3-319-97265-7_12

episodes in 24 h by 1.81 versus 0.62 episodes in the placebo arm ($p < 0.001$). Additionally, the study met secondary outcomes including decreasing episodes of urinary incontinence ($p = 0.032$), improving some measures of quality of life, and increasing the mean daytime voiding interval by 29.46 min versus 6.51 min in the placebo group ($p > 0.001$). In contrast to studies in patients with SUI, there was no improvement of bladder capacity or volume at which patients experienced DO on urodynamic follow-up. Notably, 28.1% of patients were unable to tolerate duloxetine due to adverse events including nausea, dry mouth, dizziness, constipation, and insomnia. A pilot study was performed to assess duloxetine in 23 patients with multiple sclerosis which also demonstrated statistically significant improvement in overactivity-related quality of life [5]. To date no studies have been performed comparing duloxetine to first-line anticholinergic medications. Similar agents including besipirdine, an SNRI, and escitalopram, an SSRI, have completed phase II trials, but results are not available [6, 7]. SNRIs are promising therapeutic options in patients who are able to tolerate side effects based on good evidence by the International Consultation on Incontinence (ICI) [8].

Tricyclic antidepressants increase norepinephrine and serotonin by blocking synaptic reuptake of these neurotransmitters and also have potent anticholinergic and antihistamine properties suggesting a potential role in OAB treatment. This class of drugs is no longer frequently prescribed in the treatment of depression due to side effects and overdose risks as well as the availability of multiple effective alternative agents. No randomized studies have been performed in patients with primary diagnosis of OAB. Imipramine has been studied as a combination therapy in interstitial cystitis and showed a benefit to a subset of patients with overactivity [9]. In a small study of patients with neurogenic bladder and incontinence secondary to DO, 6/10 patients had improvement in incontinence episodes and increased bladder capacity and compliance [10]. There is not adequate evidence to recommend routine use of tricyclic antidepressants in patients with OAB, but they can be considered as an option for patients unable to tolerate other agents [8].

Alpha-Adrenergic Receptor Antagonists

Alpha-adrenergic receptor antagonists are extremely effective medications for lower urinary tract symptoms caused by benign prostatic hypertrophy. Alpha 1A and 1D receptors are found predominantly in smooth muscle throughout the body, as well as in neural ganglia and the spinal cord. Activation of these G-protein-coupled receptors alters intracellular calcium content to cause muscle contraction. Targeted blocking of alpha 1A and 1D receptors in the lower urinary tract relaxes smooth muscle in the bladder neck and prostatic urethra, causing relief of obstructive symptoms with improvement of urine storage. The ubiquitous nature of these receptors accounts for generally rare but wide-ranging side effects of alpha-blockers including orthostatic hypotension, syncope, diarrhea, nausea, rhinitis, and intraoperative floppy iris syndrome [11]. These medications are especially effective in men with dual diagnoses of overactivity and lower urinary tract symptoms (LUTS) [12]. Several small RCTs have been performed in women to evaluate safety and efficacy of these medications in treating LUTS in women. A European RCT of women with at least 3 months of symptoms of OAB without stress or stress-predominant mixed incontinence or neurogenic DO compared efficacy of tamsulosin, an alpha-adrenergic receptor antagonist, tolterodine ER, and placebo [13]. After a washout period, 364 women were randomized to receive 1 of 4 doses of tamsulosin, 4 mg of tolterodine, or placebo for 6 weeks. The primary outcome measured was mean number of voids per 24 h. Secondary outcomes were mean volume per void, number of incontinence episodes, urgency episodes per 24 h, and quality of life. The study did not demonstrate any statistical difference in primary or secondary outcomes for the highest dose of tamsulosin or tolterodine compared to placebo. The lack of efficacy of tolterodine contradicts the findings of multiple prior studies, which calls into question the validity of this study. Another RCT investigated terazosin in a heterogeneous population of 83 women with International Prostate Symptom Score (IPSS) of 8 or higher seeking to measure a decrease in IPSS to less than 2 [14]. The study demonstrated improvement of IPSS scores that was statistically significant in the terazosin group. A recent meta-analysis identified 6 studies including 764 women that compared tamsulosin to placebo and prazosin or combination therapy with tolterodine [15]. Inclusion criteria were unfortunately too varied to recommend treatment with these agents, but the study did conclude that tamsulosin was safe and effective for the relief of lower urinary tract symptoms. Alpha-blockers are a promising and well-tolerated therapy, but there is not yet adequate evidence to recommend them as primary treatment of OAB particularly in females [8].

Phosphodiesterase Inhibitors

Phosphodiesterase inhibitors (PDE-Is) have a primary indication for treating erectile dysfunction. Drugs that target PDE-5 prevent the breakdown of cGMP resulting in smooth muscle relaxation and vasodilation, thereby facilitating erection. There are many PDE receptors in the bladder suggesting a role for PDE-Is in the management of OAB [16]. Initial interest in using the drugs for treatment of the bladder began in men with benign prostatic hypertrophy and LUTS. A study of tadalafil showed improvement in LUTS with significant reductions in detrusor overactivity on urodynamic assessment and moderate increases in bladder capacity [17]. Recently, the drug has been studied in women with OAB in a randomized, double-blind, placebo-controlled trial [18]. Ninety-six women were assigned to receive low-dose tadalafil or placebo for 3 months. Significant improvements were noted in patient-reported urgency, frequency, incontinence episodes, and bladder capacity ($p < 0.05$) starting at the fourth week of therapy with very low rates of adverse effects and excellent compliance. This single institution study lacked objective measures of OAB improvement and did not compare tadalafil to first-line therapy.

A small pilot study evaluated the effect of vinpocetine, a PDE-1 inhibitor, on patients who had not responded to standard therapy for OAB [19]. The cohort included patients with urgency/urge incontinence or low-compliance bladder and administered the study drug for 4 weeks with a dose increase after 2 weeks if there was no initial response. Over half the patients had symptomatic improvement, 3/19 (15.8%) with slight improvement and 8/19 (42.1%) with pronounced improvement. In the 11 patients that responded, there was a significant decrease in daytime and nighttime frequency of micturition and number of pads ($p < 0.001$, $p < 0.05$). While PDE-Is merit follow-up with larger, controlled studies with composite outcome measures, given the promising results in these trials, they are considered a recommended option by the ICI [8].

Drugs Acting on Membrane Channels

Calcium and potassium channels mediate bladder contraction and are potential therapeutic targets for pathological bladder activity [20]. Keeping potassium channels open would theoretically decrease detrusor excitability and contractility, thereby decreasing symptoms of OAB. A potassium channel opener was developed and tested in a double-blind RCT [21]. The study drug was administered to 299 women for 12 weeks who had documented frequency and urgency and had failed first-line therapy. Unfortunately, patients on the study drug did not demonstrate increase of voided volume, decrease in voiding episodes, and incontinence episodes or pad use, and did not have improvement in quality of life. The drug was well tolerated in this trial, but there is a concern that higher doses could precipitate hypotension due to the presence of potassium channels on vascular smooth muscle. Potassium channel openers are not recommended for OAB treatment based on good-quality available evidence [8].

In vivo and in vitro animal studies demonstrated that activation of vitamin D-3 receptors in bladder smooth muscle downregulates calcium channel sensitization, thereby decreasing spontaneous detrusor contractions. Elocalcitol is a synthetic vitamin D analog that was tested in a RCT of 308 women with urodynamic confirmed OAB [22]. The study did not meet the primary endpoint of increasing volume at first involuntary detrusor contraction but did significantly decrease incontinence episodes ($p = 0.02$) and showed improvement in Patient's Perception of Bladder Condition score ($p = 0.02$). Adverse effects attributable to the agent occurred in 11.7% of the study population and were mild, most commonly nausea, constipation, infection, migraine, and drowsiness. Despite the equivocal results, the drug had some effect on detrusor relaxation, so it may ultimately have a potential role in treatment of OAB in the future.

Anticonvulsants

Targeting the spinal micturition reflex pathway has led to interest in neurologic medications as potential treatments for OAB. Gabapentin is a drug used as an anticonvulsant and analgesic that is well tolerated by patients. Despite its name and chemical structure, the drug does not interact with GABA receptors or alter GABA levels but rather inhibits C-fiber nerves that are implicated in some types of dysfunctional detrusor activity [23]. Gabapentin was administered to 31 patients who had symptoms of OAB or nocturia that had not resolved with tolterodine or oxybutynin [23]. The study population was heterogeneous including 12 women with multiple sclerosis and 10 men who had previously undergone surgery for BPH. All patients continued their prior medication regimens throughout the trial. There was subjective symptom improvement in 45% of patients (14/31) with objective decrease in frequency (14.1 voids/day to 10.0 voids/day, $p = 0.01$). Another study evaluated 16 patients (15 men and 1 woman) with neurogenic OAB [24]. After 31 days of gabapentin administration, there was subjective improvement in frequency, urgency, and incontinence episodes (IPSS score 14.8 vs 8.8, $p = 0.023$), increased volume at first desire to void (121 ml vs 140 ml, $p = 0.021$), increased bladder capacity (342 ml vs 430 ml, $p = 0.05$), and decreased detrusor contractions on urodynamic evaluation (resolution in 4/16, higher volume in remaining patients). Based on these results, a double-blind RCT was performed comparing gabapentin to solifenacin and placebo [25]. Ninety-four patients with overactive bladder symptoms and bother were randomized to each treatment group for 12 weeks. The study showed significant improvement in frequency and urgency and an increase in volume voided as well as improved quality of life scores in both the gabapentin and solifenacin groups compared to placebo ($p < 0.001$). Nocturia was improved in the gabapentin group, and solifenacin increased volume per void, but the drugs were otherwise comparable. In this study gabapentin was equally efficacious as a first-line treatment option and may be an excellent and titratable alternative for patients unable to tolerate other medications.

Pregabalin has a similar mechanism to gabapentin but has higher bioavailability. Pregabalin is a federal category V controlled substance which may limit quantity and duration and which practitioners can prescribe the medication in some states [26]. Pregabalin was compared to tolterodine, in combination with tolterodine, and to placebo in women with idiopathic OAB [27]. In this study, pregabalin alone and in combination with tolterodine significantly increased mean volume voided, decreased frequency, and improved OAB-related bother scores and quality of life measures ($p < 0.028$). Patients receiving pregabalin did report more frequent moderate adverse events including dry mouth and dizziness that resulted in treatment discontinuation. Exploratory analysis did not reveal synergy of the two study medications.

Baclofen is a GABA agonist that is effective in downregulating spinal nervous activity and is used for patients with spastic neurologic disorders. After pilot studies that demonstrated a potential calming effect on involuntary detrusor contractions, a small randomized crossover trial was performed in patients with overactive bladder in 1979 [28]. Though patients on baclofen did demonstrate improvement in day- and nighttime frequency, pad use, and subjective symptom score, there was also a strong response to placebo tempering the overall results of the study. In a study of patients with dysfunctional voiding, baclofen was found to decrease voiding frequency [29]. To our knowledge no recent studies have tested baclofen in patients with OAB, but it is a treatment option for patients with incontinence based on limited evidence [8]. Other medications with similar mechanisms including a selective GABA agonist, lamotrigine, and opioids have had promising results in animal studies, but no human studies have been published to our knowledge [30, 31].

Neurokinin Receptor Antagonists

Neurokinin (NK) receptor antagonists were initially developed as treatment for depression, migraines, and chemotherapy-induced nausea. The agents have sparked interest in urology due to the role of tachykinins in the micturition reflex and in pathologic bladder contraction [32]. Aprepitant was investigated in a randomized trial of 125 women with urge urinary incontinence (UUI) [33]. Patients randomized to aprepitant were found to have a 10% decrease in frequency (−1.3 events/day, $p = 0.019$) and significantly fewer daily urgency episodes (−1.2 events/day, $p = 0.007$) though there was no effect on incontinence episodes. Patients also experienced subjective symptom improvement and decreased bother compared to placebo, but no difference in quality of life. Of note, four patients in the aprepitant group suffered serious clinical adverse effects resulting in discontinuation of the drug, and mild-moderate drug-related adverse effects were more frequent in the treatment group.

Serlopitant, which has highest affinity for the NK-1 receptor, was tested at multiple doses in comparison to tolterodine and placebo in a multicenter, randomized trial of 557 patients with OAB [34]. Both serlopitant and tolterodine significantly decreased urinary frequency compared to placebo (−1.1, −1.5, −0.5 micturitions/day, respectively). Serlopitant did not improve urgency episodes. Neupitant, another NK-1 selective agent, failed to demonstrate superiority compared to placebo in a randomized study of 325 patients with OAB [35]. Despite having some effect on urinary frequency, the results of these studies suggest NK receptor antagonists are less effective than current first-line therapy.

Cizolirtine acts via the tachykinin pathway, which is related to the NK-1 pathway. The drug decreases release of substance-P and thereby is expected to inhibit the sensory pathways involved in detrusor overactivity [36]. To examine its efficacy in OAB, cizolirtine was compared to oxybutynin and placebo in a phase II randomized, double-blind trial. Cizolirtine and oxybutynin both significantly reduced daily voids, urgency, and increased volume voided compared to placebo ($p < 0.002$). Cizolirtine also showed significant improvement in urodynamic parameters. Reported adverse effects were comparable between groups, but significantly more patients withdrew from the cizolirtine arm of the study secondary to side effects including gastrointestinal upset, vertigo, and headache. This study suggests a potential role for tachykinin-moderating drugs in the treatment of OAB.

Other Agents

Prostaglandins (PG) have been implicated in multiple studies for their role in bladder function via afferent signaling. Patients with OAB have been found to have higher urinary levels of PGE2, and OAB can be induced in normal subjects with intravesical instillation of PGE2 [37]. An EP1-receptor antagonist, ONO-8539, was developed to target this pathway by suppressing the effect of PGE2. Despite performing well in preclinical studies, this drug failed to decrease daily micturitions, urgency, and volumes per void compared to tolterodine and placebo in phase II trials.

Cannabinoids have been studied as a potential treatment for OAB. Cannabinoid-specific receptors have been found in the bladder, and activation decreases excitatory and increases inhibitory neurotransmitters, thereby relieving overactivity in animal models. Agents have been trialed in patients with OAB secondary to multiple sclerosis (MS). In a randomized controlled trial of nabiximol, a cannabinoid oromucosal spray, in patients with MS and OAB, the drug failed to meet the primary endpoint to reduce daily incontinence episodes [38]. However, there was a decrease in urgency, severity of incontinence episodes, and significant decrease in number of voids per day and subjective symptom scores. There were two reported serious adverse events. Patients in the treatment group experienced a low sense of intoxication that was comparable to the placebo group (mean 0.5 vs 0.4, scale 0–10). A small study assessing urodynamics of the same drug supported the finding of subjective improvement of symptom scores [39].

The higher prevalence of OAB in postmenopausal females suggests estrogen may have a role in OAB pathophysiology. A population-based study in Taiwan showed an adjusted hazard ratio of OAB development of 14.37 in estrogen-deprived women with breast cancer compared to non-estrogen-deprived controls [40]. However, several large epidemiologic studies have shown an association of systemic estrogen therapy with increased risk of OAB [41]. Local estrogen administration has more clearly shown positive effects on both subjective and objective measures of OAB including reduction of detrusor contractions, urgency, and frequency in meta-analyses and reviews [41]. The role and route of estrogen as a potential treatment or adjunct option remains promising but uncertain and is recommended as an option by the ICI based on limited evidence [8]. Two pilot studies investigating vaginal laser treatment in patients with vulvovaginal atrophy showed promising results with improvement of subjective and objective OAB measures [42, 43]. To our knowledge no RCTs have been performed using this treatment.

Intravesical Agents

Intravesical agents directly target the bladder mucosa and avoid systemic side effects that limit treatments but are more invasive and inconvenient than oral therapies. Intravesical chemodenervation agents such as onobotulinumtoxinA will be covered elsewhere.

Oxybutynin

Oxybutynin is an anticholinergic that is a first-line oral therapy for OAB but is not tolerated by many patients due to adverse effects. Intravesical preparations, which must be administered 2–3 times per day, have been explored to maximize clinical effect while decreasing systemic absorption owing to altered pharmacokinetics [44]. Intravesical oxybutynin was administered in a pilot study of 11 patients who previously had side effects to oral anticholinergics [45]. The ten patients who were able to tolerate intravesical infusion reported symptomatic improvement and demonstrated higher bladder capacity at lower pressure. The intravesical preparation outperformed oral oxybutynin in a recent randomized study of 35 patients with neurogenic detrusor overactivity demonstrating significantly increased bladder capacity (117 ml vs 18 ml, $p = 0.0086$) with lower rates of adverse effects (55.6% vs 82.4%) [46]. Studies in patients with non-neurogenic OAB have been mixed with subjective improvement in 50–82% of patients and consistently with few side effects [47]. Data in adult populations is limited, but this treatment is an option in patients comfortable with catheterization in order to perform the bladder instillations. A vaginal ring that releases oxybutynin is a promising alternative for female patients with OAB [48]. Phase II studies of this device showed significant improvement in frequency and incontinence episodes compared to placebo with similar rates of adverse effects; phase III studies are pending.

Atropine

Atropine is an inexpensive antimuscarinic agent that was found to be clinically ineffective in suppressing detrusor contractions when administered systemically due to significant side effects [49]. After successful animal studies with bladder instillation, an initial study was performed in 12 patients with OAB secondary to spinal cord injury. Although 5/12 patients were unable to tolerate intravesical infusion, the remaining patients had significantly increased bladder capacity (mean bladder capacity increase 301 ml, $p < 0.001$) and increased volumes at which detrusor contraction and leak occurred ($p < 0.05$) without experiencing side effects [49]. An increase in bladder capacity was confirmed in patients with OAB secondary to MS with better tolerance of intravesical therapy [50]. A double-blind, randomized, crossover study was performed comparing intravesical atropine 4 times per day to oral oxybutynin 3 times per day in 57 patients with MS. Results favored intravesical atropine with increase in bladder capacity (79.6 ± 89.6 ml vs 55.5 ± 67.2 ml, $p = 0.053$) and comparable rates of frequency and incontinence. Patients in the atropine arm had improvement in quality of life metrics and fewer anticholinergic side effects but were more likely to experience urinary retention compared to patients receiving oxybutynin [51]. Intravesical atropine can be considered in patients able to perform instillations based on limited evidence [8].

Anesthetics

Intravesical anesthetics have been researched in patients with interstitial cystitis but have had less success in patients with overactive bladder. The drugs depress afferent sensory nerves thereby allowing greater bladder relaxation and suppressing urge to void. In a study of patients with overactive bladder due to spinal cord injury or cerebrovascular disease, 20 ml of 1% or 4% lidocaine was administered intravesically and compared to saline control. The 4% solution was found to increase bladder capacity in patients with spinal cord injury >1 year significantly more than in patients with cerebrovascular disease and also to significantly decreased detrusor contractions.($p < 0.01$) [52]. Despite excellent effect in some patients without systemic absorption, the drugs have a short duration of action that has prevented routine use [44].

Vanilloids

In the healthy bladder, activation of vanilloid receptors via C-fiber afferent nerves results in detrusor contraction to expel noxious substances. In patients with spinal cord injury, there are changes in C-fiber density and response that create a new micturition reflex, which has also been implicated in the development of detrusor overactivity [53]. Intravesical administration of vanilloids desensitizes C-fibers after an initial irritating effect [54, 55]. This activity prompted research in the early 2000s on the use of intravesical capsaicin (CAP) and resiniferatoxin (RTX) in OAB. De Sèze et al. evaluated early studies of CAP and found considerable variation in doses administered but nevertheless determined there was improvement in patients with neurogenic DO with less benefit to idiopathic OAB [56]. A recent meta-analysis of vanilloids on patients with multiple sclerosis identified seven trials for consideration including four randomized controlled trials and three prospective cohort studies [54]. Meta-analysis revealed significant improvement in incontinence episodes and frequency. Several studies note that patients who respond can achieve complete continence and that a single infusion can have long-duration (6 months–1 year) effects with symptoms never returning to baseline severity [44]. A single study on RTX demonstrated improvement of bladder capacity and over 50% reduction in incontinence episodes. Unfortunately, adverse effects were reported by more than half of patients that may be partially due to the use of ethanol as the solvent. Studies of CAP in other solvents have had positive results [57].

A double-blind, randomized, controlled study compared CAP in a glucidic solvent to RTX in ethanol in patients with MS or spinal cord injury [53]. Both groups had considerable improvement in continence, frequency, and urgency (78% CAP, 80% RTX) with greater persistence of effects at 90 days in the RTX group. Side effects were temporary and tolerable but occurred in 42.9% of RTX patients and

72.2% of CAP patients. To our knowledge, no randomized studies have been performed evaluating vanilloids in patients with idiopathic OAB, but treatment with these agents can be an option based on good evidence [8].

NOP Receptor Agonists

Another target of the afferent micturition reflex pathway involved in OAB is the NOP receptor. Lazzeri et al. performed a series of studies testing nociceptin/orphanin FQ, which targets the NOP receptor, on patients with neurogenic detrusor overactivity. A pilot study in 2001 tested the intravesical infusion of nociceptin/orphanin FQ in five normal patients and nine patients with refractory OAB [58]. There was no effect on normal patients and a significant increase in bladder capacity and delay to detrusor contraction in patients with OAB. ($p < 0.05$) However, this effect did not persist on reevaluation at day 15. These findings were confirmed in a small randomized, controlled, double-blind study with no effect of the placebo solution on patients with neurogenic OAB [59]. More recently, the same group evaluated daily instillations in patients with neurogenic DO who perform CIC [60]. In addition to reaffirming the results of the first two studies, patients in the treatment group had significantly fewer incontinence episodes. To our knowledge NOP receptor agonists have not been tested in patients with non-neurogenic OAB.

Liposomes

Intravesical liposomes were found to decrease bladder hyperactivity in rats and have been studied as treatment for interstitial cystitis in humans [61]. Research in OAB has focused on the use of liposomes for drug delivery. Two contemporaneous studies compared the effect of intravesical liposomes containing botulinum toxin to normal saline on patients with OAB [62, 63]. Both studies found significant decreases in frequency and urgency without adverse effects of urinary retention or urinary tract infection.

Conclusions

Advancements in understanding normal bladder and micturition physiology and the pathophysiology of OAB have led to exploration of alternative systemic and targeted treatments. Many of these agents have been successful in randomized trials with improvements in symptoms, quality of life, and favorable side effect profiles. Despite positive results, many of these drugs are not used in routine practice and have not been compared to first-line agents. Successful treatment of patients who are refractory or intolerant to standard therapy requires further knowledge of the mechanisms and effects of these alternative agents.

References

1. Steers WD, Lee K. Depression and incontinence. World J Urol. 2001;19:351–7.
2. Kafri R, Kodesh A, Shames J, Golomb J, Melzer I. Depressive symptoms and treatment of women with urgency urinary incontinence. Int Urogynecol J. 2013;24:1953–9.
3. Millard RJ, Moore K, Rencken R, Yalcin I, Bump RC. Duloxetine vs placebo in the treatment of stress urinary incontinence: a four-continent randomized clinical trial. BJU Int. 2004;93(3):311–8.
4. Steers WD, Herschorn S, Kreder KJ, Moore K, Strohbehn K, Yalcin I, et al. Duloxetine compared with placebo for treating women with symptoms of overactive bladder. BJU Int. 2007;100(2):337–45.
5. Di Rezze S, Frasca V, Inghilleri M, Durastanti V, Cortese A, Giacomelli E, et al. Duloxetine for the treatment of overactive bladder syndrome in multiple sclerosis: a pilot study. Clin Neuropharmacol. 2012;35(5):231–4.
6. Efficacy and safety of selective serotonin reuptake inhibitor (SSRI) in overactive bladder patients [Internet]. National Library of Medicine 2009. Available from: https://clinicaltrials.gov/ct2/show/NCT00902421.
7. Besipirdine: Adis Insight Springer International; http://adisinsight.springer.com/drugs/800001339. Accessed 28 Apr 2018.
8. Andersson K-E, Cardozo L, Cruz F, Lee KS, Sahai A, Wein AJ. Incontinence. In: Abrams P, Cardozo L, Wagg A, Wein AJ, editors. Incontinence. 6th ed. Tokyo: International Consultation on Incontinence; 2016.
9. Kwon WA, Ahn SH, Oh TH, Lee JW, Han DY, Jeong HJ. Effect of low-dose triple therapy using gabapentin, amitriptyline, and a nonsteroidal anti-inflammatory drug for overactive bladder symptoms in patients with bladder pain syndrome. Int Neurourol J. 2013;17(2):78–82.
10. Cole AT, Fried FA. Favorable experiences with imipramine in the treatment of neurogenic bladder. J Urol. 1972;107(1):44–5.
11. Tamsulosin [Internet]. Truven Health Analytics, Inc. http://www.micromedexsolutions.com/. Accessed 9 Jan 2018.
12. Gacci M, Novara G, De Nunzio C, Tubaro A, Schiavina R, Brunocilla E, et al. Tolterodine extended release in the treatment of male OAB/storage luts: a systematic review. BMC Urol. 2014;14(1):84.
13. Robinson D, Cardozo L, Terpstra G, Bolodeoku J, Tamsulosin Study G. A randomized double-blind placebo-controlled multicentre study to explore the efficacy and safety of tamsulosin and tolterodine in women with overactive bladder syndrome. BJU Int. 2007;100(4):840–5.
14. Low BY, Liong ML, Yuen KH, Chee C, Leong WS, Chong WL, et al. Terazosin therapy for patients with female lower urinary tract symptoms: a randomized, double-blind, placebo controlled trial. J Urol. 2008;179(4):1461–9.
15. Zhang HL, Huang ZG, Qiu Y, Cheng X, Zou XQ, Liu TT. Tamsulosin for treatment of lower urinary tract symptoms in women: a systematic review and meta-analysis. Int J Impot Res. 2017;29(4):148–56.
16. Wein AJ, Kavoussi LR, Partin AW, Peters CA, editors. Campbell-Walsh urology. 11th ed. Philadelphia: Elsevier; 2016.
17. Matsukawa Y, Majima T, Matsuo K, Funahashi Y, Kato M, Yamamoto T, et al. Effects of tadalafil on storage and voiding function in patients with male lower urinary tract symptoms suggestive of benign prostatic hyperplasia: a urodynamic-based study. Int J Urol. 2017;198:905.

18. Chen H, Wang F, Yu Z, Zhang Y, Liu C, Dai S, et al. Efficacy of daily low-dose tadalafil for treating overactive bladder: results of a randomized, double-blind, placebo-controlled trial. Urology. 2017;100:59–64.
19. Truss MC, Stief CG, Ückert S, Becker AJ, Schultheiss D, Mchtens S, et al. Initial clinical experience with the selective phosphodiesterase-I isoenzyme inhibitor vinpocetine in the treatment of urge incontinence and low compliance bladder. World J Urol. 2000;18:439–43.
20. Darblade B, Behr-Roussel D, Oger S, Hieble JP, Lebret T, Gorny D, et al. Effects of potassium channel modulators on human detrusor smooth muscle myogenic phasic contractile activity: potential therapeutic targets for overactive bladder. Urology. 2006;68(2):442–8.
21. Chapple CR, Patroneva A, Raines SR. Effect of an ATP-sensitive potassium channel opener in subjects with overactive bladder: a randomized, double-blind, placebo-controlled study (ZD0947IL/0004). Eur Urol. 2006;49(5):879–86.
22. Digesu GA, Verdi E, Cardozo L, Olivieri L, Khullar V, Colli E. Phase IIb, multicenter, double-blind, randomized, placebo-controlled, parallel-group study to determine effects of elocalcitol in women with overactive bladder and idiopathic detrusor overactivity. Urology. 2012;80(1):48–54.
23. Kim YT, Kwon DD, Kim J, Kim DK, Lee JY, Chancellor MB. Gabapentin for overactive bladder and nocturia after anticholinergic failure. Int Braz J Urol. 2004;30(4):275–8.
24. Carbone A, Palleschi G, Conte A, Bova G, Iacovelli E, Bettolo CM, et al. Gabapentin treatment of neurogenic overactive bladder. Clin Neuropharmacol. 2006;29(4):206–14.
25. Chua ME, MCt S, Esmena EB, Balingit JC, Morales ML. Efficacy and safety of gabapentin in comparison to solifenacin succinate in adult overactive bladder treatment. Low Urin Tract Symptoms. 2017;10:135.
26. United State Department of Justice. Drug Enforcement Administration. Diversion Control Division. https://www.deadiversion.usdoj.gov/. Accessed 18 Apr 2018.
27. Marencak J, Cossons NH, Darekar A, Mills IW. Investigation of the clinical efficacy and safety of pregabalin alone or combined with tolterodine in female subjects with idiopathic overactive bladder. Neurourol Urodyn. 2011;30(1):75–82.
28. Taylor MC, Bates CP. A double-blind crossover trial of baclofen - a new treatment for the unstable bladder syndrome. BJU Int. 1979;51:504–5.
29. Xu D, Qu C, Meng H, Ren J, Zhu Y, Min Z, et al. Dysfunctional voiding confirmed by transdermal perineal electromyography, and its effective treatment with baclofen in women with lower urinary tract symptoms: a randomized double-blind placebo-controlled crossover trial. BJU Int. 2007;100(3):588–92.
30. Loutochin O, Afraa TA, Campeau L, Mahfouz W, Elzayat E, Corcos J. Effect of the anticonvulsant medications Pregabalin and lamotrigine on urodynamic parameters in an animal model of neurogenic detrusor overactivity. Neurourol Urodyn. 2012;31(7):1197–202.
31. Kalinichev M, Palea S, Haddouk H, Royer-Urios I, Guilloteau V, Lluel P, et al. ADX71441, a novel, potent and selective positive allosteric modulator of the GABA(B) receptor, shows efficacy in rodent models of overactive bladder. Br J Pharmacol. 2014;171(4):995–1006.
32. Lecci A, Maggi CA. Tachykinins as modulators of the micturition reflex in the central and peripheral nervous system. Regul Pept. 2001;101(1–3):1–18.
33. Green SA, Alon A, Ianus J, McNaughton KS, Tozzi CA, Reiss TF. Efficacy and safety of a neurokinin-1 receptor antagonist in postmenopausal women with overactive bladder with urge urinary incontinence. J Urol. 2006;176(6 Pt 1):2535–40. discussion 40.
34. Frenkl TL, Zhu H, Reiss T, Seltzer O, Rosenberg E, Green S. A multicenter, double-blind, randomized, placebo controlled trial of a neurokinin-1 receptor antagonist for overactive bladder. J Urol. 2010;184:616–22.
35. Haab F, Braticevici B, Krivoborodov G, Palmas M, Zufferli Russo M, Pietra C. Efficacy and safety of repeated dosing of netupitant, a neurokinin-1 receptor antagonist, in treating overactive bladder. Neurourol Urodyn. 2014;33(3):335–40.
36. Zat'ura F, Vsetica J, Abadias M, Pavlik I, Schraml P, Brod'ak M, et al. Cizolirtine citrate is safe and effective for treating urinary incontinence secondary to overactive bladder: a phase 2 proof-of-concept study. Eur Urol. 2010;57(1):145–52.

37. Chapple CR, Abrams P, Andersson KE, Radziszewski P, Masuda T, Small M, et al. Phase II study on the efficacy and safety of the EP1 receptor antagonist ONO-8539 for nonneurogenic overactive bladder syndrome. J Urol. 2014;191(1):253–60.
38. Kavia RB, De Ridder D, Constantinescu CS, Stott CG, Fowler CJ. Randomized controlled trial of Sativex to treat detrusor overactivity in multiple sclerosis. Mult Scler. 2010;16(11):1349–59.
39. Maniscalco GT, Aponte R, Bruzzese D, Guarcello G, Manzo V, Napolitano M, et al. THC/CBD oromucosal spray in patients with multiple sclerosis overactive bladder: a pilot prospective study. Neurol Sci. 2017;39:97.
40. Cheng CL, Li JR, Lin CH, de Groat WC. Positive association of female overactive bladder symptoms and estrogen deprivation: a nationwide population-based cohort study in Taiwan. Medicine (Baltimore). 2016;95(28):e4107.
41. Robinson D, Cardozo L, Milsom I, Pons ME, Kirby M, Koelbl H, et al. Oestrogens and overactive bladder. Neurourol Urodyn. 2014;33(7):1086–91.
42. Lin YH, Hsieh WC, Huang L, Liang CC. Effect of non-ablative laser treatment on overactive bladder symptoms, urinary incontinence and sexual function in women with urodynamic stress incontinence. Taiwan J Obstet Gynecol. 2017;56(6):815–20.
43. Perino A, Cucinella G, Gugliotta G, Saitta S, Polito S, Adile B, et al. Is vaginal fractional CO2 laser treatment effective in improving overactive bladder symptoms in post-menopausal patients? Preliminary results. Eur Rev Med Pharmacol Sci. 2016;20(12):2491–7.
44. Evans RJ. Intravesical therapy for overactive bladder. Curr Urol Rep. 2005;6:429–33.
45. Brendler CB, Radebaugh LC, Mohler JL. Topical oxybutynin chloride for relaxation of dysfunctional bladders. J Urol. 1989;141(6):1350–2.
46. Schröder A, Albrecht U, Schnitker J, Reitz A, Stein R. Efficacy, safety, and tolerability of intravesically administered 0.1% oxybutynin hydrochloride solution in adult patients with neurogenic bladder: a randomized, prospective, controlled multi-center trial. Neurourol Urodyn. 2016;35(5):582–8.
47. Lose G, Nørgaard JP. Intravesical oxybutynin for treating incontinence resulting from an overactive detrusor. BJU Int. 2001;87:767–73.
48. Gittelman M, Weiss H, Seidman L. A phase 2, randomized, double-blind, efficacy and safety study of oxybutynin vaginal ring for alleviation of overactive bladder symptoms in women. J Urol. 2014;191(4):1014–21.
49. Glickman S, Tsokkos N, Shah PJ. Intravesical atropine and suppression of detrusor hypercontractility in the neuropathic bladder. A preliminary study. Paraplegia. 1995;33(1):36–9.
50. Deaney C, Glickman S, Gluck T, Malone-Lee JG. Intravesical atropine suppression of detrusor hyperreflexia in multiple sclerosis. J Neurol Neurosurg Psychiatry. 1998;65(6):957.
51. Fader M, Glickman S, Haggar V, Barton R, Brooks R, Malone-Lee J. Intravesical atropine compared to oral oxybutynin for neurogenic detrusor overactivity: a double-blind, randomized crossover trial. J Urol. 2007;177(1):208–13. discussion 13.
52. Yokoyama O, Ishiura Y, Nakamura Y, Kunimi K, Mita E, Namiki M. Urodynamic effects of intravestical instiallation of lidocaine in patients with overactive detrusor. J Urol. 1997;157:1826–30.
53. de Seze M, Wiart L, de Seze MP, Soyeur L, Dosque JP, Blajezewski S, et al. Intravesical capsaicin versus resiniferatoxin for the treatment of detrusor hyperreflexia in spinal cord injured patients: a double-blind, randomized, controlled study. J Urol. 2004;171(1):251–5.
54. Phe V, Schneider MP, Peyronnet B, Abo Youssef N, Mordasini L, Chartier-Kastler E, et al. Intravesical vanilloids for treating neurogenic lower urinary tract dysfunction in patients with multiple sclerosis: a systematic review and meta-analysis. A report from the neuro-urology promotion Committee of the International Continence Society (ICS). Neurourol Urodyn. 2017;37:67.
55. De Ridder D, Baert L. Vanilloids and the overactive bladder. BJU Int. 2000;86:172–80.
56. de Seze M, Wiart L, Ferrière J, de Seze MP, Joseph PA, Barat M. Intravesical instillation of capsaicin in urology: a review of the literature. Eur Urol. 1999;36(4):267–177.
57. de Seze M, Gallien P, Denys P, Labat JJ, Serment G, Grise P, et al. Intravesical glucidic capsaicin versus glucidic solvent in neurogenic detrusor overactivity: a double blind controlled randomized study. Neurourol Urodyn. 2006;25(7):752–7.

58. Lazzeri M, Calo G, Spinelli M, Guerrini R, Beneforti P, Sandri S, et al. Urodynamic and clinical evidence of acute inhibitory effects of intravesical nociceptin/orphanin FQ on detrusor overactivity in humans: a pilot study. J Urol. 2001;166:2237–40.
59. Lazzeri M, Calò G, Spinelli M, Guerrini R, Salvadori S, Beneforti P, et al. Urodynamic effects of intravesical nociceptin/orphanin FQ in neurogenic detrusor overactivity: a randomized, placebo-controlled, double-blind study. Urology. 2003;61(5):946–50.
60. Lazzeri M, Calo G, Spinelli M, Malaguti S, Guerrini R, Salvadori S, et al. Daily intravesical instillation of 1 mg nociceptin/orphanin FQ for the control of neurogenic detrusor overactivity: a multicenter, placebo controlled, randomized exploratory study. J Urol. 2006;176(5):2098–102.
61. Tyagi P, Hsieh VC, Yoshimura N, Kaufman J, Chancellor MB. Instillation of liposomes vs dimethyl sulphoxide or pentosan polysulphate for reducing bladder hyperactivity. BJU Int. 2009;104(11):1689–92.
62. Chuang YC, Kaufmann JH, Chancellor DD, Chancellor MB, Kuo HC. Bladder instillation of liposome encapsulated onabotulinumtoxina improves overactive bladder symptoms: a prospective, multicenter, double-blind, randomized trial. J Urol. 2014;192(6):1743–9.
63. Kuo HC, Liu HT, Chuang YC, Birder LA, Chancellor MB. Pilot study of liposome-encapsulated onabotulinumtoxina for patients with overactive bladder: a single-center study. Eur Urol. 2014;65(6):1117–24.

Suggested Readings

Sacco E, Recupero S, Bientinesi R, Palermo G, D'Agostino D, Currò D, et al. Pioneering drugs for overactive bladder and detrusor overactivity: ongoing research and future directions. World J Obstet Gynecol. 2015;4(2):24–39.

Ellington DR, Szychowski JM, Malek JM, Gerten KA, Burgio KL, Richter HE. Combined tolterodine and vaginal estradiol cream for overactive bladder symptoms after randomized single-therapy treatment. Female Pelvic Med Reconstr Surg. 2016;22(4):254–60.

Sacco E, Bientinesi R. Innovative pharmacotherapies for women with overactive bladder: where are we now and what is in the pipeline? Int Urogynecol J. 2015;26(5):629–40.

Weber MA, Kleijn MH, Langendam M, Limpens J, Heineman MJ, Roovers JP. Local oestrogen for pelvic floor disorders: a systematic review. PLoS One. 2015;10(9):e0136265.

Chapter 13
Future Considerations in Overactive Bladder Pharmacotherapy

Karl-Erik Andersson

Background

The latest approved treatments of lower urinary tract syndrome (LUTS)/overactive bladder (OAB)—mirabegron, tadalafil, and botulinum toxin—are, together with antimuscarinics and α-adrenoceptor (AR) blockers, currently the most widely used treatments for both neurogenic and non-neurogenic LUTS/OAB [1]. Still, as monotherapies they are not effective in all patients, and new alternatives are continuously being explored. Even if much nonclinical and clinical research is ongoing, there seem to be few new principles in the pipeline. What can be expected in the future seems to be introduction of new additions to existing drug classes and combinations of existing options. However, new pharmacological principles, based on factors involved in OAB pathophysiology [1–6], may be developed. This review discusses what is currently ongoing in drug treatment of OAB/LUTS but also speculates, on the basis of promising preclinical and clinical data, what drugs can be expected to be introduced clinically within the next few years.

Drugs in the Pipeline

Antimuscarinics

Despite many different antimuscarinics being available and recommended for clinical use [1], there is still an interest in new developments [2]. Tarafenacin a novel potent antimuscarinic agent highly selective for M_3 over M_2 receptors [7], was

K.-E. Andersson
Institute of Laboratory Medicine, Lund University, Lund, Sweden
e-mail: karl-erik.andersson@med.lu.se

L. Cox, E. S. Rovner (eds.), *Contemporary Pharmacotherapy of Overactive Bladder*, https://doi.org/10.1007/978-3-319-97265-7_13

reported to have functional selectivity for the bladder over atrial tissues in the order of 200-fold in a mouse model. This may be of interest from a cardiac safety point of view. Song et al. [8] performed a multicenter, randomized controlled phase 2b trial on 235 OAB patients and showed that after 4 weeks tarafenacin at doses of 0.2 and 0.4 mg was superior to placebo in reducing the number of micturitions per day (primary endpoint). The drug showed a good safety profile, with very few cases of constipation. This may be surprising considering the profile of the highly M_3 receptor-selective darifenacin, which has constipation as a common adverse effect [1]. However, the most common side effect of tarafenacin was dry mouth, which at a dose of 0.4 mg occurred in 52 out of 76 randomized patients. It is therefore unlikely that this drug, even if proven efficacious in future studies, will offer any advantages over existing options [1, 9, 10]. OAB is a filling disorder, and even if it is well established that M_3 receptors are involved in detrusor muscle contraction, it is not necessarily by this mechanism that the beneficial effects on OAB symptoms are exerted [11].

To specifically reduce the adverse effect of tolterodine-induced dry mouth, THVD-201 (Tolenix™, twice-daily formulation) and THVD-202 (once-daily formulation) were designed. Both drugs are a combination of the muscarinic antagonist, tolterodine, with modified-release formulations of the muscarinic receptor agonist, pilocarpine, as a salivary stimulant. THVD-202 is advancing into phase 3 studies (Clinicaltrials.gov). The combination of tolterodine and pilocarpine has demonstrated efficacy comparable to twice-daily tolterodine; however, the combination showed statistically significant and clinically meaningful improvements in saliva production and dry mouth, as compared to the active-control tolterodine [12]. It is possible, but has to be demonstrated in further trials, that this advantage over tolterodine alone will be sufficient to motivate marketing of the drug.

β_3-Adrenoceptor Agonists

β_3-adrenoceptor (AR) agonists have generally been considered to improve OAB symptoms by relaxing the detrusor muscle, inhibiting spontaneous contractile activity in the detrusor, and reducing bladder afferent activity [13–15]. For example, Aizawa et al. [16] showed that single-unit afferent activities (SAAs) of both Aδ-fibers and C-fibers in response to bladder filling significantly dose-dependently decreased after mirabegron administration, the effect being more conspicuous for Aδ-fibers. During isovolumetric bladder conditions, the mean bladder pressure and the number of microcontractions decreased after mirabegron administration, whereas these parameters did not change with oxybutynin administration. However, recent evidence suggests that in addition to a direct effect on the smooth muscle, activation of prejunctional β_3-AR may result in downregulation of ACh released from cholinergic terminals, thereby exerting an additional inhibitory control of parasympathetic activity [17–20].

In addition to the only marketed β_3-AR agonist, mirabegron, there are reports on other β_3-AR agonists in development, e.g., ritobegron and solabegron. A phase 3 randomized, double-blind, placebo-controlled study of ritobegron in patients with OAB has been initiated and completed, but the results of this study have not been published, and a press release by the pharmaceutical company stated that preliminary analysis indicated that the study's primary efficacy endpoint was not met.

Efficacy and safety of solabegron (GW427353) have been recently reported in a phase 2 multicenter, randomized, proof-of-concept trial in 258 women with wet OAB [21]. Solabegron was well tolerated and at the dose of 125 mg produced a statistically significant difference in percent change from baseline to week 8 in incontinence episodes over 24 h (primary outcome) when compared with placebo ($p = 0.025$) [21]. Further studies are awaited.

There have been many early investigations of other novel and putative β_3-AR agonists for management of OAB, including CL-316243, TRK-380, AJ-9677, and BRL-37344 [22]. These agents have been reported as being in development, but no clinical data have been published. Thus, even if there are several β_3-AR agonists in the pipeline, it is uncertain which, if any, will come to market and be available for the management of OAB. A new agent, vibegron [23, 24], is a potent, selective full β_3-AR agonist across species, and it dose-dependently increased bladder capacity, decreased micturition pressure, and increased bladder compliance in rhesus monkeys [24]. The relaxation effect of vibegron was enhanced when combined with muscarinic receptor antagonists but differentially influenced by muscarinic receptor subtype selectivity. The effect was greater when vibegron was co-administered with tolterodine (nonselective antagonist), compared with co-administration with darifenacin (selective M3 receptor antagonist). Furthermore, a synergistic effect for bladder strip relaxation was observed with the combination of a β_3-AR agonist and tolterodine in contrast to simple additivity with darifenacin. The authors speculated that combination of β_3-AR agonists with non-receptor-selective antimuscarinics has the potential to redefine the standard of care for the pharmacological treatment of OAB. Yoshida et al. [25] performed a randomized, double-blind, placebo-controlled phase 3 study on 1232 patients, who were assigned to one of four 12-week treatment groups: vibegron (50 mg or 100 mg once daily), placebo, or imidafenacin (0.1 mg twice daily). The primary endpoint was change in the mean number of micturitions per day at week 12 from baseline, and secondary endpoints were changes from baselines in OAB symptom variables (daily episodes of urgency, urgency incontinence, incontinence, and nocturia and voided volume per micturition). The proportions of patients with normalization of micturition and resolution of urgency, urgency incontinence, and incontinence were significantly greater with vibegron than with placebo. Vibegron also significantly improved the quality of life (QoL), with high patient satisfaction. Incidences of drug-related adverse events with vibegron 50 mg and 100 mg were 7.6% and 5.4%, similar to placebo (5.1%) and less than with imidafenacin (10.3%). Since the duration of the study was just 12 weeks, a long-term study is needed to establish efficacy compared with other alternatives.

Even if several β_3-AR agonists have been reported as being in development, no clinical data have been published, except for solabegron and vibegron. Whether any of these agents will come to market and be available for the management of OAB remains to be established.

Botulinum Toxin A

Botulinum toxin A (BoNT-A) is a high-molecular-weight (150 kDa) neurotoxin that may not be able to gain access to the afferent nerves located immediately below the urothelium without needle injection. To improve intravesical treatment with botulinum toxins, novel therapeutic uses and formulations have been reported [26, 27]. New formulations seek to improve bioavailability at the site of action while decreasing adverse events, and several new approaches have been tested in animal models and, to some extent, in patients (e.g., increasing urothelial permeability with DMSO or protamine sulfate pretreatment, iontophoresis, low-energy shock waves, thermosensitive hydrogels and liposomes) [28].

One of the most promising approaches seems to be liposome-based [29]. Liposomes are vesicles composed of concentric phospholipid bilayers separated by aqueous compartments. Because they adsorb onto cell surfaces and fuse with cells, they are being used as vehicles for drug delivery and gene therapy. In order to have the therapeutic effects of BoNT-A on the urothelial afferent nerves without impairing detrusor contractility and to improve patients' acceptability of the treatment by overcoming the adverse effects of the cystoscope-guided needle injections, studies are ongoing exploring if liquid liposomes may deliver BoNT-A (liposome-encapsulated BoNT-A or lipotoxin) through the urothelium to the suburothelial space. In a rat model, intravesical lipotoxin cleaved SNAP-25, inhibited calcitonin gene-related peptide release from afferent nerve terminals, and blocked acetic acid-induced DO [30]. Kuo et al. [31] performed a study on 24 patients with OAB, who were nonresponsive to >3 months of therapy with traditional antimuscarinic agents. They were randomized 1:1 to receive intravesical instillation of lipotoxin or saline solution. In the lipotoxin group, 3-day urinary frequency and urgency episodes were significantly decreased at 1 month, whereas no change was reported in the control group. Importantly, no urinary tract infections or large post-void residual volumes were reported. However, only 50% of the 12 patients initially treated with lipotoxin showed a response, and only 4 had a maintained response at 3 months. Furthermore, of 12 non-responders who were subsequently treated or retreated with lipotoxin (6 from each cohort), only 1 showed a response at 3 months. Moreover, no change in urgency incontinence was found in either group, although the median baseline frequency of incontinence episodes was only 0.5 events in the lipotoxin cohort.

Chuang et al. [32] performed a prospective, multicenter, double-blind, randomized trial on 62 OAB patients inadequately managed with antimuscarinics. At 4 weeks after treatment, lipo-botulinum toxin instillation was associated with a statistically significant decrease in micturition events per 3 days and with a statistically significant decrease in urinary urgency events with respect to baseline, but not placebo. There were no statistically significant decrease in urgency severity scores compared to placebo and no increased risk of urinary retention. However, the effects of lipo-botulinum toxin on urinary urgency incontinence were inconclusive.

The combination of genetic engineering and molecular biology techniques has enabled the possibility of developing recombinant biotherapeutic proteins incorporating the light chain (endopeptidase) and the HN translocation domain of BoNT, combined with a binding domain that binds to a specific target represented by a cell surface receptor [33]. A novel-targeted BoNT-A has already completed phase 1 studies and entered proof-of-concept phase 2 studies in postherpetic neuralgia and idiopathic OAB.

Despite mildly encouraging preclinical results, significant technology refinement and clinical testing will be required in order to define the safety and efficacy profile of new BoNT formulations and engineered variants.

Combinations

Treatment of disorders with multifactorial pathophysiology with combinations of drugs seems to be a logical approach—not only can more than one underlying mechanism be influenced (if the drugs have different mechanisms of action), but also the doses of drugs can be kept low making it possible to reduce the number of side effects. LUTS/OAB in both men and women is multifactorial, and there are many examples that combined treatment can be superior to monotherapy [1]. However, which combination should be given to which patients? How much can be gained? Is there really a cost/benefit in combining currently approved drugs with respect to efficacy and side effects, or is the field open for introduction of "minor players," i.e., drugs with some efficacy, but not efficacious enough to be given as monotherapy? A variety of such combinations have been evaluated. Several randomized, controlled trials demonstrated that the combination treatment of antimuscarinic drugs and α_1-AR antagonists was more effective at reducing LUTS than α_1-AR antagonists alone in men with OAB and coexisting BPO [1, 33–42].

A large-scale, multicenter, randomized, double-blind, placebo-controlled trial (the TIMES study) demonstrated the efficacy and safety of tolterodine ER alone, tamsulosin alone, and the combination of both in 879 men with OAB and BPO [33]. In the primary efficacy analysis, 172 men (80%) receiving tolterodine ER plus tamsulosin reported treatment benefits by week 12. In the secondary efficacy analysis, patients receiving tolterodine ER plus tamsulosin compared with placebo experienced small but significant reductions in urgency incontinence, urgency episodes, daytime frequency, and nocturia. However, there were no significant differences between tamsulosin monotherapy and placebo for any diary variables at week 12. Patients receiving tolterodine ER plus tamsulosin demonstrated significant improvements in total IPSS.

The efficacy and safety of solifenacin in combination with tamsulosin were assessed in several large-scale RCTs, including the VICTOR [35], SATURN [36], and NEPTUNE [37] trials. Based on these studies, it may be concluded that the combination of antimuscarinics and α_1-AR antagonists may be the most effective therapy in men with OAB symptoms in the presence of BPO.

Abrams et al. [38] reported results of a phase 2 trial (Symphony) of combination treatment with mirabegron and solifenacin in 1306 patients with OAB. The primary endpoint was change from baseline to end of treatment in mean volume voided per micturition (MVV). The drug combinations solifenacin 5 mg plus mirabegron 50 mg, solifenacin 10 mg plus mirabegron 25 mg, and solifenacin 10 mg plus mirabegron 50 mg demonstrated significant improvements compared to both solifenacin 5 mg and placebo. No severe adverse events were reported, and treatment was generally well tolerated. Similar results were obtained by Yamaguchi et al. [37] in a multicenter, open-label, phase 4 study (MILAI study) to assess the safety and efficacy of mirabegron in combination with solifenacin in OAB patients who were being treated with solifenacin 2.5 mg or 5 mg once daily for at least 4 weeks [37] and by Drake et al. [39–41] in a phase 3b trial (BESIDE) in incontinent OAB patients. Xu et al. [42] performing a meta-analysis to evaluate the efficacy and safety of mirabegron add-on therapy to solifenacin for patients with OAB concluded that mirabegron therapy as an add-on to solifenacin provides a satisfactory therapeutic effect for OAB symptoms with a low occurrence of side effects.

Although antimuscarinic agents are the first choice of treatment for patients with OAB symptoms, these drugs do not always lead to the desired effect of detrusor stability and continence. A combined antimuscarinic regimen was evaluated as a noninvasive alternative by Amend et al. [43] for patients who had neurogenic bladder dysfunction with incontinence, reduced bladder capacity, and increased intravesical pressure. They added secondary antimuscarinics to the existing double-dose antimuscarinics for patients who previously demonstrated unsatisfactory outcomes with double-dose antimuscarinic monotherapy. The study drugs were tolterodine, oxybutynin, and trospium. After a 4-week combined regimen, incontinence episodes decreased, and reflex volume, maximal bladder capacity, and detrusor compliance increased. Side effects were comparable to those seen with normal-dose antimuscarinics. Kosilov et al. [44–46] evaluated the effectiveness of cyclic therapy of combined high-dose trospium and solifenacin depending on severity of OAB symptoms in elderly men and women. They found that this therapy of high-dose solifenacin and trospium in elderly patients with moderate or severe symptoms of OAB enabled patients to maintain a longer therapeutic effect with an acceptable level of side effects [44]. The effectiveness of combination therapy with two different antimuscarinics was also evaluated in patients with severe symptoms of OAB and BPH [46, 47]. Patients in the experimental group for 2 months received treatment with a daily combination of solifenacin 5 mg and trospium 5 mg simultaneous with tamsulosin 0.4 mg. Patients in the control group were treated only with tamsulosin. The authors concluded that combination of trospium and solifenacin in standard doses is an efficient and safe method for managing severe symptoms of OAB over the course of treatment with tamsulosin in patients with OAB/BPH [47].

However, in patients with OAB/BPH, the efficacy and side effects of combination therapy using different antimuscarinics should be further evaluated.

Based on available results, it may be concluded that combined regimens are logical and seem to be effective when monotherapy fails. However, combinations need further investigation to verify their efficacy and cost/benefit as noninvasive alternatives to third-line treatments.

Agents for Possible Future Development

As described above, animal studies and preclinical and clinical research involving modifications of existing options or directed at identifying novel pharmacological principles involved in LUTS/OAB pathophysiology are ongoing. This has been extensively discussed in several reviews [1–6]. Based on published information, the International Consultation on Incontinence (ICI) classified drugs in development depending on negative or positive proof-of-concept studies or as promising based on animal data (Table 13.1) [1]. Currently, the most promising targets seem to be purinergic receptors [48–51] and different members of the TRP channel family [52–55]. However, even if P2X3receptor antagonists have a good rationale and are currently being developed for treatment of nonbladder diseases, clinical experiences in bladder disorders have not yet been reported. Several TRP channels, including TRPV1, TRPV2, TRPV4, TRPM8, and TRPA1, are expressed in the bladder and urethra and may act as sensors of stretch and/or chemical irritation. There seem to be several links between activation of these channels and LUTS/OAB, and the therapeutic potential for TRPV1 channel agonists (capsaicin, resiniferatoxin), which

Table 13.1 Current status of possible future drugs/targets [1]

Negative proof of concept
Potassium channel openers
Prostaglandin receptor antagonists
Positive proof of concept
Neurokinin receptor antagonists
Vitamin D3 receptor agonists
Monoamine reuptake inhibitors
Opioid receptor agonists
Cox inhibitors
Promising based on animal data
Rho-kinase inhibitors
Drugs acting on GABA receptors
Purinergic system—P2X3 receptor antagonists
Cannabinoid system—exocannabinoids, FAAH inhibitors
TRP channel family—TRP channel antagonists

FAAH fatty acid amide hydrolase, *TRP* transient receptor potential inactivate the channel, has been convincingly demonstrated. Several TRP channel antagonists are in clinical development for nonbladder indications [55]. However, published clinical experiences in lower urinary tract (LUT) dysfunction are scarce, and the adverse effect of hyperthermia of the first-generation TRPV1 antagonists has delayed development. Nevertheless, TRP channels still may be most exciting targets for future LUT drugs.

References

1. Andersson KE, Cardozo L, Cruz F, Lee K-S, Suhai A, Wein AJ. Pharmacological treatment of urinary incontinence. In: Abrams P, Cardozo L, Wagg A, Wein AJ, editors. Incontinence. 6th ed. Bristol: ICI-ICS. International Continence Society; 2017. p. 805–957.
2. Yeo EK, Hashim H, Abrams P. New therapies in the treatment of overactive bladder. Expert Opin Emerg Drugs. 2013;18(3):319–37.
3. Zacche MM, Giarenis I, Cardozo L. Phase II drugs that target cholinergic receptors for the treatment of overactive bladder. Expert Opin Investig Drugs. 2014;23(10):1365–74.
4. Bechis SK, Kim MM, Wintner A, Kreydin EI. Differential response to medical therapy for male lower urinary tract symptoms. Curr Bladder Dysfunct Rep. 2015;10:177–85.
5. Sacco E, Bientinesi R. Innovative pharmacotherapies for women with overactive bladder: where are we now and what is in the pipeline? Int Urogynecol J. 2015;26(5):629–40.
6. Andersson KE. Potential future pharmacological treatment of bladder dysfunction. Basic Clin Pharmacol Toxicol. 2016;119(Suppl 3):75–85.
7. Salcedo C, Davalillo S, Cabellos J, Lagunas C, Balsa D, Pérez-Del-Pulgar S, et al. In vivo and in vitro pharmacological characterization of SVT-40776, a novel M3 muscarinic receptor antagonist, for the treatment of overactive bladder. Br J Pharmacol. 2009;156(5):807–17.
8. Song M, Kim JH, Lee KS, Lee JZ, Oh SJ, Seo JT, et al. The efficacy and tolerability of tarafenacin, a new muscarinic acetylcholine receptor M3 antagonist in patients with overactive bladder; randomised, double-blind, placebo-controlled phase 2 study. Int J Clin Pract. 2015;69(2):242–50.
9. Madhuvrata P, Cody JD, Ellis G, Herbison GP, Hay-Smith EJ. Which anticholinergic drug for overactive bladder symptoms in adults. Cochrane Database Syst Rev. 2012;1:CD005429.
10. Sebastianelli A, Russo GI, Kaplan SA, McVary KT, Moncada I, Gravas S, et al. Systematic review and meta-analysis on the efficacy and tolerability of mirabegron for the treatment of storage lower urinary tract symptoms/overactive bladder: comparison with placebo and tolterodine. Int J Urol. 2018;25(3):196–205.
11. Michel MC, Igawa Y. Therapeutic targets for overactive bladder other than smooth muscle. Expert Opin Ther Targets. 2015;19(5):687–705.
12. Dmochowski RR, Staskin DR, Duchin K, et al. Clinical safety, tolerability and efficacy of combination tolterodine/pilocarpine in patients with overactive bladder. Int J Clin Pract. 2014;68(8):986–94.
13. Biers SM, Reynard JM, Brading AF. The effects of a new selective beta3-adrenoceptor agonist (GW427353) on spontaneous activity and detrusor relaxation in human bladder. BJU Int. 2006;98(6):1310–4.
14. Andersson KE, Martin N, Nitti V. Selective β3-adrenoceptor agonists for the treatment of overactive bladder. J Urol. 2013;190(4):1173–8.
15. Igawa Y, Michel MC. Pharmacological profile of β3-adrenoceptor agonists in clinical development for the treatment of overactive bladder syndrome. Naunyn Schmiedeberg's Arch Pharmacol. 2013;386(3):177–83.

16. Aizawa N, Homma Y, Igawa Y. Effects of mirabegron, a novel β3-adrenoceptor agonist, on primary bladder afferent activity and bladder microcontractions in rats compared with the effects of oxybutynin. Eur Urol. 2012;62(6):1165–73.
17. Rouget C, Rekik M, Camparo P, Botto H, Rischmann P, Lluel P, et al. Modulation of nerve-evoked contractions by β3-adrenoceptor agonism in human and rat isolated urinary bladder. Pharmacol Res. 2014;80:14–20.
18. D' Agostino G, Maria Condino A, Calvi P. Involvement of β3- adrenoceptors in the inhibitory control of cholinergic activity in human bladder: direct evidence by [(3)H]-acetylcholine release experiments in the isolated detrusor. Eur J Pharmacol. 2015;758:115–22.
19. Gillespie JI, Rouget C, Palea S, Granato C, Korstanje C. Beta adrenergic modulation of spontaneous microcontractions and electrical field-stimulated contractions in isolated strips of rat urinary bladder from normal animals and animals with partial bladder outflow obstruction. Naunyn Schmiedeberg's Arch Pharmacol. 2015;388:719–26.
20. Andersson KE. On the site and mechanism of action of β3-adrenoceptor agonists in the bladder. Int Neurourol J. 2017;21(1):6–11.
21. Ohlstein EH, von Keitz A, Michel MC. A multicenter, double-blind, randomized, placebo-controlled trial of the β3-adrenoceptor agonist solabegron for overactive bladder. Eur Urol. 2012;62(5):834–40.
22. Thiagamoorthy G, Giarenis I, Cardozo L. Early investigational β3 adreno-receptor agonists for the management of the overactive bladder syndrome. Expert Opin Investig Drugs. 2015;24(10):1299–306.
23. Edmondson SD, Zhu C, Kar NF, Di Salvo J, Nagabukuro H, et al. Discovery of vibegron: a potent and selective β3 adrenergic receptor agonist for the treatment of overactive bladder. J Med Chem. 2016;59(2):609–23.
24. Di Salvo J, Nagabukuro H, Wickham LA, et al. Pharmacological characterization of a novel beta 3 adrenergic agonist, vibegron: evaluation of antimuscarinic receptor selectivity for combination therapy for overactive bladder. J Pharmacol Exp Ther. 2017;360(2):346–55.
25. Yoshida M, Takeda M, Gotoh M, Nagai S, Kurose T. Vibegron, a novel potent and selective β3-adrenoreceptor agonist, for the treatment of patients with overactive bladder: a randomized, double-blind, placebo-controlled phase 3 study. Eur Urol. 2018;73(5):783–90.
26. Edupuganti OP, Ovsepian SV, Wang J, Zurawski TH, Schmidt JJ, Smith L, et al. Targeted delivery into motor nerve terminals of inhibitors for SNARE-cleaving proteases via liposomes coupled to an atoxic botulinum neurotoxin. FEBS J. 2012;279(14):2555–67.
27. Kane CD, Nuss JE, Bavari S. Novel therapeutic uses and formulations of botulinum neurotoxins: a patent review (2012 - 2014). Expert Opin Ther Pat. 2015;25(6):675–90.
28. Tyagi P, Kashyap M, Yoshimura N, Chancellor M, Chermansky CJ. Past, present and future of chemodenervation with botulinum toxin in the treatment of overactive bladder. J Urol. 2017;197(4):982.
29. Janicki JJ, Chancellor MB, Kaufman J, Gruber MA, Chancellor DD. Potential effect of liposomes and liposome/encapsulated botulinum toxin and tacrolimus in the treatment of bladder dysfunction. Toxins (Basel). 2016;8(3):81.
30. Chuang YC, Tyagi P, Huang CC, Yoshimura N, Wu M, Kaufman J, Chancellor MB. Urodynamic and immunohistochemical evaluation of intravesical botulinum toxin a delivery using liposomes. J Urol. 2009;182(2):786–92.
31. Kuo HC, Liu HT, Chuang YC, Birder LA, Chancellor MB. Pilot study of liposome-encapsulated onabotulinumtoxina for patients with overactive bladder: a single-center study. Eur Urol. 2014;65(6):1117–24.
32. Chuang YC, Kaufmann JH, Chancellor DD, Chancellor MB, Kuo HC. Bladder instillation of liposome encapsulated onabotulinumtoxina improves overactive bladder symptoms: a prospective, multicenter, double-blind, randomized trial. J Urol. 2014;192(6):1743–9.
33. Keith F, John C. Targeted secretion inhibitors-innovative protein therapeutics. Toxins (Basel). 2010;2(12):2795–815.

34. Kaplan SA, Roehrborn CG, Rovner ES, Carlsson M, Bavendam T, Guan Z. Tolterodine and tamsulosin for treatment of men with lower urinary tract symptoms and overactive bladder: a randomized controlled trial. JAMA. 2006;296(19):2319.
35. Kaplan SA, He W, Koltun WD, Cummings J, Schneider T, Fakhoury A. Solifenacin plus tamsulosin combination treatment in men with lower urinary tract symptoms and bladder outlet obstruction: a randomized controlled trial. Eur Urol. 2013;63(1):158–65.
36. Van Kerrebroeck P, Haab F, Angulo JC. Efficacy and safety of solifenacin plus tamsulosin OCAS in men with voiding and storage lower urinary tract symptoms: results from a phase 2, dose-finding study (SATURN). Eur Urol. 2013;64(3):398–407.
37. Van Kerrebroeck P, Chapple C, Drogendijk T, NEPTUNE Study Group. Combination therapy with solifenacin and tamsulosin oral controlled absorption system in a single tablet for lower urinary tract symptoms in men: efficacy and safety results from the randomised controlled NEPTUNE trial. Eur Urol. 2013;64(6):1003–12.
38. Abrams P, Kelleher C, Staskin D, Rechberger T, Kay R, et al. Combination treatment with mirabegron and solifenacin in patients with overactive bladder: efficacy and safety results from a randomised, double-blind, dose-ranging, phase 2 study (symphony). Eur Urol. 2015;67(3):577–88.
39. Yamaguchi O, Kakizaki H, Homma Y, Igawa Y, Takeda M, Nishizawa O, et al. Safety and efficacy of mirabegron as 'add-on' therapy in patients with overactive bladder treated with solifenacin: a post-marketing, open-label study in Japan (MILAI study). BJU Int. 2015;116(4):612–22.
40. Drake MJ, Chapple C, Sokol R, Oelke M, Traudtner K, Klaver M et al. NEPTUNE Study Group. Long-term safety and efficacy of single-tablet combinations of solifenacin and tamsulosin oral controlled absorption system in men with storage and voiding lower urinary tract symptoms: results from the NEPTUNE study and NEPTUNE II open-label extension. Eur Urol. 2015;67(2):262–70.
41. Drake MJ, Sokol R, Coyne K, Hakimi Z, Nazir J, Dorey J, et al. NEPTUNE study group. Responder and health-related quality of life analyses in men with lower urinary tract symptoms treated with a fixed-dose combination of solifenacin and tamsulosin oral-controlled absorption system: results from the NEPTUNE study. BJU Int. 2016;117(1):165–72.
42. Xu Y, Liu R, Liu C, Cui Y, Gao Z. Meta-analysis of the efficacy and safety of mirabegron add-on therapy to solifenacin for overactive bladder. Int Neurourol J. 2017;21(3):212–9.
43. Amend B, Hennenlotter J, Schäfer T, Horstmann M, Stenzl A, Sievert KD. Effective treatment of neurogenic detrusor dysfunction by combined high-dosed antimuscarinics without increased side-effects. Eur Urol. 2008;53(5):1021–8.
44. Kosilov K, Loparev S, Iwanowskaya M, Kosilova L. Effectiveness of combined high-dosed trospium and solifenacin depending on severity of OAB symptoms in elderly men and women under cyclic therapy. Cent European J Urol. 2014;67(1):43–8.
45. Kosilov KV, Loparev SA, Ivanovskaya MA, Kosilova LV. Randomized controlled trial of cyclic and continuous therapy with trospium and solifenacin combination for severe overactive bladder in elderly patients with regard to patient compliance. Ther Adv Urol. 2014;6(6):215–23.
46. Kosilov K, Loparev S, Ivanovskaya M, Kosilova L. Additional correction of OAB symptoms by two anti-muscarinics for men over 50 years old with residual symptoms of moderate prostatic obstruction after treatment with Tamsulosin. Aging Male. 2015;18(1):44–8.
47. Kosilov KV, Loparev SA, Ivanovskaya MA, Kosilova LV. Effectiveness of solifenacin and trospium for managing of severe symptoms of overactive bladder in patients with benign prostatic hyperplasia. Am J Mens Health. 2016;10(2):157–63.
48. Ford AP, Cockayne DA. ATP and P2X purinoceptors in urinary tract disorders. Handb Exp Pharmacol. 2011;202:485–526.
49. Ford AP, Undem BJ. The therapeutic promise of ATP antagonism at P2X3 receptors in respiratory and urological disorders. Front Cell Neurosci. 2013;7:267.
50. North RA, Jarvis MF. P2X receptors as drug targets. Mol Pharmacol. 2013;83:759–69.
51. Andersson KE. Purinergic signalling in the urinary bladder. Auton Neurosci. 2015;191:78–81.

52. Avelino A, Charrua A, Frias B, Cruz C, Boudes M, de Ridder D, Cruz F. Transient receptor potential channels in bladder function. Acta Physiol (Oxf). 2013;207:110–22.
53. Deruyver Y, Voets T, De Ridder D, Everaerts W. Transient receptor potential channel modulators as pharmacological treatments for lower urinary tract symptoms (LUTS): myth or reality? BJU Int. 2015;115:686–97.
54. Franken J, Uvin P, De Ridder D, Voets T. TRP channels in lower urinary tract dysfunction. Br J Pharmacol. 2014;171:2537–51.
55. Moran MM. TRP channels as potential drug targets. Annu Rev Pharmacol Toxicol. 2018;58:309–30.

Chapter 14
Considerations in Pediatric Overactive Bladder

Alyssa Greiman and Andrew A. Stec

Introduction

Overactive bladder is a term used to describe the symptoms of urgency with or without urgency incontinence that is not the direct result of a known neurologic abnormality. This is in contrast to neurogenic detrusor overactivity which, in children, is most commonly caused by dysraphic malformations such as myelomeningocele. The treatment of non-neurogenic overactive bladder in children involves a multimodal approach including behavioral modification and biofeedback and, in refractory cases, can include pharmacotherapy with antimuscarinic medication. In the neurogenic population, there is good data that antimuscarinics increase bladder capacity and compliance and decrease involuntary detrusor contractions. However, pediatric non-neurogenic overactive bladder can be a difficult condition to diagnose and treat as children present with variable symptom profiles.

In this chapter we aim to outline the pharmacologic treatment options for pediatric overactive bladder in cases where conservative management with education, urotherapy, and biofeedback has proven unsuccessful. The focus of this chapter is the use of pharmacotherapy for pediatric non-neurogenic overactive bladder; however, as the majority of studies, especially those leading to FDA approval of oxybutynin are in children with neurogenic overactive bladder, we will also present this data for the sake of completeness.

Notable limitations in drug development for pediatric overactive bladder include the fact that pediatric overactive bladder has a different underlying etiology and pathophysiology compared to adult overactive bladder and that debate still exists regarding the most suitable endpoints for assessment of the clinical effectiveness of these medications.

A. Greiman · A. A. Stec (✉)
Department of Urology, Medical University of South Carolina, Charleston, SC, USA
e-mail: stec@musc.edu

L. Cox, E. S. Rovner (eds.), *Contemporary Pharmacotherapy of Overactive Bladder*, https://doi.org/10.1007/978-3-319-97265-7_14

Neurogenic Overactive Bladder

The goals of medical management for neurogenic bladder dysfunction are to improve continence and to achieve a bladder with normal capacity and compliance that can completely eliminate urine while protecting the kidneys. In those individuals with incomplete bladder emptying, this is primarily accomplished with clean intermittent catheterization and pharmacologic therapy. Several antimuscarinic drugs approved in adults have been evaluated for pediatric neurogenic bladder dysfunction. Oxybutynin was the first drug formally approved for use in pediatric neurogenic bladder, followed by tolterodine. Solifenacin pediatric neurogenic bladder drug trials are finished, and the drug is awaiting approval from the US Food and Drug Administration. These medications and the data supporting their use in pediatric neurogenic overactive bladder form the basis for the same medications' use in the non-neurogenic population.

Non-neurogenic Overactive Bladder

Numerous classifications are used for children presenting with functional urinary symptoms once neural and anatomic abnormalities are ruled out. In 2006, the International Children's Continence Society released standardized terminology to provide guidelines for classification and communication about lower urinary tract symptoms in children. Per this classification, overactive bladder (OAB) is "urinary urgency, usually accompanied by frequency and nocturia, with or without urinary incontinence, in the absence of urinary tract infection or other obvious pathology" [1].

The natural history of overactive bladder in children is not well understood. It was previously postulated that detrusor overactivity in children was idiopathic or due to maturational delay. Currently, causation thoughts focus on pediatric OAB being more likely associated with feed-forward loops from the generation of a high-pressure system during voiding or filling. This is in contrast to the adult population where overactive bladder is considered a chronic condition whose origin is unrelated to functional use [2]. It is difficult to assess the prevalence of overactive bladder in children due to significant variability in definitions of the condition used across pediatric studies. Primary outcome variables that are most consistent across studies are daytime versus nighttime incontinence. Associated daytime symptoms are inconsistently investigated. Nonetheless, daytime or combined daytime and nighttime incontinence at least once a week is reported to occur in about 2–4% of 7-year-old children [3, 4], with two large studies reporting overall prevalence of OAB in children as high as 15–20% [5, 6]. The prevalence of OAB appears to decrease with age from 23% at 5 years of age down to 12.2% at 13 years of age [6].

Treatment of overactive bladder in children focuses on improving voiding dynamics and storage properties of the bladder to minimize urinary symptoms and incontinence. Pharmacotherapy is used to decrease involuntary detrusor contraction and expand the child's bladder capacity. The main objectives of treatment are to normalize the micturition pattern, bladder and pelvic floor overactivity, and cure incontinence [2]. Treatment usually involves a multimodal approach starting with behavioral modifications, moving to adjunctive biofeedback and pelvic floor therapy, and in refractory cases, addition of antimuscarinic medications.

Non-pharmacologic Treatment of Overactive Bladder

The initial treatment of daytime urinary incontinence in children does not focus on medication, instead it involves a behavioral and cognitive approach. Initially, the child and parents are educated about normal bladder function and appropriate micturition schedules and techniques. They are educated on recognizing signs such as urinary urgency; and timed voiding regimens are instituted. If present, recurrent associated urinary tract infections and constipation are managed as part of a first-line therapy. The aim of urotherapy—a combination of education, timed voiding, and appropriate position for voiding, with or without physical therapy—is to normalize the micturition pattern and prevent functional disturbances.

There is no set format for urotherapy, and many clinical studies utilize different therapy regimens, making it difficult to standardize the evaluation of a treatment method's success. A Danish report of the outcomes of using standard urotherapy alone in 240 children with daytime incontinence noted achievement of dryness in 55% of children aged 4 to 16 [7]. When an alarm such as a timer watch was utilized as a reminder to void at regular intervals, up to 70% of children became dry, with equal success report using a non-contingent versus contingent alarm system [8].

Biofeedback, a technique where physiological bladder voiding and storage activity is monitored and conveyed to the patient as real-time visual or acoustic signals, can provide children with information about their unconscious physiological processes. It is commonly used to help children identify how to relax pelvic floor muscles or to recognize involuntary detrusor contractions. This technique is used to teach pelvic floor muscle relaxation with proper urethral sphincter coordination with the use of EMG electrodes and physical and visual biofeedback. While the results of biofeedback are generally positive when utilized as an adjunctive to urotherapy, there is no evidence that it is superior to urotherapy alone. Vasconcelos et al. randomized 56 children with urinary incontinence into two voiding training programs, one of which also included biofeedback. After a 3-month training program, 42.8% of children with daytime enuresis were cured at 1 month, and 72.4% were cured at 1 year. Compliance with the regimen was noted to play a large role in success. This study found that there was no difference in cure rates with the addition of biofeedback, although this group was noted to have a statistically significant decrease in PVR which was not clinically significant [9]. In the authors' opinion, biofeedback is useful and has success in patients with overactive bladder symptoms who do not respond to urotherapy alone. As it is noninvasive, it is second line in the treatment of these pediatric patients prior to initiating pharmacotherapy.

Antimuscarinic Pharmacotherapy

Antimuscarinic drugs are the primary pharmacologic treatment option available for the treatment of detrusor overactivity. Antimuscarinic medications target involuntary contractions of the detrusor muscle, which are mediated by parasympathetic stimulation of muscarinic receptors on the bladder, causing bladder overactivity [2, 10]. Most antimuscarinics are tertiary amines that are metabolized by the P450 enzyme system into active metabolites [11]. These metabolites act as competitive antagonists of the muscarinic receptors on the wall of the detrusor muscle wall, reversibly binding to M2 and M3 receptors, to relax the detrusor muscle, thereby increasing bladder capacity and compliance while decreasing detrusor contractions. Unfortunately, these drugs also bind to M1 receptors found in the brain, salivary glands, and sympathetic ganglia resulting in the side effects of blurry vision, dry mouth, dry eyes, and constipation, among others. Though these side effects are reportedly less frequent and bothersome in children compared to adults, they do impact compliance with medication therapy [12–14]. While seven different antimuscarinics are marketed for the treatment of detrusor overactivity in adults, only oxybutynin and tolterodine are currently approved for the treatment of pediatric neurogenic detrusor overactivity in North America, and only oxybutynin is approved for the treatment of pediatric overactive bladder [15]. To date, no single antimuscarinic drug has been shown to be superior to another in the adult or pediatric population [16, 17], though there is some evidence that the extended-release formulations are more efficacious than the immediate-release formulations with an improved side effect profile [18].

Oxybutynin

The immediate-release (IR) and extended-release (ER) formulations of oxybutynin are currently the only pharmacological agents approved for the treatment of OAB in children in North America [19]. Oxybutynin was first formally approved for use in children with neurogenic detrusor overactivity in 2003 [20–23]. Oxybutynin is a tertiary amine that undergoes first-pass metabolism in the liver, with N-desethyl-oxybutynin as the primary metabolite. This has a high affinity for M3 and M1 receptors, resulting in a side effect profile that limits its use [24]. More recently, the ER formulation of oxybutynin has been approved for use in children. The extended-release formulation utilizes a delivery system, whereby the medication is absorbed in the large intestine, bypassing first-pass metabolism in the liver, leading to decreased amount of active metabolite and an improved tolerability profile. Unfortunately, this delivery system requires an intact tablet that cannot be cut or crushed, making administration difficult in young children [2]. Oxybutynin IR is administered orally in a dosage of 0.2–0.6 mg/kg/day split over two to three doses, with a maximum recommended dose of 15 mg/kg/day. Oxybutynin ER is administered once daily, swallowed intact, and can be increased from 5 mg up to 20 mg/day.

Although oxybutynin is FDA approved for use in children, no studies have compared it to placebo. Its use is based on small observational studies and is extrapolated from use in adults [25]. Franco et al. evaluated the efficacy and safety of oxybutynin in children with detrusor hyperreflexia due to neurogenic bladder. This prospective open-label trial evaluated 3 formulations (tablets, syrup, and extended-release tablets) for 24 weeks in 116 children who already used oxybutynin and clean intermittent catheterization with a 3-day washout period prior to study initiation. This study found that mean urine volume per catheterization increased on average by 25.5 ml ($p < 0.001$), with a maximal cystometric capacity increase of 75.4 ml ($p < 0.001$) as well as a corresponding decrease in detrusor and intravesical pressure of −9.2 ($p < 0.001$) and − 7.5 ($p < 0.004$) cm H2O. All three formulations were well tolerated with the most common side effect being urinary tract infection in 49.1%, headache in 8.6%, and constipation in 7.8%. No patients terminated the study prematurely [23]. When evaluating 81 children diagnosed with neuropathic bladder sphincter dysfunction due to myelodysplasia on oxybutynin IR with mean follow-up duration of 4.5 years, mean cystometric capacity was increased by an average of 29 ml ($p < 0.05$), and compliance was significantly improved from a mean of 6.5 to 9.6 ml/cm H2O ($p < 0.05$) [20]. In 2002, a retrospective study on 25 children treated with oxybutynin ER, 14 of which had neurogenic bladder dysfunction and 11 of which had non-neurogenic overactive bladder, was published. This study noted 100% of patients having improvement in incontinence or voiding dysfunction on a semiquantitative questionnaire. Fifty-two percent of patients experienced side effects (dry mouth, constipation, heat intolerance, and drowsiness). Families reported better compliance using oxybutynin ER compared to the IR formulation with similar or fewer side effects and 21 of 25 patients continued to use the medication at last follow-up [21].

There are even fewer studies assessing the efficacy of oxybutynin in non-neurogenic detrusor overactivity in children, none of which are randomized or double blinded. Curran et al. conducted a retrospective review assessing the efficacy of several agents, including oxybutynin, in children with non-neurogenic detrusor overactivity confirmed by urodynamics who were refractory to behavioral therapy. In these 30 children, 18 of whom were on oxybutynin, 87% experienced complete resolution or significant improvement in their symptoms, with 38% of patients continuing on the medication after a mean follow-up of 4.7 years [26].

There is limited data on the use of the transdermal oxybutynin patch in children. This formulation comes in an adhesive patch delivering 3.9 mg of oxybutynin per day and needs to be changed twice a week to dry, intact skin. Up to two patches can be applied if the initial dose is unsatisfactory. In an open-label, dose titration, randomized, parallel group study, 57 children age 6–15 years with neurogenic detrusor overactivity were assigned randomly at a 3:1 ratio to treatment with transdermal or oral oxybutynin for 12 weeks. At the end of the 12 weeks, mean urine volume increased from 95 to 125 ml ($p < 0.001$) with transdermal oxybutynin and from 114 to 166 ml ($p < 0.002$) with oral oxybutynin. Both patient groups achieved significant increases from baseline in percentage of catheterizations without leakage (25% increase for transdermal and 24% increase for oral oxybutynin). Adherence to transdermal oxybutynin was 107% (due to changes of patch more frequently on occasion of loss of adhesion) compared to 86% to oral oxybutynin. Regarding safety, 28% of children had a mild skin reaction to the transdermal patch, and one child experienced vasodilation with oral oxybutynin [22]. In the only study to evaluate transdermal oxybutynin for the management of non-neurogenic overactive bladder in children, 35 children age 4–16 were followed for a minimum of 3 months with 97% reporting a good symptom response. Mean bladder capacity increased from 104 ml to 148 ml at 3 months. Skin irritation occurred in 35% of children, with 20% discontinuing the medication due to this irritation [27].

Intravesical oxybutynin instillation, prepared by crushing and dissolving a 5 mg tablet of oxybutynin in 30 ml of distilled water, has been studied in children with neurogenic detrusor overactivity. No data exists in patients with non-neurogenic overactive bladder, likely due to the need for catheterization. Greenfield et al. administered intravesical oxybutynin chloride to ten children with neurogenic bladder who had incontinence refractory to oral anticholinergic medications and intermittent catheterization with 50% of children becoming completely dry day and night, 30% achieving daytime continence, and 20% showing no improvement on twice daily dosing. Urodynamics revealed up to a 335% increase in bladder capacity and a 63% decrease in maximum filling pressure with no local or systemic side effects [28].

Tolterodine

Tolterodine is the first antimuscarinic agent designed specifically for use in detrusor overactivity and is felt to be more bladder selective as it acts on M2 and M3 receptors, with a greater affinity for the bladder compared to other organs and therefore is associated with fewer side effects [2]. An additional benefit is that the delivery system is such that the capsule may be cracked and sprinkled onto food for easier administration for children. While tolterodine is approved for pediatric use in neurogenic bladder, it is not yet approved for children with non-neurogenic detrusor overactivity, though there are several studies which demonstrate safety and efficacy in this patient population. Tolterodine is available as a solution, IR and ER tablets and is dosed from 0.5 to 8 mg per day. Drug formulation and dosing are based on age; children aged 4 months to 4 years are started on tolterodine oral solution 0.2 mg twice daily and can be titrated up to 2 mg twice daily as tolerated for symptom control. For children aged 5–10 years who cannot tolerate swallowing a pill, tolterodine oral solution is started at 0.5 mg twice daily and titrated up to 4 mg twice daily as needed. For children aged 11–16 who can swallow pills, the preferred formulation is tolterodine ER, starting at 2 mg daily and titrating up to 6 mg as tolerated.

Among children with neurogenic overactive bladder, three open-label, dose-escalating studies were conducted on children with neurogenic detrusor overactivity in three age groups: 1 month–4 years, 5–10 years, and 11–15 years who were prescribed tolterodine for 4 weeks. This study found a dose-related increase in volume to first detrusor contraction and cystometric capacity up to 2 mg doses, at which point thereafter, there was no dose-related improved response. Tolterodine was generally well tolerated at each dose in all age groups with the most common adverse events of constipation (9–20%) and headache (7%) not increasing in incidence with escalating doses [29]. Another group of children with neurogenic detrusor hyperreflexia aged 3 months to 15 years were prescribed tolterodine IR 0.1 mg/kg twice daily as either first-line therapy or replacing oxybutynin. The mean bladder capacity was shown to increase by 44%, with mean detrusor compliance increasing by 55% and mean maximum detrusor pressure decreasing by 46%. Additionally, 40% of incontinent children became completely or almost continent on tolterodine. There was no difference in the urodynamic effects of oxybutynin versus tolterodine; however tolterodine was noted to be better tolerated [30].

When evaluating the safety and efficacy of tolterodine in children with non-neurogenic overactive bladder, an open-label dose escalation study of 33 children treated with tolterodine IR 0.5, 1, or 2 mg twice daily for 14 days found a mean decrease of 21% in micturition frequency and a 44% decrease from baseline in the number of incontinence episodes with no associated elevation in post-void residual. The 1 mg dose was best tolerated, with 10 of the 13 adverse events occurring in the 2 mg group [31]. In a prospective crossover study of 34 children with non-neurogenic detrusor overactivity who were crossed over from oxybutynin to tolterodine 1–2 mg BID, the efficacy was found to be comparable to oxybutynin with 68% of children reporting a greater than 90% reduction in wetting episodes. Tolterodine was better tolerated, with 59% noting no side effects after previously reporting side effects on oxybutynin and 18% noting a decrease in the severity of side effects on tolterodine. Tolterodine was discontinued in 24% of children during this year-long study [32]. The results of two double-blind, placebo-controlled trials in children age 5–11 with non-neurogenic urgency urinary incontinence suggestive of detrusor overactivity randomized to 2 mg of tolterodine ER or placebo for 12 weeks did not find statistically significant improvement in difference in incontinence episodes per week, voids per 24 h, and volume of urine per voids [33]. However, secondary analysis of these patients who continued to receive tolterodine ER 2 mg daily for 12 months found that tolterodine was well-tolerated. During this study period, 12% of patients withdrew due to lack of efficacy and 3% withdrew because of side effects with an additional 8% of patients being noncompliant with taking the study medication. The most frequently reported adverse events were UTI (7%), nasopharyngitis (5%), and headaches (5%) [34]. Reinberg et al. conducted an open-label parallel group retrospective study in which children with diurnal incontinence were arbitrarily assigned to oxybutynin ER, tolterodine IR, or tolterodine ER. The children were started on the lowest dose and titrated up as needed. The study concluded that oxybutynin ER and tolterodine ER were significantly better than tolterodine IR in improving diurnal incontinence and urinary frequency and that oxybutynin ER was significantly more effective than tolterodine ER in resolving diurnal incontinence [35].

Solifenacin

Solifenacin is another once daily long-acting oral antimuscarinic that acts selectively on the M3 receptor antagonist and is associated with fewer systemic side effects than oxybutynin and is available in 5 mg or 10 mg tablets. In a prospective, open-label study of 72 children with both non-neurogenic and neurogenic overactive bladder refractory to oxybutynin or tolterodine followed for a minimum of 3 months, solifenacin was found to increase mean urodynamic bladder capacity from 146 to 311 ml and to decrease uninhibited bladder contractions from 70 to 20 cm H20. Continence improved in all patients. Four patients withdrew from the study due to intolerable side effects, with 69% of children noting no side effects [36]. Among 99 children with therapy resistant non-neurogenic overactive bladder started on solifenacin 5 mg for at least 3 months, 85% of children responded to therapy, with 45% becoming completely dry. The mean voided volume increased on average by 25%. Only 6.5% of children reported a side effect, compared to 39% on their prior antimuscarinic therapy [37].

Trospium Chloride

Trospium chloride is an alternative antimuscarinic available in tablet form and taken in twice daily doses of 10, 15, 20, or 25 mg or a once daily formulation. Trospium chloride differs from other muscarinic antagonists in that it has negligible affinity for nicotinic receptors and therapeutic doses and therefore may have fewer associated side effects. Additionally, as a quaternary ammonium cation, it stays in the periphery rather than crossing the blood-brain barrier and may have fewer neurologic side effects. It should be noted that absorption is affected by food intake and significant intraindividual and interindividual variability in bioavailability is noted in adults [2]. One single-blind, randomized control trial of 58 neurologically intact children aged 5–13 years old with urodynamically proven detrusor instability and symptoms of urinary urgency and incontinence has been performed to date. Children were randomly allocated to 10, 15, 20, or 25 mg of trospium chloride or placebo for 21 days. Response rates were assessed by incontinence episodes and urodynamic parameters. Of the 50 patients treated with trospium chloride, 82% had a positive therapeutic result versus 37.5% on placebo. On urodynamics, mean decrease in number of contractions was 54.3%, mean contraction pressure decreased by 19.3%, and mean volume at first contraction increased by 71.4%. Only four patients experienced side effects thought to be related to the medication including headache, dizziness, abdominal cramps, and dry mouth. Treatment compliance was high at 96.7% over the study period [38].

Propiverine

Propiverine, an antimuscarinic which possesses a second mode of action by inhibiting calcium influx and modulating intracellular calcium in urinary bladder smooth muscle cells in a concentration-dependent manner, is available in Europe and Asia in IR and ER formulation. Propiverine has been assessed in children in a multicenter, placebo-controlled, double-blind study where 171 children with non-neurogenic detrusor overactivity who had at least 8 or more micturition episodes per day and at least 1 incontinence episode per week were initially treated with 3 weeks of urotherapy and then were randomized to 8 weeks of medical therapy with propiverine or placebo. Voiding frequency per day was reduced by 20%, or 2 voids per day, with propiverine compared to 11%, or 1.2 voids per day, with placebo ($p < 0.0007$). A decrease of at least 1.5 voids per day was achieved in 64.3% of patients on propiverine compared to 40% with placebo ($p = 0.0018$). Incontinence episodes were decreased by 0.5 episodes with propiverine compared to 0.2 episodes per day with placebo ($p = 0.0005$). The mean voided volume increased by about 30 ml on average for propiverine compared to 5 ml for placebo ($p = 0.0001$) [39].

Fesoterodine

Fesoterodine is the newest ER antimuscarinic agent in the USA and is available in 4 mg or 8 mg tablets. This medication is similar to tolterodine but with less pharmacokinetic variability. There is no data to date on its efficacy in children; however recruitment for a randomized, double-blind, crossover study comparing fesoterodine and oxybutynin ER in children with OAB is currently underway [25].

Dual Therapy

Combination therapy with two antimuscarinic medications simultaneously has been minimally studied in children with both neurogenic and non-neurogenic detrusor overactivity with promising results. In a study of 56 children with neurogenic and non-neurogenic detrusor overactivity who had insufficient response to an optimized dose of oxybutynin or tolterodine monotherapy, dual therapy with a combination of oxybutynin, tolterodine, and/or solifenacin for a mean therapy course of 36 months was initiated. The primary end point was continence. In total, 23 patients (41%) became dry, 18 (32%) improved significantly, and 15 (27%) improved moderately. Urodynamic capacity improved from 158 mL to 359 mL. The reported overall success rate was 82%, and eight patients (14%) discontinued treatment for unsatisfactory clinical response. Of note, 50% of children experienced mild-to-moderate side effect, and two patients withdrew from the study due to their side effects [40]. More recently, a prospective study of 72 children with refractory non-neurogenic overactive bladder on oxybutynin monotherapy were treated with add-on trospium. On dual antimuscarinic therapy, 68% of children noted a good response compared to monotherapy with 22% achieving complete dryness. Treatment was discontinued in 29% of children for persistent symptoms with no improvement on dual therapy. Though 57% of children reported no adverse effects, 2.7% discontinued treatment due to intolerable side effects [41].

Novel Pharmacological Treatment of Overactive Bladder

β3-Agonists

Mirabegron is a β3-agonist that works to relax the detrusor smooth muscle during storage by activating the β3-receptor. β3-adrenoreceptors are found in urinary bladder smooth muscle and mediate detrusor muscle relaxation via a complex mechanism which includes inhibiting bladder smooth muscle cells excitability as well as having an inhibitory effect on cholinergic nerve terminals. Mirabegron is approved for the treatment of overactive bladder in adults in the USA and is available in 25 and 50 mg ER tablets. Though there is scarce data on the use of mirabegron in the pediatric population, initial results are promising. A prospective, off-label study of 28 children with non-neurogenic overactive bladder who were intolerant or refractory to antimuscarinics was treated with 25–50 mg of mirabegron for a median of 11.5 months. Median bladder capacity improved from 150 to 200 ml ($p < 0.001$), with continence improving in 90% of children, including 22% who became completely dry. Mild-to-moderate side effects were reported in 13.7% of children, with three children discontinuing mirabegron due to intolerable side effects including nasopharyngitis, nausea, and changes in behavior. There was no change in blood pressure, heart rate, or electrocardiogram [42]. There is also some emerging literature that the use of add-on regimens of mirabegron in the pediatric population with refractory overactive bladder may be well tolerated and efficacious. Morin et al. conducted a prospective off-label study of 35 children with non-neurogenic overactive bladder refractory to urotherapy and antimuscarinics. Children were prescribed 25–50 mg of mirabegron in addition to their original antimuscarinic (solifenacin, oxybutynin, or fesoterodine) for a median treatment duration of 16.4 months. All patients noted significant improvement in the continence, with 34% having complete dryness. Median voided volumes improved on average by 25% or 102 ml. Again, no change in blood pressure, heart rate, or electrocardiograms was observed.

While 80% of children did not note any adverse events, 14% had mild adverse events, 3% experienced moderate rhinitis, and two patients discontinued treatment due to either rhinitis or an elevated PVR of 50 ml [43].

Botulinum Toxin

Botulinum toxin A is a neurotoxin protein produced by the bacteria *Clostridium botulinum* that prevents the release of neurotransmitter acetylcholine at the neuromuscular junction, thereby causing flaccid paralysis.

Botulinum toxin A, while approved for adults with overactive bladder, is currently only offered as an off-label option for children with refractory overactive bladder. The most studied formulation in the pediatric population is onabotulinumtoxinA (BTX), with a suggested age threshold of 3 years dosed at 5–10 units per kilogram [44]. In 2003, children with refractory neurogenic overactive bladder and detrusor pressures over 40 cm H2O on anticholinergic therapy underwent injection of BTX 12 U/kg up to a maximum of 300 U divided over 30–50 sites. At 4-week follow-up, mean bladder capacity increased from 163 ml to 219 ml with detrusor pressure decreasing from 59.6 cm H2O to 34.9 cm H2O. The effects were noted to last approximately 6 months [45]. Among children with non-neurogenic overactive bladder, 21 children with decreased bladder capacity and urge incontinence were treated with 100 U of BTX injected into the detrusor muscle. Of the 15 children who completed long-term follow-up, 9 children (60%) had a complete response with complete resolution of urgency and incontinence with a mean increase in bladder capacity from 167 to 271 ml, and an additional 3 patients had a partial response (20%). Side effects included ten-day temporary urinary retention in one child and transient vesicoureteral reflux in another [46]. The limitation to BTX in the pediatric non-neurogenic overactive bladder population is that this procedure must be performed in many cases under general anesthesia, and, with a 2–9% risk of urinary retention, these sensate children and their families must be informed and willing to perform clean intermittent catheterization before having the procedure.

Conclusion

Overactive bladder is a common pediatric condition that can be difficult to diagnose and treat, especially due to the variability in presenting symptoms as well as underlying pathology. Initial management should include education of the parents and children on normal bladder physiology and initiation of urotherapy with timed, appropriate positioned voiding and management of constipation. Biofeedback can be added when initial conservative therapies fail. After these conservative measures, oxybutynin remains the only pharmacological treatment approved in North America for pediatric non-neurogenic overactive bladder. Though the limited number of randomized controlled trials makes assessment of the pharmacotherapy management options difficult, there are many alternatives that have been studied and may provide off-label treatment options for children OAB refractory to urotherapy. Further research with well-established clinically relevant endpoints is required to determine the optimal treatment regimen for children with refractory overactive bladder.

References

1. Austin PF, Bauer SB, Bower W, Chase J, Franco I, Hoebeke P, et al. The standardization of terminology of lower urinary tract function in children and adolescents: update report from the standardization committee of the International Children's Continence Society. Neurourol Urodyn. 2016;35(4):471–81.
2. Nijman R, Tekgul S, Chase J, Bael A, Austin P, von Gontard A. Diagnosis and management of urinary incontinence in childhood. In: Abrams P, Cardozo L, Khoury S, Wein A, editors. Incontinence, 5th ed. 5th International Consultation on Incontinence, Paris, February; 2012. p. 729–826. The International Continence Society (ICS) and the International Consultation on Urological Diseases (ICUD); 2013.
3. Järvelin MR, Vikeväinen-Tervonen L, Moilanen I, Huttunen NP. Enuresis in seven-year-old children. Acta Paediatr Scand. 1998;77(1):148–53.
4. Sureshkumar P, Craig JC, Roy LP, Knight JF. Daytime urinary incontinence in primary school children: a population-based survey. J Pediatr. 2000;137(6):814–8.
5. Kajiwara M, Inoue K, Kato M, Usui A, Kurihara M, Usui T. Nocturnal enuresis and overactive bladder in children: an epidemiological study. Int J Urol. 2006;13(1):36–41.
6. Chung JM, Lee SD, Kang DI, Kwon DD, Kim KS, Kim SY, et al.; Korean Enuresis Association. Prevalence and associated factors of overactive bladder in Korean children 5–13 years old: a nationwide multicenter study. Urology 2009;73(1):63–7; discussion 68-9.
7. Hellstrom AL, Hjalmas K, Jodal U. Rehabilitation of the dysfunctional bladder in children: method and 3-year follow-up. J Urol. 1987;138(4):847–9.
8. Halliday S, Meadow SR, Berg I. Successful management of daytime enuresis using alarm procedures: a randomly controlled trial. Arch Dis Child. 1987;62(2):132–7.
9. Vasconcelos M, Lima E, Caiafa L, Noronha A, Cangussu R, Gomes S, et al. Voiding dysfunction in children. Pelvic-floor exercises or biofeedback therapy: a randomized study. Pediatr Nephrol. 2006;21(12):1858–64.
10. Kroll P. Pharmacotherapy for pediatric neurogenic bladder. Pediatr Drugs. 2017;19(5):463–78.
11. Guay DR. Clinical pharmacokinetics of drugs used to treat urge incontinence. Clin Pharmacokinet. 2003;42(14):1243–85.
12. Blais AS, Bergeron M, Nadeau G, Ramsay S, Bolduc S. Anticholinergic use in children: persistence and patterns of therapy. Can Urol Assoc J. 2016;10(3–4):137–40.
13. Wagg A, Compion G, Fahey A, Siddiqui E. Persistence with prescribed antimuscarinic therapy for overactive bladder: a UK experience. BJU Int. 2012;110(11):1767–74.
14. Gish P, Mosholder AD, Truffa M, Johann-Liang R. Spectrum of central anticholinergic adverse effects associated with oxybutynin: comparison of pediatric and adult cases. J Pediatr. 2009;155(3):432–4.
15. Robinson D, Giarenis I, Cardozo L. New developments in the medical management of overactive bladder. Maturitas. 2013;76(3):225–9.
16. Buser N, Ivic S, Kessler TM, Kessels AG, Bachmann LM. Efficacy and adverse events of antimuscarinics for treating overactive bladder: network meta-analyses. Eur Urol. 2012;62(6):1040–60.

17. Madhuvrata P, Cody JD, Ellis G, Herbison GP, Hay-Smith EJ. Which anticholinergic drug for overactive bladder symptoms in adults. Cochrane Database Syst Rev. 2012;18(1):CD005429.
18. Novara G, Galfano A, Secco S, D'Elia C, Cavalleri S, Ficarra V, Artibani W. A systematic review and meta-analysis of randomized controlled trials with antimuscarinic drugs for overactive bladder. Eur Urol. 2008;54(4):740–63.
19. Chang SJ, Van Laecke E, Bauer SB, von Gontard A, Bagli D, Bower WF, et al. Treatment of daytime urinary incontinence: a standardization document from the International Children's Continence Society. Neurourol Urodyn. 2017;36(1):43–50.
20. Baek M, Kang JY, Jeong J, Kim DK, Kim KM. Treatment outcomes according to neuropathic bladder sphincter dysfunction type after treatment of oxybutynin chloride in children with myelodysplasia. Int Urol Nephrol. 2013;45(3):703–9.
21. Youdim K, Kogan BA. Preliminary study of the safety and efficacy of extended-release oxybutynin in children. Urology. 2002;59(3):428–32.
22. Cartwright PC, Coplen DE, Kogan BA, Volinn W, Finan E, Hoel G. Efficacy and safety of transdermal and oral oxybutynin in children with neurogenic detrusor overactivity. J Urol. 2009;182(4):1548–54.
23. Franco I, Horowitz M, Grady R, Adams RC, De Jong T, Lindert K, Albrecht D. Efficacy and safety of oxybutynin in children with detrusor hyperreflexia secondary to neurogenic bladder dysfunction. J Urol. 2005;173(1):221–5.
24. Noronha-Blob L, Kachur JF. Enantiomers of oxybutynin: in vitro pharmacological characterization at M1, M2 and m3 muscarinic receptors and in vivo effects on urinary bladder contraction, mydriasis and salivary secretion in guinea pigs. J Pharmacol Exp Ther. 1991;256(2):562–7.
25. Ramsay S, Bolduc S. Overactive bladder in children. Can Urol Assoc J. 2017;1(1–2 Suppl 1):S74–9.
26. Curran MJ, Kaefer M, Peters C, Logigian E, Bauer SB. The detrusor overactivity in childhood: long-term results with conservative management. J Urol. 2000;163(2):574–7.
27. Gleason JM, Daniels C, Williams K, Varghese A, Koyle MA, Bägli DJ, et al. Single-center experience with oxybutynin transdermal system (patch) for the management of symptoms related to non-neuropathic overactive bladder in children: an attractive, well-tolerated alternative form of administration. J Pediatr Urol. 2014;10(4):753–7.
28. Greenfield SP, Fera M. The use of intravesical oxybutynin chloride in children with neurogenic bladder. J Urol. 1991;146(2 Pt 2):532–4.
29. Ellsworth PI, Borgstein NG, Nigman RJ, Reddy PP. Use of tolterodine in children with neurogenic detrusor overactivity: relationship between dose and urodynamic response. J Urol. 2005;174(4 Pt 2):1647–51.
30. Goessl C, Sauter T, Michael T, Berge B, Staehler M, Miller K. Efficacy and tolerability of tolterodine in children with detrusor hyperreflexia. Urology. 2000;55(3):414–8.
31. Hjälmås K, Hellström AL, Mogren K, Läckgren G, Stenberg A. The overactive bladder in children: a potential future indication for tolterodine. BJU Int. 2001;87(6):569–74.
32. Bolduc S, Upadhyay J, Payton J, Bagli DJ, McLorie GA, Khoury AE, Farhat W. The use of tolterodine in children after oxybutynin failure. BJU Int. 2003;91(4):398–401.
33. Nijman RJ, Borgstein NG, Ellsworth P, Djurhuus JC. Tolterodine treatment for children with symptoms of urinary urge incontinence suggestive of detrusor overactivity: results from 2 randomized, placebo controlled trials. J Urol. 2005;173(4):1334–9.
34. Nijman RJ, Borgstein NG, Ellsworth P, Siggaard C. Long-term tolerability of tolterodine extended release in children 5–11 years of age: results from a 12-month, open-label study. Eur Urol. 2007;52(5):1511–6.
35. Reinberg Y, Crocker J, Wolpert J, Vandersteen D. Therapeutic efficacy of extended release oxybutynin chloride, and immediate release and long acting tolterodine tartrate in children with diurnal urinary incontinence. J Urol. 2003;169(1):317–9.
36. Bolduc S, Moore K, Nadeau G, Lebel S, Lamontage P, Hamel M. Prospective open label study of solifenacin for overactive bladder in children. J Urol. 2010;184(4 Suppl):1668–73.

37. Hoebeke P, De Pooter J, De Caestecker K, Raes A, Dehoorne J, Van Laecke E, Vande WJ. Solfenacin for therapy resistant overactive bladder. J Urol. 2009;182(4 Suppl):2040–4.
38. Lopez Pereira P, Miguelez C, Caffarati J, Estornell F, Anduera A. Trospium chloride for the treatment of detrusor instability in children. J Urol. 2003;170(5):1978–81.
39. Marschall-Kehrel D, Feustel C, Persson de Geeter C, Stehr M, Radmayr C, Sillén U, Strugala G. Treatment with propiverine in children suffering from non-neurogenic overactive bladder and urinary incontinence: results of a randomized, placebo-controlled, phase 3 clinical trial. Eur Urol. 2009;55(3):729–36.
40. Nadeau G, Schröder A, Moore K, Genois L, Lamontagne P, Hamel M, et al. Double anticholinergic therapy for refractory neurogenic and nonneurogenic detrusor overactivity in children: long-term results of a prospective, open-label study. Can Urol Assoc J. 2014;8(5–6):175–80.
41. Fahmy A, Youssif M, Rhashad H, Mokhless I, Mahfouz W. Combined low-dose antimuscarinics for refractory detrusor over-activity in children. J Ped Urol. 2016;12(4):219.e1–5.
42. Blais AS, Nadeau G, Moore K, Genois L, Bolduc S. Prospective pilot study of mirabegron in pediatric patients with overactive bladder. Eur Urol. 2016;70(1):9–13.
43. Morin F, Blais AS, Nadeau G, Moore K, Genois L, Bolduc S. Dual therapy for refractory overactive bladder in children: a prospective open-label study. J Urol. 2017;197(4):1158–63.
44. Apostolidis A, Dasgupta P, Denys P, Elneil S, Fowler CJ, Giannantoni A, et al.; European Consensus Panel. Recommendations on the use of onabotulinum toxin in the treatment of lower urinary tract disorders and pelvic floor dysfunctions: a European consensus report. Eur Urol 2009;55(1):100–19.
45. Schulte-Baukloh H, Michael T, Sturzebecher B, Knispel HH. Botulinum-A toxin detrusor injection as a novel approach in the treatment of bladder spasticity in children with neurogenic bladder. Eur Urol. 2003;44(1):139–43.
46. Hoebeke P, De Caestecker K, Vande Walle J, Dehoorne J, Raes A, Verleyen P, Van Laecke E. The effect of botulinum-A toxin in incontinent children with therapy resistant overactive detrusor. J Urol. 2006;176(1):328–30.

Chapter 15
Considerations in Male Overactive Bladder

Alex Gomelsky, Emily F. Kelly, and Rebecca Budish

Introduction and Definitions

As in their female counterparts, lower urinary tract symptoms (LUTS) in men are highly prevalent and impactful. In nearly 6500 men aged 40–79 from 2 population-based studies, the prevalence of LUTS (International Prostate Symptom Score (I-PSS) ≥ 8) was up to 25.6% and was similar to the reported rate of hypertension [1]. Overall, severe LUTS (I-PSS ≥20) affected 3.3% of men in this age group, a rate roughly similar to stroke (2.2%), cancer (4.5%), or heart attack (4.5%). A 10-point increase in I-PSS was associated with a 3.3-point reduction in the Medical Outcomes Study Short Form-12 (SF-12) physical health component score, which was greater than the score reduction caused by cancer, diabetes, or hypertension (2 points each).

LUTS increase as men age, and, in the UK alone, the prevalence increased from 3.5% in men aged 45–49 to >30% in men aged >85 [2, 3]. Increasing LUTS severity has also been associated with worse health-related quality of life (HRQoL) in the US Health Professionals Follow-up Study of over 8400 men [4]. The difference in mean SF-36 between those with mild and severe LUTS scores was 10.5 for the physical function domain, 24.7 for physical role, 9.6 for bodily pain, 13.5 for general health perceptions, 15.7 for vitality, 13.8 for emotional role, 7.0 for mental health, and 8.3 for social function. Comparisons of the patient group with severe LUTS with four other chronic illness groups (hypertension, diabetes, angina, and gout) showed vitality/energy, role functioning, and depressed and anxious feelings to be poorer in the severe LUTS group than in those with the other conditions.

A. Gomelsky (✉) · E. F. Kelly
Department of Urology, LSU Health – Shreveport, Louisiana State University, Shreveport, LA, USA
e-mail: agomel@lsuhsc.edu

R. Budish
LSU Health – Shreveport, Louisiana State University, Shreveport, LA, USA

L. Cox, E. S. Rovner (eds.), *Contemporary Pharmacotherapy of Overactive Bladder*, https://doi.org/10.1007/978-3-319-97265-7_15

Finally, the socioeconomic impact of LUTS diagnosis and treatment has been found to be, likewise, significant [2].

While voiding LUTS are most commonly associated with bladder outlet obstruction (BOO), the connection between storage LUTS stemming from benign prostatic enlargement/benign prostatic obstruction (BPE/BPO) and overactive bladder (OAB) is an inconsistent one. The pathophysiology of LUTS in men is not well characterized, and traditionally, both storage and voiding LUTS in men have been attributed to BOO from benign prostatic hypertrophy (BPH). However, detrusor overactivity (DO) in the absence of BOO has been shown to be a common finding. Hyman et al. found that >40% of 160 men with persistent LUTS had DO but had no evidence of BOO [5]. In another report, videourodynamic studies of 137 men ≤50 years of age with chronic voiding dysfunction revealed primary bladder neck obstruction in 54%, pseudodyssynergia in 24%, impaired bladder contractility in 17%, bladder acontractility in 5%, and DO in 49% [6]. These young men presumably did not have BPE/BPO.

The diagnosis and treatment of OAB and storage LUTS in women are relatively well-established; however, the same scenario in men may be more challenging. Is the OAB a primary phenomenon that will respond to the typical armamentarium, or is it secondary to BOO and treatment for BOO should be undertaken first? The objective of this chapter is to elucidate the pathophysiology behind BPE/BOO and OAB, as well as to evaluate the available treatment options for efficacy and safety. The common nomenclature and definitions used in this chapter are in Table 15.1 [7, 8]. For consistency, our discussion will focus on neurologically intact male, with no history of radical prostatectomy or pelvic radiation.

Table 15.1 Definitions of terms used in this chapter

Term	Abbreviation	Definition/notes
Benign prostatic enlargement [7]	BPE	Prostate gland enlargement and is usually a presumptive diagnosis based on the size of the prostate
Benign prostatic hypertrophy [7]	BPH	Histologic diagnosis that refers to the proliferation of smooth muscle and epithelial cells within the prostatic transition zone
Benign prostatic obstruction [7]	BPO	Obstruction proven by pressure flow studies, or is highly suspected from flow rates and an enlarged gland
Bladder outlet obstruction [7]	BOO	Generic term for all forms of obstruction to the bladder outlet (e.g., urethral stricture) including BPO
Detrusor overactivity [8]	DO	Urodynamic diagnosis; involuntary detrusor contractions during the filling phase; idiopathic when there is no clear cause for DO
Lower urinary tract symptoms [8]	LUTS	Divided into storage symptoms and voiding symptoms
Storage LUTS (formerly "irritative")		Includes frequency, urgency, nocturia, UUI
Voiding LUTS (formerly "obstructive")		Includes weak urinary stream, hesitancy, intermittency, straining to void, feeling of incomplete emptying
Overactive bladder [8]	OAB	Characterized by the storage symptoms of urgency with or without UUI, usually with frequency and nocturia
Urgency urinary incontinence [8]	UUI	Storage symptom; complaint of involuntary leakage accompanied by or immediately preceded by urgency

Relationship Between BOO and OAB

The relationship between BOO and OAB is incompletely understood, as storage LUTS may result from BOO, OAB, or a contribution from both. Accordingly, there may be more than one mechanism responsible for LUTS in men. In men with BPE, LUTS are frequently caused by some element of partial BOO which leads to changes in bladder function [9, 10]. Through animal studies, it is believed that the initial response of the detrusor to BOO is smooth muscle hypertrophy [11, 12]. In turn, hypertrophy leads to significant intra- and extracellular changes in the smooth muscle cell that result in DO and, in some cases, hypocontractility. Additionally, in both animal models and in humans, unrelieved BOO is associated with the development of significant increases in detrusor extracellular matrix [11–13]. Finally, normal aging independent of BOO may produce some of the same changes in bladder function, histology, and cellular function, indicating a multifactorial etiology [14, 15]. Both BOO and detrusor hypocontractility may present with similar voiding symptoms such as hesitancy, intermittency, and a decreased force of stream.

When BOO-induced detrusor changes lead to DO or decreased compliance, associated symptoms may include urinary frequency and urgency. Several hypotheses have been proposed for development of DO, thought to be the linchpin of OAB [16]. The neurogenic hypothesis suggests that DO arises from nerve-mediated excitation of the detrusor, while the myogenic hypothesis espouses a combination of the increased possibility of spontaneous smooth muscle excitation and enhanced spreading of this activity to a majority of the bladder wall. Finally, the integrative hypothesis proposes that a spectrum of triggers can generate DO, predominantly through exaggerated micromotion of the detrusor and propagation.

A decreased ability to accommodate increasing urinary volumes during bladder filling appears to be the link between storage LUTS from BPE/BPO and OAB. Although the etiology of OAB is not completely understood, the impaired accommodation may lead to heightened sensation, which may present with urinary urgency, frequency, and UUI. Several studies support the contention that OAB is a factor in male storage LUTS. Abrams et al. found that approximately one-third of men continue to have predominantly storage symptoms attributed to DO after elective prostatectomy to relieve BOO [17]. Additionally, Van Venrooij et al. found that only 50% of men with preoperative, urodynamically proven DO had resolution of their DO after transurethral resection of the prostate (TURP) [18].

Workup of Male LUTS

Standard Workup

The AUA Guideline on the management of BPH recommends the following tests prior to initiating basic management of LUTS in men: relevant medical history, assessment of LUTS, severity and bother (i.e., I-PSS), physical examination with digital rectal exam (DRE), urinalysis, serum prostate specific antigen (PSA) in appropriately selected patients, and a frequency/volume chart [7]. The guidelines panel suggested that the I-PSS, quality of life (QoL) question, and the BPH Impact Index (BII) are excellent, validated, quantitative assessment tools to evaluate symptoms and bother. Detailed management was recommended in the setting of a suspicious DRE, hematuria, abnormal PSA, pain with urination or pelvic pain, urinary tract infection (UTI), palpable bladder on abdominal examination, and evidence of neurological disease [7].

For those men with minimal to no bother from their LUTS, reassurance and follow-up can be safely recommended [7]. For those men with bothersome LUTS, standard treatment consisting of altering modifiable factors such as fluid/food intake, modifying concurrent medications, and lifestyle advice should be offered to all men. Medications such as alpha-adrenergic antagonists (α-blockers) and 5-α reductase inhibitors (5-αRIs) may also be initiated at this time.

For those men with persistent bothersome LUTS despite vigilant attempts at initial "conservative" management, the panel recommended a detailed additional evaluation in the form of validated questionnaires (e.g., I-PSS or BII) and a frequency/volume chart [7]. The I-PSS asks the participant to best describe the frequency of seven symptoms on a scale of zero (not at all) to five (almost always). The questions encompass voiding (incomplete emptying, intermittency, weak stream, straining to void) and storage LUTS (frequency, urgency, nocturia). Symptom scores of 0–7 are considered mild, 8–19 moderate, and 20–35 severe. Also, a QoL question asks "How would you feel if you had to live with your urinary condition the way it is now for the rest of your life?" The answers may range from zero (delighted) to six (terrible). The AUA BPH Guideline considers a three-point improvement in the I-PSS as meaningful. The BII consists of four questions on patient well-being and social implications of LUTS [19].

Optional Tests

Optional tests at this stage include urinary flow rate (Q) and post-void residual urine determination (PVR) [7]. Both tests are noninvasive and may provide useful information regarding storage and emptying that may help guide further management, workup, or invasive therapy. Maximum urinary flow rate (Q_{max}) may serve as a useful surrogate for obstruction, as 90% of men with a $Q_{max} < 10$ mL/sec have BOO [20]. It is important to note that a low Q_{max} does not distinguish between urodynamic obstruction and detrusor hypocontractility. Furthermore, Q_{max} may vary significantly from void to void and may be highly dependent on voided volume. Thus, multiple voids and voided volumes ≥150 mL are recommended before definitive interpretation. PVR performed by noninvasive ultrasonography may also have significant intraindividual variability, and obtaining multiple values may be beneficial before making significant changes to the treatment plan.

We believe that both of these tests are invaluable in the evaluation of male LUTS. Since both are objective and noninvasive measures, there is virtually no downside to performing them in a serial manner to monitor the progression of a patient's condition from baseline. Furthermore, a reasonable Q_{max} and/or low PVR may grant the physician more confidence in focusing their treatment on options that may impact detrusor activity.

Other diagnostic modalities may be indicated in selected cases. Cystoscopy is indicated in cases of LUTS associated with painful urination and/or hematuria, while upper tract imaging may be indicated in cases with hematuria. Cystoscopy may also rule out other sources of BOO, such as urethral stricture disease, and better delineate prostate morphology, such as the presence of a large median lobe or a high bladder neck. Transrectal prostate ultrasound with biopsy may be performed in cases of elevated PSA or abnormal DRE, and TRUS alone may also be beneficial in estimating prostate size when planning potentially invasive bladder outlet procedures.

Role of Urodynamics in Male LUTS

The utility of urodynamics (UDS) , and specifically pressure flow studies (PFS), is controversial in the setting of male LUTS. The AUA Urodynamic Guidelines made three statements relating to OAB and five statements relating to urodynamic evaluation in men with voiding LUTS [21]. The highest level of evidence was B for statement 17, and this was viewed as a standard: "Clinicians should perform PFS in men when it is important to determine if urodynamic obstruction is present in men with LUTS, particularly when invasive, potentially morbid or irreversible treatments are considered." Statement 6 addressing the utility of multichannel UDS in OAB was classified as an option, with a Grade C level of evidence: "Clinicians may perform multi-channel filling cystometry when it is important to determine if altered compliance, DO or other urodynamic abnormalities are present (or not) in patients with urgency incontinence in whom invasive, potentially morbid or irreversible treatments are considered." Likewise, Statement 8 was a clinical principle: "Clinicians should counsel patients with urgency incontinence and mixed incontinence that the absence of DO on a single urodynamic study does not exclude it as a causative agent for their symptoms." Thus, the absence of DO on filling CMG does not exclude a diagnosis of idiopathic OAB and should not preclude the offering of OAB treatment options. Performing PVR was a clinical principle and, as mentioned previously, should not be argued against.

On the one hand, these series of tests are the only tests that directly measure the contribution of detrusor and outlet to LUTS, and a high-pressure, low flow pattern on PFS is pathognomonic for BOO. On the other hand, the testing is invasive and has inherent potential for discomfort, local trauma, and UTI. A recent critical evaluation of the UDS guidelines suggested that, while UDS and PFS may provide objective data that corresponds to the patient's symptoms, these tests may not be necessary to begin empiric therapy for LUTS [22]. UDS may be useful if initial treatment fails or potentially invasive or irreversible treatment is planned. The guidelines do not discuss the presence of detrusor underactivity (DUA), which may impact outcomes after BOO surgery. A recent systematic review by Kim et al. showed that preoperative DUA correlated with poorer I-PSS and Q_{max} improvement in 10 studies encompassing 1113 patients undergoing TURP and laser surgery [23].

Treatment Algorithm

Several authors have proposed algorithms to guide treatment for men with LUTS, and these are all relatively similar [7, 24, 25]. Prior to offering treatment options, the algorithms typically echo the statements of the AUA BPH Guideline. In addition, we will also typically obtain Q/PVR in our patients, as the benefits of obtaining these two noninvasive studies outweigh any risks. Furthermore, findings of a $Q_{max} < 10$ mL/sec and/or PVR exceeding 150 mL may help guide the treatment discussion and plan. The algorithm suggested by Chapple appears to be the simplest: treat the predominant bothersome symptoms first, be they storage or emptying [24]. The author recommends treatment with an α-blocker for voiding-predominant LUTS, an anticholinergic for storage-predominant LUTS, and combination therapy for those with failure of symptom resolution on initial therapy. We agree with this approach but would emphasize that behavioral and lifestyle modification should be first-line therapy for all men. This is likewise advocated by both the AUA guidelines on BPH and OAB [7, 26].

Treatment Options

As mentioned previously, one treatment approach is to treat the BPE/BPO first ("treat the outlet"). This may be accomplished with pharmacological measures (α-blockers, 5-αRIs, phosphodiesterase type 5 inhibitors (PDE5Is), and combination therapy) or surgical maneuvers. These procedures include simple prostatectomy, TURP, and minimally invasive procedures, such as holmium laser enucleation (HoLEP), photoselective vapoenucleation (PVP), prostatic urethral lift, and convective thermal therapy. The second treatment approach is to treat the OAB symptoms first ("treat the bladder"). The options are pharmacological (e.g., anticholinergics, β-3 agonists, or combination therapy) and surgical (intravesical onabotulinumtoxinA injection, sacral nerve neuromodulation (SNS), percutaneous tibial nerve stimulation (PTNS)). While chronic indwelling urethral/suprapubic catheters and bladder augmentation/urinary diversion are potential treatment options for severe and refractory symptoms, they will not be discussed here. The following discussion of safety and efficacy will focus on the impact of the aforementioned treatments on storage LUTS in men.

Measurement of Outcomes

Outcomes after treatment for LUTS are typically separated into several categories. Micturition diary variables per 24 h include total, daytime and nighttime voids, urgency and UUI episodes, and incontinence episodes. Validated questionnaires include I-PSS (total, voiding (I-PSS-V), and storage (I-PSS-S) subsets),

BII, and Overactive Bladder Symptom Score (OABSS). QoL is commonly represented by I-PSS-QoL. Urodynamic indices include Q_{max} and PVR, and common adverse events are represented by study dropout rates and urinary retention episodes.

Pharmaceutical Treatment Options for BPO

Pharmacologic options for men with BPE/BPO and symptomatic LUTS include alpha-blockers that address heightened bladder outlet tone and 5-ARIs that decrease the size of the prostate through hormonal routes. While PDE5Is have been shown to have a beneficial effect on the voiding symptoms associated with BPE/BPO, there are no specific data describing their impact on urinary storage LUTS.

The data regarding the impact of α-blockers and 5-ARIs on storage LUTS is sparse, since storage symptoms are rarely a primary or secondary outcome of most of these studies. The most relevant data comes from the Medical Therapy of Prostatic Symptoms (MTOPS) study which compared the effects of placebo, doxazosin, finasteride, and combination therapy in 3047 men [27]. At 4-year follow-up, the I-PSS (a secondary outcome) improved significantly in all active treatment groups vs. the placebo group ($p < 0.001$ for doxazosin, $p = 0.001$ for finasteride and $p < 0.001$ for combination therapy). The 4-year mean reduction in I-PSS was 4.9 in the placebo group, 6.6 in the doxazosin group, 5.6 in the finasteride group, and 7.4 in the combination therapy group. Combination therapy was associated with a superior improvement in I-PSS compared to either doxazosin ($p = 0.006$) or finasteride ($p < 0.001$) alone. It must be noted that the improvement in I-PSS was not subcategorized by storage vs. voiding subsets.

Surgical Options for BPO

Transurethral Resection of the Prostate (TURP) Monopolar TURP (M-TURP) has long been considered the gold standard for surgical management of BPO/BOO. The procedure is associated with a ~70% reduction in I-PSS, ~45% reduction in prostate volume, ~12 mL/sec increase in Q_{max}, and ~76% reduction in PVR volume [28]. TURP may also improve storage LUTS. Van Venrooij et al. correlated urodynamic changes with changes in LUTS in 93 men available 6 months following TURP [18]. Improvements after TURP were significantly associated with decreased BOO ($p < 0.01$); however, 32 men who were unobstructed or equivocal preoperatively also benefited moderately from resection. Bladder capacity increased by 45% postoperatively, contributing to a significant decrease in symptoms and bother and improvement in well-being. Ninety percent of the men with a urodynamically proven stable bladder maintained a stable bladder after TURP, while 50% of those with preoperative DO became stable postoperatively.

Bipolar TURP (B-TURP) allows for resection using normal saline irrigant, thus minimizing TUR syndrome seen with the monopolar TURP (M-TURP). Al-Rawashdah et al. compared 36-month outcomes of M-TURP versus B-TURP in a randomized prospective study of 497 patients [29]. The authors found no significant difference between treatment modalities in reference to PVR, I-PSS, and I-PSS-QoL, with men in both groups having statistically significant improvements in all of the aforementioned outcomes criteria ($p < 0.0001$). Men undergoing B-TURP had a smaller drop in serum hemoglobin levels, decreased need for blood transfusion, and decreased risk of TUR syndrome (0 vs. 7 men after M-TURP).

Minimally Invasive Surgical Therapy for the Prostate (MIST) Endoscopic techniques began to emerge in the early 1990s that served as an alternative to the TURP. These techniques used various ablative technologies that theoretically improved hemostasis, hospitalization time, and post-procedural catheterization time and could be performed in an outpatient or office setting.

De Nunzio et al. enrolled 150 consecutive patients with LUTS from BPE/BOO and performed prostate photoselective vaporization with the 80 W potassium titanyl phosphate (KTP) laser [30]. Mean parameters were: age 69.6 years, prostate volume 52 mL, I-PSS 22.3, and Q_{max} 9 mL/sec. Storage symptoms decreased by 54.5%, 63.6%, 72.7%, and 81.8% at 1, 3, 6, and 12 months of follow-up, respectively ($p < 0.001$). Voiding symptoms decreased 63.6%, 72.7%, 81.8%, and 90.9% at the same follow-up intervals, respectively ($p < 0.001$). Retrograde ejaculation was reported in 67% of patients.

Lee et al. enrolled 331 patients with a mean prostate volume of 69.5 mL to undergo HoLEP [31]. At 6 months after surgery, the following statistically significant changes ($p < 0.001$) were seen vs. baseline: decreased total I-PSS (5.1 vs. 18.5), decreased I-PSS storage subset (3.3 vs. 7.5), decreased I-PSS-QoL (1.1 vs. 4.0), and decreased OABSS (2.8 vs. 6.2). As expected, significant improvements in Q_{max} and PVR were also observed.

Saito et al. specifically investigated improvement in storage LUTS after HoLEP in 74 men [32]. Blood flow measurements within the bladder mucosa were obtained before and after the procedure. The median I-PSS improved significantly from 20 to 3 ($p < 0.001$), and the I-PSS storage subset decreased from 13 to 3 ($p < 0.001$). Median bladder blood flow increased at the trigone from 9.57 mL/s to 17.60 mL/s, with 48 of 74 men (65%) having significant blood flow improvement. The authors felt the potential of increased perfusion post-HoLEP to be a key factor in the improvement of storage symptoms.

Fifteen centers enrolled and randomized 197 men I-PSS ≥ 13, $Q_{max} \leq 15$ mL/s, and prostate volume of 30–80 mL to convective radiofrequency thermal therapy (Rezūm; NxThera, Maple Grove, MN, USA) or control [33]. At 3 months, men in the active treatment arm experienced a 160% I-PSS improvement compared to controls ($p < 0.0001$), while a $\geq 50\%$ improvement in I-PSS, QoL, Q_{max}, and BII remained durable throughout the 3-year follow-up ($p < 0.0001$). No de novo erectile dysfunction was reported and the surgical retreatment rate was 4.4%. Transient adverse effects include dysuria (16.9%), hematuria (11.8%), and frequency/urgency (5.9%), and men with enlarged median lobes experienced similar efficacy to those with predominantly lateral lobe hyperplasia.

In a prostatic urethral lift (PUL; UroLift®, Neotract, Pleasanton, CA, USA) permanent implants are placed to hold open the lateral prostatic lobes. Nineteen centers enrolled and randomized 206 men with I-PSS >12, $Q_{max} \leq 12$ mL/s, and prostate volume of 30–80 mL to the PUL or blinded sham control [34]. At 3 months, men who underwent PUL experienced an 88% greater I-PSS improvement than those in the sham group. Improvement in I-PSS, QoL, BII, and Q_{max} were durable through 5-year follow-up with improvements of 36%, 50%, 52%, and 44%, respectively. There was no de novo, sustained erectile or ejaculatory dysfunction reported, and surgical retreatment was 13.6%.

Pharmaceutical Treatment Options for OAB

Monotherapy with Antimuscarinics The outcomes of studies evaluating anticholinergic monotherapy for LUTS are summarized in Table 15.2 [35–44]. There has been some concern that anticholinergics may decrease detrusor contractility and theoretically increase PVR, especially in men with significant BOO. Subsequently, the risk of increasing PVR might lead to UR and infection. In practice, improvements in voiding diary parameters and I-PSS scores are seen, with minimal incidence of UR or change in PVR. Studies focusing on patient-reported outcomes (PROs) likewise report excellent outcomes. Staskin et al. found an improvement in urgency on Patient Perception of Bladder Condition (PPBC) questionnaire in 369 men who used the oxybutynin transdermal system (OXY-TDS; Oxytrol®, Watson Laboratories, Morristown, NJ) [45]. Mean scores on the King's Health Questionnaire decreased significantly ($p \leq 0.0196$) from baseline to study end in eight of ten domains, indicating improved HRQoL. Likewise, after 12 weeks of flexibly dosed solifenacin, Kaplan et al. cited significant improvement in mean PPBC ($p < 0.0001$) and Overactive Bladder Questionnaire ($p \leq 0.001$) scores [46]. In men without presumed BOO, solifenacin significantly improved PRO measures of symptom bother, HRQoL, and overall perception of bladder problems. Finally, Ginsberg et al. saw significant improvements from baseline on the PPBC after 12-week treatment with either daily fesoterodine 8 mg or tolterodine extended-release (ER) 4 mg compared with placebo [41].

A recent network meta-analysis demonstrated that tolterodine ER was significantly better than placebo in reducing micturitions/24 h (−0.76, $p < 0.001$), incontinence episodes (−0.36, $p < 0.001$), urgency episodes (−0.77, $p < 0.001$), and UUI episodes (−0.34, $p < 0.001$) [47]. Furthermore, in a review of tolterodine ER for the treatment of male OAB, Gacci et al. found that the ER formulation was associated with a 71% mean reduction in UUI episodes vs. a 60% reduction in the immediate release (IR) group ($p < 0.05$) [48].

Table 15.2 Anticholinergic monotherapy for male storage lower urinary tract symptoms

Author/year	Treatment	N/N*	Study period	Micturition indices (mean) Δ Total voids/24 h	Δ Incont/24 h	Δ Nocturnal voids/24 h	Mean Δ total I-PSS	% UR	Mean ΔPVR (mL)
Kaplan 2006 [35], Dmochowski 2007 [36]	Placebo	374	12 w	−8.0	NR	−4.4	NR	0.5%	NR
	Tolterodine ER 4	371		−11.0 (s)		−4.4 (ns)		1.1%	
Roehrborn 2006 [37]	Placebo	86	12 w	NR	−5.9	NR	NR	0%	NR
	Tolterodine ER 4	77			−11.9 (s)			1.3%	
Herschorn 2010 [38]	Placebo	124	12 w	−0.8	−1.1	NR	NR	0.8%	−0.6
	Fesoterodine 4	120		−1.6 (s)	−1.8			0.8%	9.6
	Fesoterodine 8	114		−2.1 (s)	−2.4 (s)			5.3%	20.2 (s)
MacDiarmid 2011 [39]	Placebo	82/71	12 w	−1.5	−1.4	−0.5	NR	0%	NR
	Trospium ER	94/82		−2.5 (s)	−2.3 (s)	−0.9 (s)		2.1%	
Burgio 2011 [40]	Behavioral therapy	73/64	8 w	−2.2 (ns)	−1.6 (ns)	−0.7 (s)	−3.4 (ns)	NR	NR
	Oxybutynin ER 5-30	70/60		−2.0	−1.1	−0.3	−3.2		
Ginsberg 2013 [41]	Placebo	133/116	12 w	−1.3	−1.4	−0.3	NR	2%	NR
	Fesoterodine 8	265/227		−2.1 (s)	−1.4	−0.4		2%	
	Tolterodine ER 4	275/254		−2.0 (s)	−1.4 (ns)	−0.5 (s)		<1%	
van Kerrebroeck 2013a [42]	Placebo	92/89	12 w	−0.9	−1.0	NR	−6.3	0%	4.6
	Solifenacin 3	43/42		−1.0	−1.4		−7.4	0%	8.1
	Solifenacin 6	43/42		−1.1	−0.8		−6.0	0%	26.8
	Solifenacin 9	44/42		−1.3	−0.8		−6.3	2.3%	31.8
Burger 2014 [43]	Solifenacin 5, 10	799/786	12 w	−3.6	−1.7	−1.4	−6.0	0%	−0.9
Yokoyama 2015 [44]	Placebo	381/230	12 w	−1.1	NR	−0.5	NR	NR	−0.1
	Oxybutynin TDS	573/346		−1.5 (s)		−0.7 (s)			0.3 (ns)

*N/N** number of patients recruited/completed study, *Δ* change, *h* hours, *incont* incontinence episodes, *I-PSS* International Prostate Symptom Score, *UR* urinary retention, *PVR* post-void residual, *NR* not recorded, *ER* extended-release, *w* weeks, (*s*) statistically significant, (*ns*) not statistically significant, *TDS* transdermal system

Known, urodynamically proven BOO does not appear to be a contraindication to the use of anticholinergics for storage LUTS, with a significant impact on the Q_{max}, voiding pressure, and PVR vs. placebo [49]. Median treatment differences in Q_{max} and $P_{det}Q_{max}$ were comparable in men >40 years of age with BOO/confirmed DO who were randomized to 12 weeks of tolterodine IR 2 mg twice daily or placebo. The volume to first detrusor contraction and maximum cystometric bladder capacity was significantly higher in the tolterodine group, while PVR (25 mL vs. 0 mL) significantly favored placebo. Urinary retention developed in one patient in the placebo group, and the incidence of treatment-emergent adverse events (TEAEs) was not significantly different between groups.

Combination Therapy with α-Blockers and Antimuscarinics This category of treatment is unique in that it has ample Level 1 evidence to support the use of combination therapy for men with OAB (Table 15.3) [50–68, 69]. Clear improvement is seen in voiding diary variables and I-PSS, while the impact on efficient emptying is minimal, at best. Several meta-analyses and systematic reviews have reached the same conclusions [70–72]. The conclusion held up regardless of medication combination or dosing. One caveat regarding data interpretation is the relative lack of long-term outcomes. In light of the significant discontinuation rates seen with anticholinergics, adherence to medication is an important outcome variable in this population. Rates of discontinuation found in medical claim studies suggest that 43–83% of patients discontinue medication within the first 30 days and rates continue to rise over time [73].

To date, Liao et al. were the first to perform a 12-week, prospective, randomized study of first-line anticholinergic and α-blocker monotherapy for men with storage-predominant LUTS [74]. The authors included men with an I-PSS ≥8, I-PSS-S ≥ I-PSS-V, and PVR ≤ 250 mL and randomized them to receive daily tolterodine 4 mg ($n = 89$) or doxazosin 4 mg ($n = 74$). The I-PSS, I-PSS-S, and QoL index decreased significantly in both groups. An improved outcome (global response assessment (GRA) ≥ 1) at 4 weeks was reported in 69% of men receiving doxazosin and 78% of those receiving tolterodine. Patients with tolterodine treatment failure (GRA < 1) had higher baseline I-PSS-V and I-PSS intermittency domain, whereas patients with doxazosin treatment failure had a higher baseline I-PSS urgency domain. The rate of improved outcome was comparable between first-line tolterodine and doxazosin monotherapy for male storage LUTS. The authors suggested anticholinergic monotherapy for men with smaller prostate volume and higher urgency symptom scores and α-blocker monotherapy for those with higher voiding symptom scores.

B-Adrenoceptor Agonists Much of the data regarding daily mirabegron for OAB is derived from three large studies with <30% of participants being male. In a pooled analysis of >3500 patients randomized to placebo, mirabegron 50 mg, and mirabegron 100 mg, Nitti et al. cited significant improvements in micturition diary variables and PROs with both doses of mirabegron [75]. The efficacy profile of daily mirabegron 50 mg was maintained over 12 months of treatment [76]. However, the

Table 15.3 Combination therapy with α-blockers and anticholinergics

Author/year	Treatment		N/N*	Study period	Micturition indices (mean)			Mean Δ total IPSS	% UR	Mean Δ PVR (mL)
	α-Bl	Anti-Chol			Δ Total voids/24 h	Δ Incont/24 h	Δ Noct voids/24 h			
Athanasopoulos 2003 [50]	Tam		25	12 w	NR	NR	NR	NR	0%	−8.2
	Tam	Tolt 2	25						0%	−4.2
Kaplan 2006 [51]	Placebo		222/188	12 w	−1.4	−0.3	−0.4	−6.0	1.3%	−3.6
		eTolt	217/189		−1.6	−0.8 (s)	−0.4	−6.9	0.9%	+5.3 (ns)
	Tam		215/186		−1.7	−0.7	−0.5	−7.9 (s)	0%	+0.1 (ns)
	Tam	eTolt	225/191		−2.5 (s)	−0.9 (s)	−0.6 (s)	−8.0 (s)	0.9%	+6.4 (ns)
McDiarmid 2008 [52]	Tam	Plac	209/206	12 w	NR	NR	NR	−5.2	0%	+7.8
	Tam	eOxy	209/203					−6.9 (s)	0%	+18.2 (s)
Chapple 2009 [53]	α-Bl	Plac	323/292	12 w	−1.2	−0.8	−0.3	−4.3	1.8%	+1.0
	α-Bl	eTolt	329/283		−1.8 (s)	−0.7 (ns)	−0.5 (s) (NU)	−4.7 (ns)	1.8% (ns)	+13.6 (s)
Kaplan 2009 [54]	Tam	Plac	195/174	12 w	−0.7	NR	NR	−4.9	0%	−13.5
	Tam	Soli 5	203/167		−1.1 (ns)			−5.4 (ns)	3.0%	0
Kaplan 2011 [55]	α-Bl	Plac	472/424	12 w	−1.5	−0.8	−0.9	−4.4	0.2%	
	α-Bl	Feso	471/401		−1.9 (s)	−0.9 (ns)	−0.9 (ns) (NU)	−4.4 (ns)	0.2% (ns)	+9 (s) (vs. α-Bl-Plac)
Takeda 2013 [56]	Tam		154/123	12 w	−0.4	−0.5	−0.1	−3.4	0	+3.2
	Tam	Imida	154/123		−1.8 (s)	−1.1 (s)	−0.4 (s)	−5.4 (s)	0	+4.9 (ns)
van Kerrebroeck 2013a [42]	Placebo		92/89	12 w	−0.9	−1.0	NR	−6.3	0%	+4.6
	Tam		179/176		−1.0	−0.7		−7.7	0.6%	−4.0
	Tam	Soli 3	180/179		−1.7	−0.9		−7.8	1.1%	+6.4
	Tam	Soli 6	180/176		−1.7	−1.5		−7.7	0%	+16.9
	Tam	Soli 9	176/173		−1.7 (s)	−0.5 (ns)		−6.6 (ns)	1.1%	+16.5

Author/year	Treatment		N/N*	Study period	Micturition indices (mean)			Mean Δ total IPSS	% UR	Mean Δ PVR (mL)
	α-Bl	Anti-Chol			Δ Total voids/24 h	Δ Incont/24 h	Δ Noct voids/24 h			
van Kerrebroeck 2013b [57]	Placebo		341/315	12 w	−1.1	+0.1	−0.3	−5.4	0%	−6.1
	Tam		327/294		−1.7 (s)	−0.2	−0.4	−6.2 (s)	0.3%	−5.0
	Tam	Soli 6	339/298		−2.3 (s)	0.0	−0.5 (s)	−7.0 (s)	0%	+3.8
	Tam	Soli 9	327/292		−1.9 (s)	+0.1	−0.4	−6.5 (s)	1%	+12.3
Lee 2014 [58]	Tam 0.2		71/69	4 w	NR	NR	NR	−6.2	1.4%	−29.7
	Tam 0.2	Soli 5		8 w						
	Tam 0.2	Soli 5	71/70	12 w				−6.8 (ns)	0%	+9.7 (ns)
Singh, 2015 [59]	Tam	Plac	30/30	8 w	−3.9	−1.1	−1.9	−6.3	3%	−16.9 (s)
	Tam	Dari	30/26		−4.8 (s)	−1.5 (s)	−2.2 (s)	−7.9 (s)	13% (ns)	+10.8 (s)
Kim 2016 [60]	α-Bl	Tolt 2	47/40	12 w	−1.3	−0.7	−0.4	−5.5	0%	+0.5
	α-Bl	Tolt 4	48/39		−1.7 (ns)	−3.9 (ns)	−0.4 (ns)	−6.3 (ns)	0%	+43.6 (s)
Kosilov 2016 [61]	Tam	Plac	81	8 w	−0.4	−0.7	−0.5	−6.0[a]	NR	+0.9
	Tam	Soli + Tros	91		−3.5 (s)	−2.5 (s)	−2.2 (ns)	−6.3[a]		+3.1
Cai 2016 [62]	Plac	Plac	38/30	12 w	NR	NR	NR	−5.8	2.6%	−11.2
				24 w				−7.2		−16.7
	Tam	Plac	38/32	12 w				−9.2 (s)	0%	−31.1
				24 w				−9.6 (s)		−32.4
	Plac	eTolt	38/27	12 w				−6.8 (s)	7.9%	+10.4
				24 w				−5.7		+12.9
	Tam	eTolt	38/29	12 w				−12.2 (s)	2.6%	−27
				24 w				−14.7 (s)		−27.9
Cao 2016 [63]	Doxa4	eTolt	110/97	12 w	NR	NR	NR	−8.9 (s)	0%	−19.1
	Tam	eTolt	110/95					−5.4	0%	−17.3 (ns)

(continued)

Table 15.3 (continued)

	Treatment				Micturition indices (mean)					
Author/year	α-Bl	Anti-Chol	N/N*	Study period	Δ Total voids/24 h	Δ Incont/24 h	Δ Noct voids/24 h	Mean Δ total IPSS	% UR	Mean Δ PVR (mL)
Drake 2016 [64]	Tam	Soli 6 Soli 9	1066/970	52 w	−2.5	−1.4	NR	−9.0	0.7%	+6.0
Cho 2017 [65]	α-Bl		111/93	12 w	−1.9	NR	−0.5	−9.9	0%	−4.6
	α-Bl	Imida	110/93		−2.1 (s)		−0.5 (ns)	−8.8 (ns)	0%	+2.6 (ns)
Matsukawa 2017 [66]	Silo		60/56	12 w	NR	NR	NR	−6.2	0%	−21
	Silo	Prop	60/53					−6.6 (ns)	0%	+23 (s)
	Silo		60/56	52 w				−5.3	0%	−17
	Silo	Prop	60/53					−7.5 (ns)	0%	+20 (s)
Lee 2017 [67]	Tam 0.2		44/38	12 w	NR	NR	NR	−11.9	0%	−3.8
	Tam 0.2	Soli 5	55/50					−9.3	0%	+8.2
	Tam 0.2	Soli 10	47/38					−6.6 (ns)	4%	+26.7 (ns)
Wang 2017 [68]	Tam 0.2		62	12 w	−5.3 (s)	−0.5	−1.2	−5.3	0%	−15.3
	Tam 0.2	Soli 5	62		−7.6 (s)	−1.1 (s)	−2.1 (s)	−8.5 (s)	0%	−19.6 (ns)

From Gomelsky et al. [69], with permission

α-Bl alpha-adrenergic blocker, *Anti-chol* anticholinergic medication, *N/N** number of patients recruited/completed study, *h* hours, *Δ* change, *Incont* incontinence episodes, *Noct* nocturnal, *IPSS* International Prostate Symptom Score, *UR* urinary retention episodes, *PVR* post-void residual (mL), *Tam* tamsulosin, *w* weeks, *NR* not recorded, *Tolt* tolterodine, *eTolt* extended-release tolterodine, (*s*) statistically significant, (*ns*) not statistically significant, *eOxy* extended-release oxybutynin, *NU* nocturnal urgency episodes, *Plac* placebo, *Soli* solifenacin, *Feso* fesoterodine, *Imida* imidafenacin, *Dari* darifenacin, *Tros* trospium, *Doxa* doxazosin, *Silo* silodosin, *Prop* propiverine

[a]Authors excluded urgency and frequency subscores from IPSS analysis

outcomes in either manuscript were not stratified by patient sex. Nitti et al. randomized 200 men with BOO/LUTS to placebo, mirabegron 50 mg, or 100 mg and performed urodynamics [77]. Treatment with either dose of mirabegron was non-inferior to placebo for impact on Q_{max} and $P_{det}Q_{max}$. The study's primary outcomes were urodynamic parameters, and the impact on storage symptoms was not evaluated.

Tubaro et al. performed a critical analysis of the efficacy and safety of daily mirabegron 50 mg in male OAB patients from five phase III studies that included placebo or anticholinergic as a comparator [78]. Three reports were 12-week placebo-controlled studies; one was a 12-week non-inferiority phase IIIb study (BEYOND; mirabegron vs. solifenacin 5 mg), and the other was a 52-week active-controlled phase III safety study (mirabegron vs. tolterodine ER 4 mg). Male patients with concomitant voiding LUTS, BPE/BPO, and α-blocker use were included in the analysis. In the pooled studies, mirabegron demonstrated superiority vs. placebo for reducing micturition frequency, while improvements in urgency and incontinence were not significantly different. In the BEYOND study, mirabegron was comparable to solifenacin for reducing micturition frequency, urgency, and incontinence episodes. In the safety analyses, mirabegron was well tolerated at 12 and 52 weeks, and TEAEs were similar to those of placebo.

Additional OAB Treatments

The AUA/SUFU OAB Guideline stated that additional treatment options may be presented to the patient if "treatment goals (are) not met after appropriate duration, patient desires further treatment, is willing to engage in treatment, and/or further treatment (is) in patient's best interests" [26]. These options include intradetrusor onabotulinumtoxinA injection (standard), PTNS (recommendation), and SNS (recommendation) [26]. Unfortunately, as with most OAB treatments, most trials of onabotulinumtoxinA for idiopathic OAB include predominantly women. Hsiao et al. reported on 60 patients available for 6-month follow-up, 29 of whom were male (48%) [79]. Compared to baseline, OABSS decreased (11.7 vs. 8.4, $p < 0.001$), and the urgency severity scale decreased (3.8 vs. 3.1, $p = 0.001$). On a 3-day micturition diary, the number of micturitions (32.9 vs. 38.3), urgency episodes (21.9 vs. 30), and UUI episodes (5.0 vs. 8.2) all decreased significantly ($p < 0.001$) when compared to baseline.

One of the most common side effects of onabotulinumtoxinA injection is urinary retention, which, depending on the definition, patient population, and injection dosage, may be 5–43% [80]. Risk factors for retention include preoperative elevated PVR (≥100 mL) and retention after the previous injection procedures. A recent study addressed men with persistent OAB refractory to medications after surgical intervention for BOO. Chughtai et al. performed a double-blinded pilot study where 15 men received 200 units of onabotulinumtoxinA and 13 men received placebo [81]. Men receiving onabotulinumtoxinA demonstrated significantly improved QoL scores at 180 and 270 days after treatment ($p = 0.02$ and 0.03, respectively) as well as significantly lower International Consultation on Incontinence Questionnaire (ICIQ) scores ($p < 0.05$). Daily urinary frequency improved from 11 to 8 episodes in the treatment arm, and the response was durable for up to 90 days. I-PSS, PVR, and urgency were unchanged postoperatively in both groups.

In a recent review of the literature, de Wall and Heesakkers concluded that PTNS led to an overall subjective symptom improvement in ~60% of the patients and ~50% improvement in voiding diary parameters with sustainable outcome on the long run [82]. Of interest, there was a ~20% placebo effect (subjective improvement measured by patients who actually received sham treatment). PTNS was safe without any significant side effects but was time-consuming and not cost-effective as a primary treatment.

Likewise, long-term outcomes after SNS are also from studies which enrolled mostly women. Siegel et al. reported long-term results in 272 implanted patients, of whom only 24 (9%) were male [83]. At 5-year follow-up, mean reduction in UUI episodes from baseline was 2 leaks/day, and reduction in urgency/frequency was 5.4 voids/day. There was a significant improvement in all ICIQ-OAB symptoms and QoL measures.

Conclusions

Storage and voiding LUTS often coexist in men, and one or both types of LUTS may become bothersome. While the pathophysiology is incompletely understood, both types of LUTS may occur secondary to BOO. In such situations, addressing BOO either pharmacologically or surgically may improve storage and voiding LUTS. On the other hand, storage LUTS and OAB may occur without attendant BOO, and thus, DO can be effectively and safely addressed with pharmaceutical and surgical means. Urinary retention, once thought to be a major detriment of OAB treatment in men, does not appear to be as common as once thought. Combination therapy may be used in those men where both categories of LUTS are bothersome, and this treatment regimen is well-supported by Level 1 evidence. Other treatment regimens also appear to be safe and effective but lack concrete supportive evidence. For example, studies of medications and surgical interventions for BPE/BPO rarely have storage LUTS as a primary or secondary outcome. Likewise, many of the studies of third-tier OAB treatments, such as onabotulinumtoxinA, SNS, or PTNS, enroll predominantly women, and outcomes in men are largely absent. When approaching the male with LUTS, it is prudent to treat the bothersome symptoms first and to begin with the most conservative option. Fortunately, multiple options are available for those men with significant TEAEs or those with insufficient symptoms improvement.

References

1. Robertson C, Link CL, Onel E, Mazzetta C, Keech M, Hobbs R, et al. The impact of lower urinary tract symptoms and comorbidities on quality of life: the BACH and UREPIK studies. BJU Int. 2007;99(2):347–54.
2. Speakman M, Kirby R, Doyle S, Ioannou C. Burden of male lower urinary tract symptoms (LUTS) suggestive of benign prostatic hyperplasia (BPH)—focus on the UK. BJU Int. 2015;115(4):508–19.
3. Logie J, Clifford GM, Farmer RD. Incidence, prevalence and management of lower urinary tract symptoms in men in the UK. BJU Int. 2005;95(4):557–62.
4. Welch G, Weinger K, Barry MJ. Quality-of-life impact of lower urinary tract symptom severity: results from the Health Professionals Follow-up Study. Urology. 2002;59(2):245–50.
5. Hyman MJ, Groutz A, Blaivas JG. Detrusor instability in men: correlation of lower urinary tract symptoms with urodynamic findings. J Urol. 2001;166(2):550–2; discussion 553.
6. Kaplan SA, Ikeguchi EF, Santarosa RP, D'Alisera PM, Hendricks J, Te AE, Miller MI. Etiology of voiding dysfunction in men less than 50 years of age. Urology. 1996;47(6):836–9.
7. McVary KT, Roehrborn CG, Avins AL, Barry MJ, Bruskewitz RC, Donnell RF, et al. Update on AUA guideline on the management of benign prostatic hyperplasia. J Urol. 2011;185(5):1793–803.
8. Abrams P, Andersson KE, Birder L, Brubaker L, Cardozo L, Chapple C, et al. Members of Committees; Fourth International Consultation on Incontinence. Fourth International Consultation on Incontinence Recommendations of the International Scientific Committee: evaluation and treatment of urinary incontinence, pelvic organ prolapse, and fecal incontinence. Neurourol Urodyn. 2010;29(1):213–40.
9. Roehrborn CG. Benign prostatic hyperplasia: etiology, pathophysiology, epidemiology, and natural history. In: Wein AJ, Kavoussi LR, Partin AW, Peters CA, editors. Campbell-Walsh Urology. 11th ed. Philadelphia: Elsevier; 2016. p. 2435.
10. Moss MC, Rezan T, Karaman UR, Gomelsky A. Treatment of concomitant OAB and BPH. Curr Urol Rep. 2017;18(1):1–7.
11. Levin RM, Monson FC, Haugaard N, Buttyan R, Hudson A, Roelofs M, et al. Genetic and cellular characteristics of bladder outlet obstruction. Urol Clin North Am. 1995;22(2):263–83.
12. Levin RM, Haugaard N, O'Connor L, Buttyan R, Das A, Dixon JS, Gosling JA. Obstructive response of human bladder to BPH vs. rabbit bladder response to partial outlet obstruction: a direct comparison. Neurourol Urodyn. 2000;19(5):609–29.
13. Gosling JA, Gilpin SA, Dixon JS, Gilpin CJ. Decrease in the autonomic innervation of human detrusor muscle in outflow obstruction. J Urol. 1986;136(2):501–4.
14. Nordling J. The aging bladder—a significant but underestimated role in the development of lower urinary tract symptoms. Exp Gerontol. 2002;37(8–9):991–9.
15. Chai TC, Andersson KE, Tuttle JB, Steers WD. Altered neural control of micturition in the aged f344 rat. Urol Res. 2000;28(5):348–54.
16. Drake JM. Overactive bladder. In: Wein AJ, Kavoussi LR, Partin AW, Peters CA, editors. Campbell-Walsh urology. 11th ed. Philadelphia: Elsevier; 2016. p. 1796.
17. Abrams PH, Farrar DJ, Turner-Warwick RT, Whiteside CG, Fenneley RC. The results of prostatectomy: a symptomatic and urodynamic analysis of 152 patients. J Urol. 1979;121(5):640–2.
18. Van Venrooij GE, Van Melick HH, Eckhardt MD, Boon TA. Correlations of urodynamic changes with changes in symptoms and well-being after transurethral resection of the prostate. J Urol. 2002;168(2):605–9.
19. Barry MJ, Fowler FJ Jr, O'Leary MP, Bruskewitz RC, Holtgrewe HL, Mebust WK. Measuring disease-specific health status in men with benign prostatic hyperplasia. Measurement Committee of the American Urological Association. Med Care. 1995;33(4 Suppl):AS145–55.

20. Blaivas JG. Multichannel urodynamic studies in men with benign prostatic hyperplasia. Indications and interpretation. Urol Clin North Am. 1990;17(3):543–52.
21. Winters JC, Dmochowski RR, Goldman HB, Herndon CD, Kobashi KC, Kraus SR, et al.; American Urological Association; Society of Urodynamics, Female Pelvic Medicine & Urogenital Reconstruction. Urodynamic studies in adults: AUA/SUFU guideline. J Urol 2012;188(6 Suppl):2464–72.
22. Gomelsky A, Khaled D, Krlin R. A critical appraisal of the AUA Urodynamics guidelines. AUA Update Series 2017, Vol. 36, Lesson 12. Linthicum: American Urological Association.
23. Kim M, Jeong CW, Oh SJ. Effect of preoperative urodynamic detrusor underactivity on transurethral surgery for benign prostatic hyperplasia: a systematic review and meta-analysis. J Urol. 2018;199(1):237–44.
24. Chapple C. Systematic review of therapy for men with overactive bladder. Can Urol Assoc J. 2011;5(5 Suppl 2):S143–5.
25. Wang CC, Liao CH, Kuo HC. Clinical guidelines for male lower urinary tract symptoms associated with non-neurogenic overactive bladder. Urol Sci. 2015;26(1):7–16. Review
26. Gormley EA, Lightner DJ, Burgio KL, Chai TC, Clemens JQ, Culkin DJ, et al.; American Urological Association; Society of Urodynamics, Female Pelvic Medicine & Urogenital Reconstruction. Diagnosis and treatment of overactive bladder (non-neurogenic) in adults: AUA/SUFU guideline. 2012; amended 2014. http://www.auanet.org/guidelines/overactive-bladder-(oab)-(aua/sufu-guideline-2012-amended-2014). Accessed 27 Apr 2018.
27. McConnell JD, Roehrborn CG, Bautista OM, Andriole GL Jr, Dixon CM, Kusek JW, et al.; Medical Therapy of Prostatic Symptoms (MTOPS) Research Group. The long-term effect of doxazosin, finasteride, and combination therapy on the clinical progression of benign prostatic hyperplasia. N Engl J Med 2003;349(25):2387–98.
28. Cornu JN. Bipolar, monopolar, photovaporization of the prostate, or Holmium laser enucleation of the prostate: how to choose what's best? Urol Clin N Am. 2016;43(3):377–84.
29. Al-Rawashdah SF, Pastore AL, Salhi YA, Fuschi A, Petrozza V, Maurizi A, et al. Prospective randomized study comparing monopolar with bipolar transurethral resection of prostate in benign prostatic obstruction: 36-month outcomes. World J Urol. 2017;35(10):1595–601.
30. De Nunzio C, Miano R, Trucchi A, Miano L, Franco G, Squillacciotti S, et al. Photoselective prostatic vaporization for bladder outlet obstruction: 12-month evaluation of storage and voiding symptoms. J Urol. 2010;183(3):1098–103.
31. Lee YJ, Oh SA, Kim SH, Oh SJ. Patient satisfaction after holmium laser enucleation of the prostate (HoLEP): a prospective cohort study. PLoS One. 2017;12(8):e0182230.
32. Saito K, Hisasue S, Ide H, Aoki H, Muto S, Yamaguchi R, et al. The impact of increased bladder blood flow on storage symptoms after holmium laser enucleation of the prostate. PLoS One. 2015;10(6):e0129111.
33. McVary KT, Roehrborn CG. Three-year outcomes of the prospective, randomized controlled Rezūm System study: convective radiofrequency thermal therapy for treatment of lower urinary tract symptoms due to benign prostatic hyperplasia. Urology 2018;111:1–9, 1.
34. Roehrborn CG, Barkin J, Gange SN, Shore ND, Giddens JL, Bolton DM, et al. Five year results of the prospective randomized controlled prostatic urethral L.I.F.T. study. Can J Urol. 2017;24(3):8802–13.
35. Kaplan SA, Roehrborn CG, Dmochowski R, Rovner ES, Wang JT, Guan Z. Tolterodine extended release improves overactive bladder symptoms in men with overactive bladder and nocturia. Urology. 2006;68(2):328–32.
36. Dmochowski R, Abrams P, Marschall-Kehrel D, Wang JT, Guan Z. Efficacy and tolerability of tolterodine extended release in male and female patients with overactive bladder. Eur Urol. 2007;51(4):1054–64; disscussion 1064.
37. Roehrborn CG, Abrams P, Rovner ES, Kaplan SA, Herschorn S, Guan Z. Efficacy and tolerability of tolterodine extended-release in men with overactive bladder and urgency urinary incontinence. BJU Int. 2006;97(5):1003–6.

38. Herschorn S, Jones JS, Oelke M, MacDiarmid S, Wang JT, Guan Z. Efficacy and tolerability of fesoterodine in men with overactive bladder: a pooled analysis of 2 phase III studies. Urology. 2010;75(5):1149–55.
39. MacDiarmid SA, Ellsworth PI, Ginsberg DA, Oefelein MG, Sussman DO. Safety and efficacy of once-daily trospium chloride extended-release in male patients with overactive bladder. Urology. 2011;77(1):24–9.
40. Burgio KL, Goode PS, Johnson TM, Hammontree L, Ouslander JG, Markland AD, et al. Behavioral versus drug treatment for overactive bladder in men: the Male Overactive Bladder Treatment in Veterans (MOTIVE) Trial. J Am Geriatr Soc. 2011;59(12):2209–16.
41. Ginsberg D, Schneider T, Kelleher C, Van Kerrebroeck P, Swift S, Creanga D, et al. Efficacy of fesoterodine compared with extended-release tolterodine in men and women with overactive bladder. BJU Int. 2013;112(3):373–85.
42. van Kerrebroeck P, Haab F, Angulo JC, et al. Efficacy and safety of solifenacin plus tamsulosin OCAS in men with voiding and storage lower urinary tract symptoms: results from a phase 2, dose-finding study (SATURN). Eur Urol. 2013;64(3):398–407.
43. Burger M, Betz D, Hampel C, Vogel M. Efficacy and tolerability of solifenacin in men with overactive bladder: results of an observational study. World J Urol. 2014;32(4):1041–7.
44. Yokoyama O, Yamaguchi A, Yoshida M, Yamanishi T, Ishizuka O, Seki N, et al. Once-daily oxybutynin patch improves nocturia and sleep quality in Japanese patients with overactive bladder: post-hoc analysis of a phase III randomized clinical trial. Int J Urol. 2015;22(7):684–8.
45. Staskin DR, Rosenberg MT, Dahl NV, Polishuk PV, Zinner NR. Effects of oxybutynin transdermal system on health-related quality of life and safety in men with overactive bladder and prostate conditions. Int J Clin Pract. 2008;62(1):27–38.
46. Kaplan SA, Goldfischer ER, Steers WD, Gittelman M, Andoh M, Forero-Schwanhaeuser S. Solifenacin treatment in men with overactive bladder: effects on symptoms and patient-reported outcomes. Aging Male. 2010;13(2):100–7.
47. Buser N, Ivic S, Kessler T, Kessels A, Bachmann L. Efficacy and adverse events of antimuscarinics for treating overactive bladder: network meta-analyses. Eur Urol. 2012;62(6):1040–60.
48. Gacci M, Novara G, De Nunzio C, et al. Tolterodine extended release in the treatment of male OAB/storage LUTS: a systematic review. BMC Urol. 2014;14:84.
49. Abrams P, Kaplan S, De Koning Gans HJ, Millard R. Safety and tolerability of tolterodine for the treatment of overactive bladder in men with bladder outlet obstruction. J Urol. 2006;175(3 Pt 1):999–1004; discussion 1004.
50. Athanasopoulos A, Gyftopoulos K, Giannitsas K, Fisfis J, Perimenis P, Barbalias G. Combination treatment with an alpha-blocker plus an anticholinergic for bladder outlet obstruction: a prospective, randomized, controlled study. J Urol. 2003;169(6):2253–6.
51. Kaplan SA, Roehrborn CG, Rovner ES, Carlsson M, Bavendam T, Guan Z. Tolterodine and tamsulosin for treatment of men with lower urinary tract symptoms and overactive bladder. JAMA. 2006;296(19):2319–28.
52. MacDiarmid SA, Peters KM, Chen A, Armstrong RB, Orman C, Aquilina JW, Nitti VW. Efficacy and safety of extended-release oxybutynin in combination with tamsulosin for treatment of lower urinary tract symptoms in men: randomized, double-blind, placebo-controlled study. Mayo Clin Proc. 2008;83(9):1002–10.
53. Chapple C, Herschorn S, Abrams P, Sun F, Brodsky M, Guan Z. Tolterodine treatment improves storage symptoms suggestive of overactive bladder in men treated with alpha-blockers. Eur Urol. 2009;56(3):534–41.
54. Kaplan SA, McCammon K, Fincher R, Fakhoury A, He W. Safety and tolerability of solifenacin add-on therapy to alpha-blocker treated men with residual urgency and frequency. J Urol. 2009;182(6):2825–30.
55. Kaplan SA, Roehrborn CG, Gong J, Sun F, Guan Z. Add-on fesoterodine for residual storage symptoms suggestive of overactive bladder in men receiving α-blocker treatment for lower urinary tract symptoms. BJU Int. 2011;109(12):1831–40.

56. Takeda M, Nishizawa O, Gotoh M, Yoshida M, Takahashi S, Masumori N. Clinical efficacy and safety of imidafenacin as add-on treatment for persistent overactive bladder symptoms despite α-blocker treatment in patients with BPH: the ADDITION STUDY. Urology. 2013;82(4):887–93.
57. van Kerrebroeck P, Chapple C, Drogendijk T, Klaver M, Sokol R, Speakman M, et al.; NEPTUNE Study Group. Combination therapy with solifenacin and tamsulosin oral controlled absorption system in a single tablet for lower urinary tract symptoms in men: efficacy and safety results from the randomised controlled NEPTUNE trial. Eur Urol. 2013;64(6):1003–12.
58. Lee SH, Byun SS, Lee SJ, Kim KH, Lee JY. Effects of initial combined tamsulosin and solifenacin therapy for overactive bladder and bladder outlet obstruction secondary to benign prostatic hyperplasia: a prospective, randomized, multicenter study. Int Urol Nephrol. 2014;46(3):523–9.
59. Singh I, Agarwal V, Garg G. 'Tamsulosin and darifenacin' versus 'tamsulosin monotherapy' for 'BPH with accompanying overactive bladder'. J Clin Diagn Res. 2015;9:PC08–11.
60. Kim TH, Jung W, Suh YS, Yook S, Sung HH, Lee KS. Comparison of the efficacy and safety of tolterodine 2 mg and 4 mg combined with an α-blocker in men with lower urinary tract symptoms (LUTS) and overactive bladder: a randomized controlled trial. BJU Int. 2016;117(2):307–15.
61. Kosilov KV, Loparev SA, Ivanovskaya MA, Kosilova LV. Effectiveness of solifenacin and trospium for managing of severe symptoms of overactive bladder in patients with benign prostatic hyperplasia. Am J Mens Health. 2016;10(2):157–63.
62. Cai JL, Zhou Z, Yang Y, Yan YF, Jing S, Na YQ. Efficacy and safety of medium-to-long-term use of tolterodine extended release with or without tamsulosin in patients with benign prostate hyperplasia and larger prostate size: a double-blind, placebo-controlled, randomized clinical trial. Chin Med J. 2016;129(24):2899–906.
63. Cao Y, Wang Y, Guo L, Yang X, Chen T, Niu H. A randomized, open-label, comparative study of efficacy and safety of tolterodine combined with tamsulosin or doxazosin in patients with benign prostatic hyperplasia. Med Sci Monit. 2016;22:1895–902.
64. Drake MJ, Sokol R, Coyne K, Hakimi Z, Nazir J, Dorey J, et al.; NEPTUNE study group. Responder and health-related quality of life analyses in men with lower urinary tract symptoms treated with a fixed-dose combination of solifenacin and tamsulosin oral-controlled absorption system: results from the NEPTUNE study. BJU Int. 2016;117(1):165–72.
65. Cho S, Kwon SS, Lee KW, Yoo TK, Shin DG, Kim SW, et al. A multicenter real-life study of the efficacy of an alpha-blocker with or without anticholinergic agent (imidafenacin) treatment in patients with lower urinary tract symptoms/benign prostatic hyperplasia and storage symptoms. Int J Clin Pract. 2017;71(5):e12938.
66. Matsukawa Y, Takai S, Funahashi Y, Kato M, Yamamoto T, Gotoh M. Long-term efficacy of a combination therapy with an anticholinergic agent and an α1-blocker for patients with benign prostatic enlargement complaining both voiding and overactive bladder symptoms: a randomized, prospective, comparative trial using a urodynamic study. Neurourol Urodyn. 2017;36(3):748–54.
67. Lee KW, Hur KJ, Kim SH, Cho SY, Bae SR, Park BH, et al. Initial use of high-dose anticholinergics combined with alpha-blockers for male lower urinary tract symptoms with overactive bladder: a prospective, randomized preliminary study. Low Urin Tract Symptoms. 2017;9(3):129–33.
68. Wang H, Chang Y, Liang H. Tamsulosin and solifenacin in the treatment of benign prostatic hyperplasia in combination with overactive bladder. Pak J Med Sci. 2017;33(4):988–92.
69. Gomelsky A, Kelly EF, Dalton DC. Combination treatment for male lower urinary tract symptoms with anticholinergic and alpha-blockers. Curr Opin Urol. 2018;28(3):277–83.
70. Filson CP, Hollingsworth JM, Clemens JQ, Wei JT. The efficacy and safety of combined therapy with α-blockers and anticholinergics for men with benign prostatic hyperplasia: a meta-analysis. J Urol. 2013;190(6):2153–60.

71. Hao N, Tian Y, Liu W, Wazir R, Wang J, Liu L, et al. Antimuscarinics and α-blockers or α-blockers monotherapy on lower urinary tract symptoms—a meta-analysis. Urology. 2014;83(3):556–62.
72. Gong M, Dong W, Huang G, Gong Z, Deng D, Qiu S, Yuan R. Tamsulosin combined with solifenacin versus tamsulosin monotherapy for male lower urinary tract symptoms: a meta-analysis. Curr Med Res Opin. 2015;31(9):1781–92.
73. Sexton CC, Notte SM, Maroulis C, Dmochowski RR, Cardozo L, Subramanian D, Coyne KS. Persistence and adherence in the treatment of overactive bladder syndrome with anticholinergic therapy: a systematic review of the literature. Int J Clin Pract. 2011;65(5):567–85.
74. Liao CH, Kuo HC. How to choose first-line treatment for men with predominant storage lower urinary tract symptoms: a prospective randomised comparative study. Int J Clin Pract. 2015;69(1):124–30.
75. Nitti VW, Khullar V, van Kerrebroeck P, Herschorn S, Cambronero J, Angulo JC, et al. Mirabegron for the treatment of overactive bladder: a prespecified pooled efficacy analysis and pooled safety analysis of three randomised, double-blind, placebo-controlled, phase III studies. Int J Clin Pract. 2013;67(7):619–32.
76. Chapple CR, Kaplan SA, Mitcheson D, Blauwet MB, Huang M, Siddiqui E, Khullar V. Mirabegron 50 mg once-daily for the treatment of symptoms of overactive bladder: an overview of efficacy and tolerability over 12 weeks and 1 year. Int J Urol. 2014;21(10):960–7.
77. Nitti VW, Rosenberg S, Mitcheson DH, He W, Fakhoury A, Martin NE. Urodynamics and safety of the β3-adrenoceptor agonist mirabegron in males with lower urinary tract symptoms and bladder outlet obstruction. J Urol. 2013;190(4):1320–7.
78. Tubaro A, Batista JE, Nitti VW, Herschorn S, Chapple CR, Blauwet MB, et al. Efficacy and safety of daily mirabegron 50 mg in male patients with overactive bladder: a critical analysis of five phase III studies. Ther Adv Urol. 2017;9(6):137–54.
79. Hsiao S-M, Lin H-H, Kuo H-C. Factors associated with therapeutic efficacy of intravesical onabotulinumtoxinA injection for overactive bladder syndrome. PLoS One. 2016;11(1):e0147137.
80. Osborn DJ, Kaufman MR, Mock S, Guan MJ, Dmochowski RR, Reynolds WS. Urinary retention after intravesical onabotulinumtoxinA injection for idiopathic overactive bladder in clinical practice and predictors of this outcome. Neurourol Urodyn. 2015;34(7):675–8.
81. Chughtai B, Dunphy C, Lee R, Lee D, Sheth S, Marks L, et al. Randomized, double-blind, placebo controlled pilot study of intradetrusor injections of onabotulinumtoxinA for the treatment of refractory overactive bladder persisting following surgical management of benign prostatic hyperplasia. Can J Urol. 2014;21(2):7217–21.
82. de Wall LL, Heesakkers JP. Effectiveness of percutaneous tibial nerve stimulation in the treatment of overactive bladder syndrome. Res Rep Urol. 2017;9:145–57.
83. Siegel S, Noblett K, Mangel J, Bennett J, Griebling TL, Sutherland SE, et al. Five-year followup results of a prospective, multicenter study of patients with overactive bladder treated with sacral neuromodulation. J Urol. 2018;199(1):229–36.

Chapter 16
Considerations in the Medically Complex and Frail Elderly

Adrian Wagg

Why Might OAB in the Elderly Be Different?

People in late life may be no different from those of a younger chronological age; they constitute the robust elderly, ageing with neither significant comorbid disease nor physical or cognitive disability. Canadian estimates of successful ageing, assuming older people (65+) living in institutions have aged unsuccessfully, suggest the prevalence of successful ageing is 35.3% [1]. For the majority of older people, however, late life is characterised by comorbid disease and cognitive or functional decline, often coexisting. This, plus the impact of physiological and pathological change both within and outside the lower urinary tract, means that the assessment and treatment of overactive bladder (OAB) in the frail or medically complex elderly require a different approach from that in the robust elderly.

Physiology, Pathophysiology and Epidemiology

There is a paucity of longitudinal data regarding the physiological changes in the function and control of the lower urinary tract (LUT) that are associated with normal ageing. Therefore, separating the effects of ageing from those of pathology is often difficult, especially as studies typically involve symptomatic patients or those who have received treatment. Likewise, the effects of changes in the availability and use of different treatments over time confound efforts to obtain reliable long-term

A. Wagg
Department of Medicine, University of Alberta, Edmonton, AB, Canada
e-mail: adrian.wagg@ualberta.ca

L. Cox, E. S. Rovner (eds.), *Contemporary Pharmacotherapy of Overactive Bladder*, https://doi.org/10.1007/978-3-319-97265-7_16

data. By the time people reach later life, typically over the age of 70, the age of the older cohort in large epidemiological studies in this area [2], natural attrition often renders the retention of patient cohorts with a sufficient size difficult. The prevalence of several LUTS, and urinary urgency, the hallmark symptom of overactive bladder (OAB), nocturia, and urgency incontinence, is known to increase in association with advancing age. Furthermore, in older persons over the age of 65 years fulfilling the Fried criteria for frailty, the prevalence of LUTS is higher than for any group of individuals, other than those with spinal cord injuries [3]. In the EPIC multinational cohort study, an age-associated rise was observed in the prevalence of urinary urgency, from 7.1% (95%CI 6.3–8) in men and 9.7% (95%CI 8.8–10.7) in women <40 years of age to 19.1% (95%CI 17.5–20.7) and 18.3% (95%CI 16.9–19.6), respectively, in those ≥60 years of age, and the prevalence of incontinence (of any cause) increased from 2.4% (95%CI 1.9–2.9) and 7.3% (95%CI 6.5–8.1) in men and women <40 years of age to 5.4% (95%CI 4.9–5.9) and 19.5% (95%CI 18.7–20.3) in those >60 years of age. What is clear is that urinary urgency, nocturia and urgency incontinence become dominant symptoms in older patients with LUTS. Functional MRI studies in older people (≥60 years of age) suggest that failure of activation in areas of the brain relating to continence, such as the orbitofrontal regions and the insula, might lessen the ability to suppress urgency [4].

The accumulation of white matter hyperintensities (WMH) within the brain is well recognised to be associated with ageing, and such features are more common in those with vascular risk factors including hypertension, diabetes mellitus and hypercholesterolaemia [5].

Available evidence suggests that WMH correlate with geriatric syndromes including falls [6, 7], cognitive impairment [6, 8] and incontinence and an association exists between the severity of LUTS and the degree of WMH on MRI [6, 9]. Conceivably, a high WMH burden may impair suppression of the ability of the pontine micturition centre to maintain the bladder in the storage phase and increase the likelihood of urgency and urgency incontinence. People with a higher white matter hyperintensity load show a greater prevalence of detrusor overactivity and increased difficulty maintaining continence during cystometry than those persons with a lesser degree of white matter hyperintensity load [10].

OAB, Multimorbidity and Frailty

Older people with OAB, whether in the community or in nursing homes, appear to have greater comorbidity and more impairments in activities of daily living than those without OAB [11, 12]. OAB and urgency incontinence may also be an early marker of frailty, with a shared, common pathway to the geriatric syndromes of later life. In a Taiwanese study of UI and its association with frailty among 440 men aged 80 years and older using the clinical frailty scale [13], the prevalence of UI was 19.1%. Frailty was more common among subjects with UI than those without (60.7% vs 32.3%). Men with UI also had more comorbidity, poorer physical function and were more likely to have depressive symptoms, impaired cognitive function, poorer nutritional status, more polypharmacy and a higher likelihood of faecal incontinence than those men who were not frail [14]. In a population-based study of older Mexican Americans, UI was associated with functional decline in ADLs, IADLs and physical performance [15]. A Portuguese study showed that older people who presented with either "slowness" or "exhaustion" had a risk of UI almost five times greater than those without [16]. In the majority of these individuals, the UI is epidemiologically likely to be of the urgency type, although often the authors did not report the classification. There may then be something about multimorbidity, frailty and OAB in older persons all of which are the end result of shared pathophysiological mechanisms.

Age-Related Changes in Pharmacology

There are numerous factors potentially affecting drug clearance in medically complex older patients. Specific age-related changes occur in pharmacokinetics, drug absorption, distribution, metabolism and clearance. These changes are illustrated in Table 16.1.

Lower Doses

Until recently, medically complex older persons were either overtly or unintentionally excluded from OAB drug studies. The age-related changes in pharmacology suggest that some UI drugs may be effective at lower than standard doses in frail or medically complex older persons with concomitant decreased adverse effects [17]. There are some data supporting the effective use of low-dose oxybutynin in older persons [18, 19]. A single study has assessed low standard doses of trospium chloride and solifenacin in combination in older people of average age 69.4 years in comparison to higher doses and showed higher efficacy of lower dose combination therapy [20]. However, data from pooled analyses of solifenacin [21] and fesoterodine [22] comparing data from younger (<65) and older (>65) adults suggest that older people are more likely to require higher doses of medication than younger people to achieve the same degree of symptom relief. Data from prospective randomised controlled trials of fesoterodine showed that the majority of older people elected to increase their dose of medication during the trial [23, 24].

Polypharmacy

Approximately 60% of people over age 65 take at least one prescribed medication, and about one-third take more than five prescribed drugs. In addition, many older persons take over-the-counter, naturopathic or herbal agents and dietary

Table 16.1 Age-related changes in pharmacology

	Changes	OAB drugs potentially affected
Absorption	Minimal quantitative change despite decreased gastric motility, yet little known regarding effect on slow-release agents	Extended release preparations – probably no clinically relevant effect
	Decreased skin thickness – increased absorption	Transdermal preparations
Distribution	Decrease in lean body mass leads to decreased volume of distribution and half-life for hydrophilic drugs and increased volume of distribution and increased half-life for lipophilic agents	Lipophilic agents, tricyclic antidepressants
	Decreased protein binding in patients with low albumin, leading to higher concentration of free drug	Tolterodine
Hepatic metabolism	Decrease in Phase I reactions (oxidation/reduction)	Tricyclic antidepressants (use not recommended)
	Decreased hepatic blood flow and hepatic mass, leading to reduced clearance for agents with first-pass metabolism	Oxybutynin Tolterodine Solifenacin darifenacin
	Cytochrome P450	Oxybutynin Tolterodine Solifenacin Darifenacin Mirabegron 5-HMT (clearance only)
Clearance	Decrease in renal clearance	Tolterodine Fesoterodine (5-HMT)

5-HMT 5-hydroxymethyl tolterodine

supplements, with the rate of use varying across countries and cultures. In 2010–2011, approximately 15.1% of older adults were at risk for a potential major drug-drug interaction compared with an estimated 8.4% in 2005–2006 [25].The likelihood of adverse drug events and drug-drug interactions rises exponentially as the number of medications increases above four, the conventional, but now rather outdated, limit of determination of polypharmacy. In a study of patients seeking care for their incontinence, those taking more than five medications are almost five times more likely to be taking a medication contributing to urinary symptoms, when adjusting for age, sex and comorbidity (OR = 4.9, 95% CI = 3.1–7.9); in this series there was neither association between age or sex and the use of medications potentially contributing to urinary symptoms nor between class of medication, type or severity of incontinence [26]. A medication review should be mandatory in any medically complex or frail older person before considering pharmacological therapy for two reasons:

- Removal of any medications which may impair the probability of successful toileting
- Minimisation of excessive anticholinergic load (see below)

Adverse Drug Events

Adverse drug events (ADEs) are extremely common in older persons [27], with rates up to 35% among community-dwelling persons aged >65 in the United States. Factors associated with higher ADEs are higher drug doses, age-related pharmacological changes, polypharmacy, comorbid conditions and the interactions between them and female sex [28, 29]. Older people are at higher risk of ADEs from antimuscarinics because of age- and comorbidity-related changes in muscarinic receptor number and distribution, blood-brain barrier transport and drug metabolism [30]. In the medically complex elderly antimuscarinic ADEs can result in sedation, delirium and falls, although there are few data specifically on the bladder antimuscarinics. Xerostomia is also common in older people [31] and was the subject of an FDA warning regarding oxybutynin and dental decay in older people. A sub-cut analysis of a Canadian randomised controlled trial of solifenacin, 5 mg/day, versus oxybutynin 5 mg tid, examined the tolerability of both drugs in subjects under and over the age of 65 years; the study found that dry mouth was no more common among those over the age of 65 but was more common and more severe with oxybutynin [32]. In those over 75 years of age treated with 8 mg versus 4 mg of fesoterodine from a pooled analysis of data from registration trials, dry mouth was more common in the older sample; this finding was duplicated in a prospective trial of fesoterodine in older patients [22, 24].

Another antimuscarinic ADE to which the medically complex older person may be predisposed is decreased visual accommodation, but this has been specifically evaluated only in young healthy volunteers [33] and a single prospective cohort including patients up to the age of 60 years [34]. Drug trials typically report only "blurred vision". In an analysis of adverse events in association with fesoterodine exposure, data from all patients with OAB from all fesoterodine trials were analysed, showing both the rate of ADE and the likelihood of experiencing an ADE depending upon the number of comorbid conditions or the number of coexistent medications at trial entry. Additionally, the study reported on the number of CNS adverse events stratified by age and fesoterodine dose. At baseline, 1546 (55%) of patients aged 65–74 years were taking more than 5 medications versus 696 (45%) of patients aged ≥75 years. However, 944 (61%) of those in the group ≥75 years of age had more than 5 concomitant conditions at baseline versus 1469 (52%) of those in the younger age group ($p < 0.0001$). There was a significant increase in the likelihood of reporting a treatment emergent AE in association with an increase in the number of coexistent medications; the OR increased by a factor 1.028 per medication increase (95% CI, 1.0143–1.044, $p < 0.0003$). For the number of concomitant diseases, the OR of having a TEAE level increase in the number of concomitant diseases was 1.058 (95% CI, 1.044–1.072, $p < 0.0001$). The number of CNS-related adverse events was not associated with fesoterodine dose, and there was no consistent effect of age on the likelihood of a CNS-related adverse event being reported [35].

Anticholinergic Medication and Cognitive Impairment

There have been a number of reports linking anticholinergic medication burden to cognitive impairment, an increase in incident dementia diagnosis and a possible increase in mortality [36–39]. These papers use scales and scores based upon literature review and consensus. This is because in randomised studies there is no relationship between the serum anticholinergic activity of each drug and cognitive impairment [40]. Medications with anticholinergic properties are commonly used by older persons. As much as there is a reported increase in overall medication prescribing for older persons, temporal trends also reveal an increase in anticholinergic medication prescribing [41]. Due to the nature of the cohorts of persons studied, data on medications used for overactive bladder and urgency incontinence are limited to identifying immediate release oxybutynin and tolterodine as a factor in exposure. In the study of Gray [42], over 10 years, those with the highest cumulative burden of oxybutynin exposure had a significant association with cognitive impairment. In the recent study of Richardson, a small effect size, with odds ratios between the prescription of any drug with an ACB score of 1, 2 or 3 (increasing potency) and an incident dementia diagnosis of between 1.06 and 1.11, was found between anticholinergic cognitive burden and the risk of an incident dementia diagnosis with no clear increase in association with anticholinergic potency. The risk persisted with exposures up to 20 years prior to diagnosis [39]. Cognitive effects may be underdetected because they are clinically subtle, neither asked about nor reported by the patient, or mistaken for age-related diseases and ageing [43, 44].

It is clear that duration and extent of exposure to medications with anticholinergic properties are significant factors in the observed associations with cognition, but the data are, to some extent, conflicting with one study suggesting that global cognition was significantly greater in the group receiving either moderate to high exposure to anticholinergic agents versus those who received none. The authors suggested that older adults might experience some beneficial cognitive effects from anticholinergic drugs, possibly due to the therapeutic effects of these medications in controlling comorbidities, outweighing any adverse effects on cognition. Persons with pre-existing cognitive impairment (especially from conditions known to affect central cholinergic pathways) may be at greater risk for cognitive impairment although there are also some data to suggest that those with established dementia may not experience cognitive decline following therapy with anticholinergic agents [45, 46].

OAB in Those with a Dementia Diagnosis

The likelihood of incontinence increases in association with the severity of dementia, but until recently longitudinal studies did not identify an association with incident cases [47, 48]. One longitudinal study of 6349 community-dwelling women found that a decrease in mental functioning as measured by a modified Mini-Mental

Status Exam (MMSE) was not associated with increased frequency of urinary incontinence over 6 years but did predict a greater impact [49]. Despite strong associations with baseline incontinence in the Canadian Study of Health and Aging, moderate or severe cognitive impairment, measured by the same modified MMSE, was not associated with incident UI over 10 years [50]. However, in a longitudinal study of 12,432 women aged between 70 and 75 years with a 3-year follow-up, there was a strong association with a dementia diagnosis (OR 2.34) [51]. Similarly, over a 9-year follow-up of 1453 women aged 65, dementia was strongly associated with incident urinary incontinence (RR 3.0) [52]. Likewise, in a Scottish study, the prevalence of urinary incontinence increased with decreasing Mini-Mental State Scores and was notably more common in those with impairments of attention and orientation, verbal fluency, agitation and disinhibition [53]. In a UK General Practitioner database, when compared with those without a dementia diagnosis, dementia was associated with approximately three times the rate of diagnosis of urinary incontinence. The incidence rates of first diagnosis per 1000 person-years at risk (95% confidence interval) for urinary incontinence in the dementia cohort, among men and women, respectively, were 42.3 (40.9–43.8) and 33.5 (32.6–34.5) [54]. When assessed urodynamically, the majority of incontinence associated with dementia appears to be related to detrusor overactivity, resulting in urgency incontinence [55, 56]. Incontinence in dementia adds to caregiver burden [57] and influences decisions to relocate people to care homes [52]. Whether successful management of incontinence is able to reduce either this associated burden or alter decisions to institutionalise these people is unknown, evidence is limited to case reports and anecdotal evidence. Evidence on pharmacological treatment for UI in those with dementia is lacking; that which does exist is considered in the sections on individual drugs. One matter that is apparent, and which was never reported in the registration trials for the cholinesterase inhibitor drugs (CEI), was the association between their prescription and new onset urgency incontinence [58]. This finding has not been replicated in a large Dutch dataset analysis [59]. Further evidence for an interaction between antimuscarinics and CEI comes from a report on nursing home residents from the United States [60]. Residents with a dementia diagnosis, newly treated with cholinesterase inhibitors, were more likely to then be prescribed a bladder antimuscarinic than those with a dementia diagnosis not on a CEI, an example of the geriatric "prescribing cascade" [61]. In a study to determine the proportion of nursing home residents with OAB or UI with potential contraindications to antimuscarinic treatment, CEI and bladder antimuscarinics were prescribed concurrently in 24% [62]. Co-prescription of both a bladder antimuscarinic and cholinesterase inhibitor can lead to acceptable continence outcomes and no diminution of cognition, but the evidence supporting this is of low to moderate quality [63–65]. More studies are needed, but clearly a discussion on the relative merits of continuation and cessation of the cholinesterase inhibitor should be held before initiating an antimuscarinic agent; the addition of mirabegron may be an attractive alternative in this scenario. The potential for antimuscarinic agents to either cause or worsen cognitive impairment depends on the individual drug's potential to cross the blood-brain barrier (BBB). In older people, and in those with comorbid inflammatory conditions, the permeability of the BBB is increased. Data for the common antimuscarinic agents' ability to cross the BBB are derived from models; both this and their affinity for M1 muscarinic receptors are shown in Table 16.2 [66–73].

Pharmacotherapy for the Medically Complex and Frail Older Person

Until relatively recently there was a dearth of data regarding the pharmacological treatment of OAB – urgency incontinence in older people. The majority of available data came from post hoc analyses of pooled data from patients, over the age of 65y, who had been included in registration trials. Typically, older people comprised around 30% of the total patient sample. There was little information on comorbid conditions or coexisting medication, common in older individuals. Such trials demonstrated overall efficacy and tolerability of the medication under question, with no unexpected adverse events, but failed to report adverse events of interest in older populations [74]. The quality of trials in older people has been assessed in a recent systematic review. Of 1380 records that were screened according to predefined inclusion/exclusion criteria, only 8 papers were suitable for inclusion. Published

Table 16.2 Pharmacological characteristics of commonly used OAB anticholinergics

Anticholinergic	Chemical structure (amine)	Molecular weight of the base compound (kDa)	Lipophilicity	pKi for M1 receptors	pKi for M3 receptors
Oxybutynin (desethyl oxybutynin) [66, 67]	Tertiary	357.5	High	9.9 6.0	12.3 5.5
Darifenacin [68]	Tertiary	426.6	Moderate	8.2	9.1
Solifenacin [69, 70]	Tertiary	362.5	Low to moderate	7.6	8.0
Tolterodine[a] [69]	Tertiary	325.5	Low to moderate	8.5	7.9
Fesoterodine[a] [71]	Tertiary	411.6	Low to moderate	6.2	<6.0
5-HMT hydroxymethyl tolterodine[a] [71]	Tertiary	341.49 (not applicable)	Low to moderate	8.7	8.2
Trospium [68]	Quaternary	392.1	Very low	9.1	9.3
Propiverine [72]		403.9		6.6	6.4
Imidafenacin [73]	Tertiary	319.4	High		

pK data collated from references as shown – studies may not be directly comparable
[a]Fesoterodine and tolterodine are both rapidly hydrolysed to 5-hydroxymethyl tolterodine (5-HMT)

reports were incomplete, and there was inconsistent reporting of subject attrition, patient characteristics, inclusion/exclusion criteria and other details. Only three of the eight included OAB trials received quality ratings equating to strong or fair [75]. The following section considers the available evidence for existing drugs, in alphabetical order.

Darifenacin

Darifenacin was the subject of the first prospectively designed trial in persons aged ≥65 (mean age 72 y). There was no statistically significant difference between drug and placebo for the primary end point, UI frequency, but there were statistically significant improvements versus placebo in urinary frequency (−25.3% vs.−18.5% with placebo; $p < 0.01$) and quality of life, as measured by OAB-q and patient perception of bladder condition [76]. There is also a 2-year extension study in subjects >65, showing maintenance of OAB symptom improvement over the 2 years with 44.4% patients achieving ≥90% reduction in incontinence episodes at 2 years for the 64% (137/214) subjects remaining in the study [77]. Both studies likely recruited robust community-dwelling elderly, the extent to which these individuals had multimorbidity was not reported. The cognitive effects of darifenacin have been prospectively studied in a series of trials. The first was a 3-period crossover RCT in 129 older subjects (mean age 71), 88% of whom had comorbid medical conditions and 93% were on other medications [78]. Darifenacin at 7.5 and 15 mg doses did not adversely affect cognition compared to placebo. A subsequent study in cognitively intact older persons ($n = 49$, mean age 66 y) compared titrated darifenacin and oxybutynin ER with placebo over a period of 3 weeks [79]. Oxybutynin ER, but not darifenacin or placebo, adversely affected the primary end point and delayed a recall on the Name-Face Association Test. However, oxybutynin was titrated 1 week earlier than darifenacin and to a final dose (20 mg daily) much higher than that most commonly used in clinical practice.

Fesoterodine

The majority of prospectively gathered data relevant to either the medically complex or frail older person come from trials of fesoterodine, a prodrug which is rapidly and completely converted into 5-hydroxymethyl tolterodine, one of the major active metabolites of tolterodine. There is a pooled analysis demonstrating efficacy of fesoterodine in subjects over the age of 65, stratified into >65 and > 75 year age groups from all prospective registration studies, a large prospective study which reported the efficacy of fesoterodine in subjects stratified by age (>65 and > 75 y) and a prospective study in the medically complex or vulnerable elderly [22, 80, 81]. In a European trial of 794 elderly men and women with OAB [24], 47% of whom were men, 46% of subjects reported urgency incontinence episodes at baseline and 64% had prior treatment with antimuscarinics. At week 12, the improvement from baseline in urgency episodes (−1.92 v − 3.47, $p < 0.001$), micturitions (−0.93 v − 1.91, $p < 0.001$), nocturnal micturition (−0.27 v − 0.51, $p = 0.003$), severe urgency episodes (−1.55, −2.40, $p < 0.001$) and incontinence pad use was statistically significantly greater with fesoterodine (pooled 4 and 8 mg) than with placebo. The responses on the treatment benefit scales, OAB-S, PPBC and UPS, were also significantly greater in those in the fesoterodine group versus placebo. The results of the open-label extension study [82] confirmed the efficacy and tolerability of active drug further over 12 weeks. A *post hoc* analysis from participants in the study investigated factors associated with dose escalation and identified at baseline body mass index (OR, 1.06, 95% CI 1.01, 1.12; P = 0.0222) and male sex (OR, 2.06, 95% CI 1.28, 3.32; P = 0.0028) and at week 4, change from baseline in urgency episodes (OR, 1.12, 95% CI 1.05, 1.20; P = 0.0008) and patient perception of bladder control (PPBC) (OR, 1.44, 95% CI 1.12, 1.84; P = 0.004) as significantly affecting the likelihood of dose escalation at week 4 [83]. A 12-week double-blind, placebo-controlled study examined the effect of fesoterodine in vulnerable older people as assessed by the Vulnerable Elders Survey [84], which identifies those at risk of death or decline in the following 2 years. This included 562 people of mean age 75 years and resulted in mean reductions in UUI episodes at week 12 versus placebo (−0.65 (0.21), $p < 0.0018$) and 24 h micturition frequency (−0.84 (0.23), $p < 0.0003$) [85]. In this study, over 50% of patients described themselves as exhausted during activities of daily living and 47% had an impaired Timed Up and Go test, suggesting some aspect of frailty.

Fesoterodine 8 mg has been compared to tadalafil 5 mg in a small study evaluating efficacy on OAB symptoms, impact on quality of life and sexual function in older men. All were over 65 years of age, and 65% of them were over 75 years of age. The most common comorbidities were hypertension 37.8% (39/103), diabetes mellitus 18.4% (19/103), heart disease 16.5% (17/103) and depression 10.6% (11/103). Fesoterodine was effective in treating OAB symptoms in this group of multimorbid older men, whilst tadalafil showed superior efficacy in improving total IPSS and sexual function scores [86]. There were no statistically significant changes in performance on a computer-assisted battery of cognitive tests versus placebo in a single small study of cognitively intact older subjects, using alprazolam as an active control [87].

Imidafenacin

Although only available in Asia, imidafenacin has been assessed in older people regarding its pharmacokinetic oral clearance which is decreased with advancing age, increasing hepatic function parameters (AST and ALP), food intake and itraconazole co-administration [88]. The absorption rate is also decreased with food intake [89]. There have been reports of reversible cognitive impairment in two older

Japanese patients (age 79 y), although a causal link was not proven [90]. A study of cognitive change in 62 patients (age range 25–86 y) with OAB and neurological disease (including dementia) found no cognitive impairment measured by MMSE Alzheimer's Disease Assessment Scale-Cognitive or Frontal Assessment Battery over the 12 weeks of the study [91].

Mirabegron

Mirabegron is the first commercially available beta-3-agonist for the treatment of OAB. Theoretically, mirabegron acts by improving relaxation of the detrusor during filling, a perhaps over simplistic view of its mechanism of action which is slowly being clarified [92]. Although mirabegron is a weak inhibitor of the p-glycoprotein system, which might therefore lead to raised central levels of antimuscarinics which are p-glycoprotein substrates which are actively removed from the CNS (darifenacin, 5-hydroxymethyl tolterodine [5-HMT], trospium), there is unlikely to be any mechanism whereby mirabegron might adversely affect cognition although direct data are, as yet, lacking.

A pooled analysis examining the short-term efficacy and longer term safety of mirabegron from patients >65 and >75 years of age included in the four major registration trials of mirabegron demonstrated a reduction in mean numbers of incontinence episodes and micturitions/24 h from baseline to final visit in patients aged ≥65 and ≥75 years. The drug was well tolerated in both age groups and withdrawals from treatment were low. Hypertension and urinary tract infection were among the most common TEAEs over 12 weeks and 1 year. As might be expected, the incidence of dry mouth, a typical anticholinergic TEAE, was up to sixfold higher among the older patients randomised to tolterodine than any dose of mirabegron [93]. A recent non-randomised, open-label study examining the effectiveness and safety of solifenacin (10 mg) and mirabegron (50 mg) in combination versus the single drugs over 6 weeks in 143 women and 95 men over 65 (average age, 71.2) reported a statistically significant additional effect of dual therapy versus monotherapy in terms of a reduction in incontinence episodes [94]. In an open-label single-centre study involving 60 patients with a mean age of 72.3 years (50–86 years) using urodynamic variables and the overactive bladder symptom score to assess efficacy, mirabegron, 50 mg once daily over 12 weeks was associated with a reduction in mean OAB symptom score (9.4 to 6.2 points [$P < 0.001$]), a statistically significant increase in volume at first desire to void and maximum cystometric capacity and an absence in detrusor overactivity in 14 of 35 patients compared with that at baseline ($P < 0.01$). There was no change in observed voiding function variables. There was neither age-stratified reporting of results nor any indication of the frailty status of older persons in this study [95]. Approximately 1/3 patients in a prospective multi-armed trial of mirabegron at either the 25 mg or 50 mg dose, in combination with solifenacin, at either the 5 mg or 10 mg dose, were ≥ 65 years of age [96]. In this study, likewise there was neither reporting of comorbidity and coexisting medication status, nor were results stratified by age. In general, however, in patients with OAB and UUI, whether or not they had received previous treatment, combined therapy with solifenacin 5 mg and mirabegron 25 mg and solifenacin 5 mg with mirabegron 50 mg produced additive improvements in efficacy compared with monotherapies. Approximately 30% of patients across all treatment groups experienced a treatment emergent adverse effect. Unfortunately, for such a large trial, statistical superiority of combined therapy for the primary end point of the study was not met.

In a pre-planned analysis of older (>65y) patients participating in the BESIDE study (approx 30% of 2110) of combination mirabegron and solifenacin showed that the combination of mirabegron 50 mg and solifenacin 5 mg was marginally better than either solifenacin 5 mg or 10 mg in achieving improvements in disease-related variables. There was no mention of either comorbidity or coexistent medication. There were no unexpected safety concerns, and treatment emergent adverse events were similar across each group. The authors concluded that combination therapy might achieve a reduction in anticholinergic load, but the significance of this reduction is purely conjectural [97].

A trial of mirabegron with considerable relevance to the medically complex elderly addressed the effects of β3-adrenoreceptor stimulation on the left ventricular ejection fraction of patients with heart failure, albeit this trial was in relatively young patients. Normally, β3 agonists might be expected to worsen heart failure by a deleterious effect on cardiac myocyte function in the failing heart, but by reduction in sodium overload, β3-agonism might also be protective. Mirabegron was given at a dose of 150 mg by titration over 26 weeks to 70 patients of mean (SD) age 58 ± 12 years. There was no difference over the duration of the trial in left ventricular ejection fraction (LVEF) between the mirabegron- and placebo-treated groups. In a subsequent exploratory analysis, those patients with the lowest LVEF appeared to benefit from treatment [98].

Mirabegron's effect on treatment of detrusor hyperactivity and impaired contractile function (DHIC) compared to its effect on detrusor overactivity has been studied in a small sample of elderly Japanese patients' mean (SD) age of 79.3 (9.6) years [99]. A within-group analysis showed that mirabegron 25 mg was associated with an improvement in the OAB symptom score, urgency severity scale and a global response assessment but not on the International Prostate Symptom Score. Patients with large (volume not stated) post-void residual volumes (PVR) were more likely than those without to develop PVR > 180 mL following treatment with mirabegron.

The results of a prospective placebo-controlled randomised controlled trial (NCT02216214) of mirabegron's efficacy and safety in patients over the age of 65 years, with one-third expected to be over the age of 75 are expected to be released in 2018.

Oxybutynin

The majority of older studies in older people used immediate release oxybutynin (oxybutynin IR). The study by Szonyi et al. examined the effects of low-dose oxybutynin plus bladder training compared to placebo and bladder retraining in the treatment of detrusor instability (as it was then termed) in frail elderly patients living independently in the community. Frailty was implied, but not defined; bladder retraining was defined as postponement of voiding. The study reported a statistically significant reduction in daytime frequency in the oxybutynin exposed group over the duration of the study which did not extend to change in incontinence episodes, nocturnal incontinence episodes or nocturia. At the end of the study, 79% of oxybutynin- versus 55% placebo-exposed patients described a benefit of treatment. Five of 30 patients on placebo and 8/30 patients on oxybutynin withdrew early; the proportion of patients reporting common antimuscarinic side effects was not different between the groups [100]. There are three studies of extended release oxybutynin (oxybutynin ER), one examining cognitive effects in nursing home residents with dementia and urgency UI [101], the other reporting on the effect in cognitively impaired nursing home residents [102] and the last involving cognitively intact community-dwelling women over age 65 [103]. The latter trial aimed to compare the efficacy of oxybutynin extended release three times per day administration of oxybutynin IR in reducing symptoms of OAB in a community-dwelling female population over the age of 65. Unfortunately, the study was discontinued because of poor patient recruitment; over 3 years only 23% of the sample size was recruited, and additionally, an interim analysis of results revealed that the anticipated difference in responses to treatment, upon which the sample size was determined, was not achieved. Published trials of the efficacy of transdermal oxybutynin included subjects up to age 100 and in institutional care settings but did not stratify results by age or comorbidity [104]. An older small ($n = 15$) trial of oxybutynin IR and habit training in nursing home residents showed no effect on UI episodes [105]. In a larger follow-up study in nursing home residents who had failed prompted voiding, the addition of titrated oxybutynin IR resulted in a significant but modest reduction versus placebo [106]. Wet checks decreased from 27% at baseline to 20% on drug and 24% on placebo, leading the authors to conclude that the improvement was not clinically significant especially given the continuing requirement for nursing intervention. However, their a priori definition of "clinically significant improvement" (one or fewer episodes of daytime UI) was achieved by 40% on drug but only 18% on placebo ($p < 0.05$). The dose generally associated with improvement was 2.5 mg three times daily. In a short-term, controlled study of UI in nursing home residents ($n = 24$), there was little effect of oxybutynin IR 5 mg twice daily [107]. Transdermal oxybutynin gel has been reported to have no effect on cognitive function in healthy older people [108]. Unfortunately, the Phase III trial of the preparation [109] reported no efficacy data from older patients. Due to concern regarding the association between anticholinergic drugs and cognition (see above), a number of articles [110, 111] and national [112] and European guidelines [113] have counselled against the use of oxybutynin immediate release in frail older adults.

Propiverine

In 46 patients with dementia (mean age 81 y), there was a 40% decrease in urgency UI with propiverine 20 mg/day for 2 weeks [114], similar to 2 small Japanese trials [115, 116] and a German trial in 98 patients [117], but these trials are of generally low quality. Propiverine's high protein-binding, extensive first-pass metabolism and renal clearance [116] need to be considered when used in frail or medically complex older people. This is borne out by the LUTS-FORTA classification for the drug [118]. Propiverine's impact on intraocular pressures has been described in a small study of older patients, 1 in 24 patients with open-angle glaucoma treated with topical β-blockers and 1 in 24 patients with narrow-angle glaucoma treated with pilocarpine with or without topical β-blockers. Over a week's treatment with propiverine, this study found no increase in intraocular pressures in either group, regardless of previous surgery for their glaucoma. In a trial examining the effect of propiverine on Mini-Mental State Examination (MMSE) Scores in patients over the age of 70 y (range, 70–93 y), published only in abstract, no effect on cognition could be found over 12 weeks of propiverine therapy. The authors stratified the results by baseline MMSE; there was no effect observed in the lowest scoring group [119].

Solifenacin

A study comparing placebo, solifenacin in addition to mirabegron and solifenacin, included older people of mean age 71.2 years. All patients had urodynamically diagnosed detrusor overactivity [86, 120]. All subjects were assessed using validated questionnaires, bladder diaries and post-treatment urodynamics. Overall combined therapy led to more pronounced improvements compared to the monotherapy and placebo groups. Assessment of severity was significantly improved with combination therapy. No safety differences were observed. No mention was either made of comorbidity or frailty, but patients who suffered from chronic active diseases including hypertension were excluded from the study. A secondary analysis of pooled Phase III data in patients aged 65 and older (all community dwelling and fit, mean age 72) found similar efficacy to that reported for younger- and middle-aged persons [21]. However, direct comparison with subjects <65 yrs. from the same pooled trials was not done. Adverse effects in older frailer patients have not been specifically reported. However, data from an open-label, 12-week trial in patients treated by community urologists found that overall treatment-emergent adverse events were more likely in patients aged >80 years (OR 3.9 [95% CI 1.3–11.5]) and those taking concomitant medications (OR 1.8 [95% CI 1.2–2.6]) [121]. Patients with concurrent medications were more likely to be male and on average about 12–14 years older, have comorbid disease, and be administered higher doses of solifenacin. There was no increase in heart rate or blood pressure associated with solifenacin exposure. The cognitive safety of 10 mg solifenacin versus placebo and 10 mg oxybutynin IR was tested in an exploratory study in 12 cognitively intact older subjects without OAB. Solifenacin showed no evidence of impaired cognition or self-ratings of mood and alertness versus placebo [122]. In a 3-way crossover design, chronic dosing of 5 mg solifenacin, placebo and 5 mg bid of oxybutynin were compared using a similar battery of tests in 23 older subjects with mild cognitive impairment. There was no statistically significant effect on cognition of solifenacin versus placebo. In this study, oxybutynin 5 mg bid was associated with impairment in power and speed of attention in a post hoc analysis at 1 + 2 h post dose [123].

Tolterodine

Data from tolterodine studies in older patients allow no judgement to be made about their frailty, medical complexity or "geriatric" status. Tolterodine has more recently been used as an active descriptive comparator in mirabegron trials, but there has been little other research activity. Patients included in RCTs of tolterodine ER were usually community dwelling, able to complete the requirements of the trial and appear to have relatively low, where reported, distributions of common comorbid conditions unlike most frail older persons [124]. Although several trials included patients in their ninth and tenth decades [124–126], the mean age (approximately 64 years) was much lower, and no results have been stratified by age. In a secondary analysis of a large, open-label German trial of tolterodine IR 2 mg twice daily, higher age was significantly associated with "less favourable efficacy", but the absolute difference in odds was only 0.019 and probably insignificant [127]. In a non-randomised study, tolterodine was given to 48 nursing home residents who did not respond to toileting alone; 31 of these patients had a 29% increase in dryness (versus 16% in residents on toileting alone) [128]. There are no prospective data on tolerability in frail older patients. There have been case reports of hallucinations (73-year-old woman with dementia [129]) and worsening memory [130], including in a 65-year-old cognitively intact woman [131]. There is also a case report of delirium when tolterodine was given with a cholinesterase inhibitor [132].

Trospium Chloride

Although often promoted for use in the elderly because of the reduced likelihood that the drug crosses the blood-brain barrier, and because of a low propensity for drug-drug interactions, there is only one study assessing trospium in older people, none in the frail elderly and one in what might constitute the medically complex elderly. There is also a small study in cognitively intact older people assessing cognitive safety. The first was a subgroup analysis of pooled data for 143 subjects (85 trospium ER, 58 placebo; mean age 79 years and ranging up to 90 years; 73% female) receiving once-daily trospium 60 mg extended release (ER) or placebo for 12 weeks, followed by 9-month open-label extension periods during which all subjects received trospium ER [133]. At week 12 of the double-blind period, trospium ER produced greater improvements from baseline than placebo in voiding diary variables, global assessment and quality-of-life indices. Efficacy and tolerability persisted among subjects receiving open-label trospium ER for up to 1 year. There was 10% occurrence of both dry mouth and constipation associated with trospium exposure. The trial in what might constitute medically complex people on account of their coexisting medications examined the safety and efficacy outcomes with trospium chloride XR 60 mg in patients with OAB who were taking seven or more concomitant medications at baseline. Of all 1135 included patients, 427 were taking 7 or more medications. Among these, there was no significant difference between trospium chloride XR and placebo in the proportion of subjects experiencing one or more TEAEs (64.5% vs 58.3%). The odds of experiencing a TEAE were influenced by concomitant medication use, but not by randomization to either trospium or placebo. For those taking ≥7 concomitant medications, compared to those taking 1–2 concomitant medications, the adjusted odds ratio (OR) for experiencing any TEAE was 3.39 (95% CI 2.39, 4.80) [134]. The effect of 60 mg trospium chloride once daily over 10 days on either learning or memory in 12 cognitively intact older people (>65–75 years) resulted in no change in standardised testing. Additionally, no trospium was detectable in the CSF of the subjects at day 10 [135, 136].

Potentially Inappropriate Drugs for Older Persons

There are a number of frameworks which consider appropriate prescribing for older people. The generation of such guidance is often consensus driven, given the nature of underlying evidence, but they do, in general, have clinical utility. A revised Beer's criteria was introduced in 2015 [137]. These guidelines focus on drugs with lower risk-benefit ratios and higher potential for drug-drug and drug-disease interactions and are used for nursing home regulation and quality performance measurement. The concerns regarding oxybutynin and tolterodine in causing urinary retention have been removed. All bladder antimuscarinics are included with respect to their anticholinergic properties. More recently, a system for prescribing appropriate medications for older persons, the *F*it f*or t*he *A*ged (FORTA) criteria, has been published with respect to drugs for lower urinary tract symptoms [118]. These guidelines systematically review available evidence for the use of medications in the population studied (in this case adults >65y with multimorbidity) and assign levels of appropriateness according to the available data. A Delphi process is used to assign drugs into Absolutely, Beneficial, Caution and Don't criteria. Of all lower urinary tract drugs, fesoterodine achieves a Beneficial grade. The majority of drugs were placed into the Caution category, reflecting either deficiencies in, or absence of, available data.

Conclusion

Whilst there is still a relative dearth of pharmacotherapeutic studies in either medically complex or frail older men and women, things are slowly improving. The quality of trials has improved as an effect of time, as much as anything else. Practitioners should be aware of factors in the management of this group of individuals that need to be taken into account when prescribing for OAB and urgency incontinence including LUT and non-LUT factors. As with any of the drugs for OAB, a chronic disease management approach, including regular review and counselling, should be adopted to maximise adherence to treatment and to give realistic expectations of symptom resolution.

References

1. Meng X, D'Arcy C. Successful aging in Canada: prevalence and predictors from a population-based sample of older adults. Gerontology. 2014;60(1):65–72.
2. Irwin DE, Milsom I, Hunskaar S, Reilly K, Kopp Z, Herschorn S, et al. Population-based survey of urinary incontinence, overactive bladder, and other lower urinary tract symptoms in five countries: results of the EPIC study. Eur Urol. 2006;50(6):1306–14; discussion 14-5.
3. Wagg A, Gibson W, Ostaszkiewicz J, Johnson T 3rd, Markland A, Palmer MH, et al. Urinary incontinence in frail elderly persons: report from the 5th International Consultation on Incontinence. Neurourol Urodyn. 2015;34(5):398–406.
4. Griffiths D, Tadic SD, Schaefer W, Resnick NM. Cerebral control of the bladder in normal and urge-incontinent women. NeuroImage. 2007;37(1):1–7.
5. Ylikoski A, Erkinjuntti T, Raininko R, Sarna S, Sulkava R, Tilvis R. White matter hyperintensities on MRI in the neurologically nondiseased elderly. Analysis of cohorts of consecutive subjects aged 55 to 85 years living at home. Stroke. 1995;26(7):1171–7.
6. Wakefield DB, Moscufo N, Guttmann CR, Kuchel GA, Kaplan RF, Pearlson G, et al. White matter hyperintensities predict functional decline in voiding, mobility, and cognition in older adults. J Am Geriatr Soc. 2010;58(2):275–81.
7. Enzinger C, Linortner P, Schmidt R, Ropele S, Pendl B, Petrovic K, et al. White matter hyperintensities alter the functional organization of the motor system with ageing—first evidence from FMRI (Oral Communication). 19th European Stroke Conference; 2010 May 26–29; Barcelona, Spain. Cerebrovascular Diseases 2010; 29(Suppl):79.
8. Prins ND, Scheltens P. White matter hyperintensities, cognitive impairment and dementia: an update. Nat Rev Neurol. 2015;11(3):157–65.
9. Sakakibara R, Panicker J, Fowler CJ, Tateno F, Kishi M, Tsuyuzaki Y, et al. Vascular incontinence: incontinence in the elderly due to ischemic white matter changes. Neurol Int. 2012;4(2):e13.
10. Tadic SD, Griffiths D, Murrin A, Schaefer W, Aizenstein HJ, Resnick NM. Brain activity during bladder filling is related to white matter structural changes in older women with urinary incontinence. NeuroImage. 2010;51(4):1294–302.
11. Ganz ML, Liu J, Zou KH, Bhagnani T, Luo X. Real-world characteristics of elderly patients with overactive bladder in the United States. Curr Med Res Opin. 2016;32(12):1997–2005.
12. Zarowitz BJ, Allen C, O'Shea T, Tangalos E, Berner T, Ouslander JG. Clinical burden and nonpharmacologic management of nursing facility residents with overactive bladder and/or urinary incontinence. Consult Pharm. 2015;30(9):533–42.
13. Rockwood K, Song X, MacKnight C, Bergman H, Hogan DB, McDowell I, et al. A global clinical measure of fitness and frailty in elderly people. CMAJ. 2005;173(5):489–95.
14. Wang CJ, Hung CH, Tang TC, Chen LY, Peng LN, Hsiao FY, et al. Urinary incontinence and its association with frailty among men aged 80 years and older in Taiwan: a cross-sectional study. Rejuvenation Res. 2017;20(2):111–7.
15. Miles TP, Palmer RF, Espino DV, Mouton CP, Lichtenstein MJ, Markides KS. New-onset incontinence and markers of frailty: data from the Hispanic Established Populations for Epidemiologic Studies of the Elderly. J Gerontol A Biol Sci Med Sci. 2001;56(1):M19–24.
16. Silva VA, Souza KL, D'Elboux MJ. Urinary incontinence and the criteria of frailness among the elderly outpatients. Rev Esc Enferm USP. 2011;45(3):672–8.
17. Rochon PA, Anderson GM, Tu JV, Gurwitz JH, Clark JP, Shear NH, et al. Age- and gender-related use of low-dose drug therapy: the need to manufacture low-dose therapy and evaluate the minimum effective dose. J Am Geriatr Soc. 1999;47(8):954–9.
18. Bemelmans BL, Kiemeney LA, Debruyne FM. Low-dose oxybutynin for the treatment of urge incontinence: good efficacy and few side effects. Eur Urol. 2000;37(6):709–13.
19. Malone-Lee J, Lubel D, Szonyi G. Low dose oxybutynin for the unstable bladder. BMJ. 1992;304(6833):1053.

20. Kosilov KV, Loparev SA, Ivanovskaya MA, Kosilova LV. Comparative effectiveness of combined low- and standard-dose trospium and solifenacin for moderate overactive bladder symptoms in elderly men and women. Urol Int. 2014;93(4):470–3.
21. Wagg A, Wyndaele JJ, Sieber P. Efficacy and tolerability of solifenacin in elderly subjects with overactive bladder syndrome: a pooled analysis. Am J Geriatr Pharmacother. 2006;4(1):14–24.
22. Kraus SR, Ruiz-Cerda JL, Martire D, Wang JT, Wagg AS. Efficacy and tolerability of fesoterodine in older and younger subjects with overactive bladder. Urology. 2010;76(6):1350–7.
23. Dubeau CE, Kraus SR, Griebling TL, Newman DK, Wyman JF, Johnson TM 2nd, et al. Effect of fesoterodine in vulnerable elderly subjects with urgency incontinence: a double-blind, placebo-controlled trial. J Urol. 2014;191(2):395–404.
24. Wagg A, Khullar V, Marschall-Kehrel D, Michel MC, Oelke M, Darekar A, et al. Flexible-dose fesoterodine in elderly adults with overactive bladder: results of the randomized, double-blind, placebo-controlled study of fesoterodine in an aging population trial. J Am Geriatr Soc. 2013;61(2):185–93.
25. Qato DM, Wilder J, Schumm LP, Gillet V, Alexander GC. Changes in prescription and over-the-counter medication and dietary supplement use among older adults in the United States, 2005 vs 2011. JAMA Intern Med. 2016;176(4):473–82.
26. Kashyap M, Tu le M, Tannenbaum C. Prevalence of commonly prescribed medications potentially contributing to urinary symptoms in a cohort of older patients seeking care for incontinence. BMC Geriatr. 2013;13:57.
27. Cresswell KM, Fernando B, McKinstry B, Sheikh A. Adverse drug events in the elderly. Br Med Bull. 2007;83:259–74.
28. Hofer-Dueckelmann C, Prinz E, Beindl W, Szymanski J, Fellhofer G, Pichler M, et al. Adverse drug reactions (ADRs) associated with hospital admissions—elderly female patients are at highest risk. Int J Clin Pharmacol Ther. 2011;49(10):577–86.
29. Rodenburg EM, Stricker BH, Visser LE. Sex differences in cardiovascular drug-induced adverse reactions causing hospital admissions. Br J Clin Pharmacol. 2012 Dec;74(6):1045–52.
30. Feinberg M. The problems of anticholinergic adverse effects in older patients. Drugs Aging. 1993;3(4):335–48.
31. Hopcraft MS, Tan C. Xerostomia: an update for clinicians. Aust Dent J. 2010;55(3):238–44; quiz 353.
32. Herschorn S, Pommerville P, Stothers L, Egerdie B, Gajewski J, Carlson K, et al. Tolerability of solifenacin and oxybutynin immediate release in older (> 65 years) and younger (</= 65 years) patients with overactive bladder: sub-analysis from a Canadian, randomized, double-blind study. Curr Med Res Opin. 2011;27(2):375–82.
33. Chapple CR, Nilvebrant L. Tolterodine: selectivity for the urinary bladder over the eye (as measured by visual accommodation) in healthy volunteers. Drugs R D. 2002;3(2):75–81.
34. Altan-Yaycioglu R, Yaycioglu O, Aydin Akova Y, Guvel S, Ozkardes H. Ocular side-effects of tolterodine and oxybutynin, a single-blind prospective randomized trial. Br J Clin Pharmacol. 2005;59(5):588–92.
35. Wagg A, Arumi D, Herschorn S, Angulo Cuesta J, Haab F, Ntanios F, et al. A pooled analysis of the efficacy of fesoterodine for the treatment of overactive bladder, and the relationship between safety, co-morbidity and polypharmacy in patients aged 65 years or older. Age Ageing. 2017;46(4):620–6.
36. Fox C, Richardson K, Maidment ID, Savva GM, Matthews FE, Smithard D, et al. Anticholinergic medication use and cognitive impairment in the older population: the medical research council cognitive function and ageing study. J Am Geriatr Soc. 2011;59(8):1477–83.
37. Gray SL, Anderson ML, Dublin S, Hanlon JT, Hubbard R, Walker R, Yu O, Crane PK, Larson EB. Cumulative use of strong anticholinergics and incident dementia: a prospective cohort study. JAMA Intern Med. 2015;175(3):401–7.
38. Carriere I, Fourrier-Reglat A, Dartigues JF, Rouaud O, Pasquier F, Ritchie K, et al. Drugs with anticholinergic properties, cognitive decline, and dementia in an elderly general population: the 3-city study. Arch Intern Med. 2009;169(14):1317–24.

39. Richardson K, Fox C, Maidment I, Steel N, Loke YK, Arthur A, et al. Anticholinergic drugs and risk of dementia: case-control study. BMJ. 2018;361:k1315.
40. Salahudeen MS, Chyou TY, Nishtala PS. Serum anticholinergic activity and cognitive and functional adverse outcomes in older people: a systematic review and meta-analysis of the literature. PLoS One. 2016;11(3):e0151084.
41. Sumukadas D, McMurdo ME, Mangoni AA, Guthrie B. Temporal trends in anticholinergic medication prescription in older people: repeated cross-sectional analysis of population prescribing data. Age Ageing. 2014;43(4):515–21.
42. Gray SL, Anderson ML, Dublin S, Hanlon JT, Hubbard R, Walker R, et al. Cumulative use of strong anticholinergics and incident dementia: a prospective cohort study. JAMA Intern Med. 2015;175(3):401–7.
43. Kay GG, Abou-Donia MB, Messer WS Jr, Murphy DG, Tsao JW, Ouslander JG. Antimuscarinic drugs for overactive bladder and their potential effects on cognitive function in older patients. J Am Geriatr Soc. 2005;53(12):2195–201.
44. Wagg A. The cognitive burden of anticholinergics in the elderly—implications for the treatment of overactive bladder. Eur Urol Rev. 2012;7(1):42–9.
45. Fox C, Livingston G, Maidment ID, Coulton S, Smithard DG, Boustani M, et al. The impact of anticholinergic burden in Alzheimer's dementia-the LASER-AD study. Age Ageing. 2011;40(6):730–5.
46. Whalley LJ, Sharma S, Fox HC, Murray AD, Staff RT, Duthie AC, et al. Anticholinergic drugs in late life: adverse effects on cognition but not on progress to dementia. J Alzheimers Dis. 2012;30(2):253–61.
47. Ouslander JG, Uman GC, Urman HN, Rubenstein LZ. Incontinence among nursing home patients: clinical and functional correlates. J Am Geriatr Soc. 1987;35(4):324–30.
48. Østbye T, Borrie MJ, Hunskaar S. The prevalence of urinary incontinence in elderly Canadians and its association with dementia, ambulatory function, and institutionalization. Norsk Epidemiologi. 2009;8(2):177–82.
49. Huang AJ, Brown JS, Thom DH, Fink HA, Yaffe K, Study of Osteoporotic Fractures Research G. Urinary incontinence in older community-dwelling women: the role of cognitive and physical function decline. Obstet Gynecol. 2007;109(4):909–16.
50. Ostbye T, Seim A, Krause KM, Feightner J, Hachinski V, Sykes E, et al. A 10-year follow-up of urinary and fecal incontinence among the oldest old in the community: the Canadian Study of Health and Aging. Can J Aging. 2004;23(4):319–31.
51. Byles J, Millar CJ, Sibbritt DW, Chiarelli P. Living with urinary incontinence: a longitudinal study of older women. Age Ageing. 2009;38(3):333–8. discussion 251
52. Thom DH, Haan MN, Van Den Eeden SK. Medically recognized urinary incontinence and risks of hospitalization, nursing home admission and mortality. Age Ageing. 1997;26(5):367–74.
53. Alcorn G, Law E, Connelly PJ, Starr JM. Urinary incontinence in people with Alzheimer's disease. Int J Geriatr Psychiatry. 2014;29(1):107–9.
54. Grant RL, Drennan VM, Rait G, Petersen I, Iliffe S. First diagnosis and management of incontinence in older people with and without dementia in primary care: a cohort study using The Health Improvement Network primary care database. PLoS Med. 2013;10(8):e1001505.
55. Resnick NM, Yalla SV, Laurino E. The pathophysiology of urinary incontinence among institutionalized elderly persons. N Engl J Med. 1989;320(1):1–7.
56. Lee SH, Cho ST, Na HR, Ko SB, Park MH. Urinary incontinence in patients with Alzheimer's disease: relationship between symptom status and urodynamic diagnoses. Int J Urol. 2014;21(7):683–7.
57. Cassells C, Watt E. The impact of incontinence on older spousal caregivers. J Adv Nurs. 2003;42(6):607–16.
58. Starr JM. Cholinesterase inhibitor treatment and urinary incontinence in Alzheimer's disease. J Am Geriatr Soc. 2007;55(5):800–1.
59. Kroger E, Van Marum R, Souverein P, Carmichael PH, Egberts T. Treatment with rivastigmine or galantamine and risk of urinary incontinence: results from a Dutch database study. Pharmacoepidemiol Drug Saf. 2015;24(3):276–85.

60. Siegler EL, Reidenberg M. Treatment of urinary incontinence with anticholinergics in patients taking cholinesterase inhibitors for dementia. Clin Pharmacol Ther. 2004;75(5):484–8.
61. Gill S, Mamdani M, Naglie G, Streiner DL, Bronskill SE, Kopp A, Shulman KI, Lee PE, Rochon PA. A prescribing cascade involving cholinesterase inhibitors and anticholinergic drugs. Arch Intern Med. 2005;165(7):808–13.
62. Zarowitz BJ, Allen C, O'Shea T, Tangalos EG, Berner T, Ouslander JG. Challenges in the pharmacological management of nursing home residents with overactive bladder or urinary incontinence. J Am Geriatr Soc. 2015;63(11):2298–307.
63. Isik AT, Celik T, Bozoglu E, Doruk H. Trospium and cognition in patients with late onset Alzheimer disease. J Nutr Health Aging. 2009;13(8):672–6.
64. Sink KM, Thomas J 3rd, Xu H, Craig B, Kritchevsky S, Sands LP. Dual use of bladder anticholinergics and cholinesterase inhibitors: long-term functional and cognitive outcomes. J Am Geriatr Soc. 2008;56(5):847–53.
65. Sakakibara R, Ogata T, Uchiyama T, Kishi M, Ogawa E, Isaka S, et al. How to manage overactive bladder in elderly individuals with dementia? A combined use of donepezil, a central acetylcholinesterase inhibitor, and propiverine, a peripheral muscarine receptor antagonist. J Am Geriatr Soc. 2009;57(8):1515–7.
66. WebMD L. Rx List: the internet drug index: Web MD; 2012. Available from: http://www.rxlist.com/toviaz-drug.htm. Accessed 28 May 2018.
67. Reitz AB, Gupta SK, Huang Y, Parker MH, Ryan RR. The preparation and human muscarinic receptor profiling of oxybutynin and N-desethyloxybutynin enantiomers. Med Chem. 2007;3(6):543–5.
68. Napier C, Gupta P. Darifenacin is selective for the human recombinant M3 receptor subtype (abstract). Neurourol Urodyn. 2002;21:A445.
69. Ikeda K, Kobayashi S, Suzuki M, Miyata K, Takeuchi M, Yamada T, et al. M(3) receptor antagonism by the novel antimuscarinic agent solifenacin in the urinary bladder and salivary gland. Naunyn Schmiedeberg's Arch Pharmacol. 2002;366(2):97–103.
70. Kobayashi S1, Ikeda K, Miyata K. Comparison of in vitro selectivity profiles of solifenacin succinate (YM905) and current antimuscarinic drugs in bladder and salivary glands: a Ca2+ mobilization study in monkey cells. Life Sci. 2004;74(7):843–53.
71. Wagg A, Verdejo C, Molander U. Review of cognitive impairment with antimuscarinic agents in elderly patients with overactive bladder. Int J Clin Pract. 2010;64(9):1279–86.
72. Wuest M, Weiss A, Waelbroeck M, Braeter M, Kelly LU, Hakenberg OW, et al. Propiverine and metabolites: differences in binding to muscarinic receptors and in functional models of detrusor contraction. Naunyn Schmiedeberg's Arch Pharmacol. 2006;374(2):87–97.
73. Kobayashi F, Yageta Y, Yamazaki T, Wakabayashi E, Inoue M, Segawa M, et al. Pharmacological effects of imidafenacin (KRP-197/ONO-8025), a new bladder selective anticholinergic agent, in rats. Comparison of effects on urinary bladder capacity and contraction, salivary secretion and performance in the Morris water maze task. Arzneimittelforschung. 2007;57(3):147–54.
74. Paquette A, Gou P, Tannenbaum C. Systematic review and meta-analysis: do clinical trials testing antimuscarinic agents for overactive bladder adequately measure central nervous system adverse events? J Am Geriatr Soc. 2011;59(7):1332–9.
75. Kistler KD, Xu Y, Zou KH, Ntanios F, Chapman DS, Luo X. Systematic literature review of clinical trials evaluating pharmacotherapy for overactive bladder in elderly patients: an assessment of trial quality. Neurourol Urodyn. 2018;37(1):54–66.
76. Chapple C, DuBeau C, Ebinger U, Rekeda L, Viegas A. Darifenacin treatment of patients >or= 65 years with overactive bladder: results of a randomized, controlled, 12-week trial. Curr Med Res Opin. 2007;23(10):2347–58.
77. Hill S, Elhilali M, Millard RJ, Dwyer PL, Lheritier K, Kawakami FT, et al. Long-term darifenacin treatment for overactive bladder in patients aged 65 years and older: analysis of results from a 2-year, open-label extension study. Curr Med Res Opin. 2007;23(11):2697–704.
78. Lipton RB, Kolodner K, Wesnes K. Assessment of cognitive function of the elderly population: effects of darifenacin. J Urol. 2005;173(2):493–8.

79. Kay G, Crook T, Rekeda L, Lima R, Ebinger U, Arguinzoniz M, et al. Differential effects of the antimuscarinic agents darifenacin and oxybutynin ER on memory in older subjects. Eur Urol. 2006;50(2):317–26.
80. Malhotra BK, Wood N, Sachse R. Influence of age, gender, and race on pharmacokinetics, pharmacodynamics, and safety of fesoterodine. Int J Clin Pharmacol Ther. 2009;47(9):570–8.
81. Sand PK, Heesakkers J, Kraus SR, Carlsson M, Guan Z, Berriman S. Long-term safety, tolerability and efficacy of fesoterodine in subjects with overactive bladder symptoms stratified by age: pooled analysis of two open-label extension studies. Drugs Aging. 2012;29(2):119–31.
82. Wagg A, Khullar V, Michel MC, Oelke M, Darekar A, Bitoun CE. Long-term safety, tolerability and efficacy of flexible-dose fesoterodine in elderly patients with overactive bladder: open-label extension of the SOFIA trial. Neurourol Urodyn. 2014;33(1):106–14.
83. Wagg A, Darekar A, Arumi D, Khullar V, Oelke M. Factors associated with dose escalation of fesoterodine for treatment of overactive bladder in people >65 years of age: a post hoc analysis of data from the SOFIA study. Neurourol Urodyn. 2015;34(5):438–43.
84. Min L, Yoon W, Mariano J, Wenger NS, Elliott MN, Kamberg C, et al. The vulnerable elders-13 survey predicts 5-year functional decline and mortality outcomes in older ambulatory care patients. J Am Geriatr Soc. 2009;57(11):2070–6.
85. Dubeau CE, Kraus SR, Griebling TL, Newman DK, Wyman JF, Johnson TM 2nd, et al. Effect of fesoterodine in vulnerable elderly subjects with urgency incontinence: a double-blind, placebo controlled trial. J Urol. 2014;191(2):395–404.
86. Dell'Atti L. Efficacy of Tadalafil once daily versus Fesoterodine in the treatment of overactive bladder in older patients. Eur Rev Med Pharmacol Sci. 2015;19(9):1559–63.
87. Kay GG, Maruff P, Scholfield D, Malhotra B, Whelan L, Darekar A, et al. Evaluation of cognitive function in healthy older subjects treated with fesoterodine. Postgrad Med. 2012;124(3):7–15.
88. Ohno T, Nakayama K, Nakade S, Kitagawa J, Ueda S, Miyabe H, et al. Effect of itraconazole on the pharmacokinetics of imidafenacin in healthy subjects. J Clin Pharmacol. 2008;48(3):330–4.
89. Ohno T, Nakade S, Nakayama K, Kitagawa J, Ueda S, Miyabe H, et al. Absolute bioavailability of imidafenacin after oral administration to healthy subjects. Br J Clin Pharmacol. 2008;65(2):197–202.
90. Shiota T, Torimoto K, Momose H, Nakamuro T, Mochizuki H, Kumamoto H, et al. Temporary cognitive impairment related to administration of newly developed anticholinergic medicines for overactive bladder: two case reports. BMC Res Notes. 2014;7:672.
91. Sakakibara R, Tateno F, Yano M, Takahashi O, Sugiyama M, Ogata T, et al. Imidafenacin on bladder and cognitive function in neurologic OAB patients. Clin Auton Res. 2013;23(4):189–95.
92. Michel MC, Korstanje C. beta3-Adrenoceptor agonists for overactive bladder syndrome: role of translational pharmacology in a repositioning clinical drug development project. Pharmacol Ther. 2016;159:66–82.
93. Wagg A, Cardozo L, Nitti VW, Castro-Diaz D, Auerbach S, Blauwet MB, et al. The efficacy and tolerability of the beta3-adrenoceptor agonist mirabegron for the treatment of symptoms of overactive bladder in older patients. Age Ageing. 2014;43(5):666–75.
94. Kosilov K, Loparev S, Ivanovskaya M, Kosilova L. A randomized, controlled trial of effectiveness and safety of management of OAB symptoms in elderly men and women with standard-dosed combination of solifenacin and mirabegron. Arch Gerontol Geriatr. 2015;61(2):212–6.
95. Matsukawa Y, Takai S, Funahashi Y, Yamamoto T, Gotoh M. Urodynamic evaluation of the efficacy of mirabegron on storage and voiding functions in women with overactive bladder. Urology. 2015;85(4):786–90.
96. Herschorn S, Chapple CR, Abrams P, Arlandis S, Mitcheson D, Lee KS, et al. Efficacy and safety of combinations of mirabegron and solifenacin compared with monotherapy and placebo in patients with overactive bladder (SYNERGY study). BJU Int. 2017;120(4):562–75.
97. Gibson W, MacDiarmid S, Huang M, Siddiqui E, Stolzel M, Choudhury N, et al. Treating overactive bladder in older patients with a combination of Mirabegron and Solifenacin: a Prespecified analysis from the BESIDE study. Eur Urol Focus. 2017;3(6):629–38.

98. Bundgaard H, Axelsson A, Hartvig Thomsen J, Sorgaard M, Kofoed KF, Hasselbalch R, et al. The first-in-man randomized trial of a beta3 adrenoceptor agonist in chronic heart failure: the BEAT-HF trial. Eur J Heart Fail. 2017;19(4):566–75.
99. Lee CL, Kuo HC. Efficacy and safety of mirabegron, a beta3 -adrenoceptor agonist, in patients with detrusor hyperactivity and impaired contractility. Low Urin Tract Symptoms. 2018. Apr 26. https://doi.org/10.1111/luts.12224.
100. Szonyi G, Collas DM, Ding YY, Malone-Lee JG. Oxybutynin with bladder retraining for detrusor instability in elderly people: a randomized controlled trial. Age Ageing. 1995;24(4):287–91.
101. Lackner TE, Wyman JF, McCarthy TC, Monigold M, Davey C. Randomized, placebo-controlled trial of the cognitive effect, safety, and tolerability of oral extended-release oxybutynin in cognitively impaired nursing home residents with urge urinary incontinence. J Am Geriatr Soc. 2008;56(5):862–70.
102. Lackner TE, Wyman JF, McCarthy TC, Monigold M, Davey C. Efficacy of oral extended-release oxybutynin in cognitively impaired older nursing home residents with urge urinary incontinence: a randomized placebo-controlled trial. J Am Med Dir Assoc. 2011;12(9):639–47.
103. Minassian VA, Ross S, Sumabat O, Lovatsis D, Pascali D, Al-Badr A, et al. Randomized trial of oxybutynin extended versus immediate release for women aged 65 and older with overactive bladder: lessons learned from conducting a trial. J Obstet Gynaecol Can. 2007;29(9):726–32.
104. Sand P, Zinner N, Newman D, Lucente V, Dmochowski R, Kelleher C, et al. Oxybutynin transdermal system improves the quality of life in adults with overactive bladder: a multicentre, community-based, randomized study. BJU Int. 2007;99(4):836–44.
105. Ouslander JG, Blaustein J, Connor A, Pitt A. Habit training and oxybutynin for incontinence in nursing home patients: a placebo-controlled trial. J Am Geriatr Soc. 1988;36(1):40–6.
106. Ouslander JG, Schnelle JF, Uman G, Fingold S, Nigam JG, Tuico E, et al. Does oxybutynin add to the effectiveness of prompted voiding for urinary incontinence among nursing home residents? A placebo-controlled trial. J Am Geriatr Soc. 1995;43(6):610–7.
107. Zorzitto ML, Holliday PJ, Jewett MA, Herschorn S, Fernie GR. Oxybutynin chloride for geriatric urinary dysfunction: a double-blind placebo-controlled study. Age Ageing. 1989;18(3):195–200.
108. Kay GG, Staskin DR, Macdiarmid S, McIlwain M, Dahl NV. Cognitive effects of oxybutynin chloride topical gel in older healthy subjects: a 1-week, randomized, double-blind, placebo- and active-controlled study. Clin Drug Investig. 2012;32(10):707–14.
109. Staskin DR, Dmochowski RR, Sand PK, Macdiarmid SA, Caramelli KE, Thomas H, et al. Efficacy and safety of oxybutynin chloride topical gel for overactive bladder: a randomized, double-blind, placebo controlled, multicenter study. J Urol. 2009;181(4):1764–72.
110. Gibson W, Athanasopoulos A, Goldman H, Madersbacher H, Newman D, Spinks J, et al. Are we shortchanging frail older people when it comes to the pharmacological treatment of urgency urinary incontinence? Int J Clin Pract. 2014;68(9):1165–73.
111. Biardeau X, Campeau L, Corcos J. We should not use oxybutynin chloride in OAB. Neurourol Urodyn. 2017;36(3):822–3.
112. National Collaborating Centre for Women's and Children's Health (UK). Urinary incontinence in women: the management of urinary incontinence in women. London: Royal College of Obstetricians and Gynaecologists (UK); 2013. National Institute for Health and Care Excellence: Clinical Guidelines.
113. Lucas MG, Bedretdinova D, Berghmans LC, Bosch JLHR, Burkhard FC, Cruz AK, et al. Guidelines on urinary incontinence. European Association of Urology Web site. http://uroweb.org/wp-content/uploads/20-Urinary-Incontinence_LR1.pdf. Updated 2015. Accessed 28 May 2018.
114. Madersbacher H, Murtz G. Efficacy, tolerability and safety profile of propiverine in the treatment of the overactive bladder (non-neurogenic and neurogenic). World J Urol. 2001;19(5):324–35.

115. Mori S, Kojima M, Sakai Y, Nakajima K. Bladder dysfunction in dementia patients showing urinary incontinence: evaluation with cystometry and treatment with propiverine hydrochloride. Nippon Ronen Igakkai Zasshi. 1999;36(7):489–94 [Article in Japanese].
116. Otomo E, Maruyama S, Kobayashi I, et al. Clinical evaluation of propiverine hydrochloride (P-4) on urinary disturbances due to neurological diseases. Jpn J Pharmacol. 1990;18:1731.
117. Dorschner W, Stolzenburg JU, Griebenow R, Halaska M, Brunjes R, Frank M, et al. The elderly patient with urge incontinence or urge-stress incontinence—efficacy and cardiac safety of propiverine. Aktuelle Urol. 2003;34(2):102–8.
118. Oelke M, Becher K, Castro-Diaz D, Chartier-Kastler E, Kirby M, Wagg A, et al. Appropriateness of oral drugs for long-term treatment of lower urinary tract symptoms in older persons: results of a systematic literature review and international consensus validation process (LUTS-FORTA 2014). Age Ageing. 2015;44(5):745–55.
119. Oelke M, Murgas S, Schneider T, Heßdörfer E. Influence of propiverine er 30 mg once daily on cognitive function in elderly female and male patients with overactive bladder: a noninterventional study to assess real life data (abstract). Proceedings of the International Continence Society Annual Scientific Meeting Barcelona; 2013. 2013:201.
120. Kosilov KV, Loparev SA, Ivanovskaya MA, Kosilova LV. Effectiveness of solifenacin and trospium for managing of severe symptoms of overactive bladder in patients with benign prostatic hyperplasia. Am J Mens Health. 2016;10(2):157–63.
121. Michel MC, Wetterauer U, Vogel M, de la Rosette JJ. Cardiovascular safety and overall tolerability of solifenacin in routine clinical use: a 12-week, open-label, post-marketing surveillance study. Drug Saf. 2008;31(6):505–14.
122. Wesnes KA, Edgar C, Tretter RN, Bolodeoku J. Exploratory pilot study assessing the risk of cognitive impairment or sedation in the elderly following single doses of solifenacin 10 mg. Expert Opin Drug Saf. 2009;8(6):615–26.
123. Wagg A, Dale M, Tretter R, Stow B, Compion G. Randomised, multicentre, placebo-controlled, double-blind crossover study investigating the effect of solifenacin and oxybutynin in elderly people with mild cognitive impairment: the SENIOR study. Eur Urol. 2013;64(1):74–81.
124. Zinner NR, Mattiasson A, Stanton SL. Efficacy, safety, and tolerability of extended-release once-daily tolterodine treatment for overactive bladder in older versus younger patients. J Am Geriatr Soc. 2002;50(5):799–807.
125. Millard R, Tuttle J, Moore K, Susset J, Clarke B, Dwyer P, et al. Clinical efficacy and safety of tolterodine compared to placebo in detrusor overactivity. J Urol 1999;161(5):1551–5.
126. Drutz HP, Appell RA, Gleason D, Klimberg I, Radomski S. Clinical efficacy and safety of tolterodine compared to oxybutynin and placebo in patients with overactive bladder. Int Urogynecol J Pelvic Floor Dysfunct. 1999;10(5):283–9.
127. Michel MC, Schneider T, Krege S, Goepel M. Does gender or age affect the efficacy and safety of tolterodine? J Urol. 2002;168(3):1027–31.
128. Ouslander JG, Maloney C, Grasela TH, Rogers L, Walawander CA. Implementation of a nursing home urinary incontinence management program with and without tolterodine. J Am Med Dir Assoc. 2001;2(5):207–14.
129. Tsao JW, Heilman KM. Transient memory impairment and hallucinations associated with tolterodine use. N Engl J Med. 2003;349(23):2274–5.
130. Womack KB, Heilman KM. Tolterodine and memory: dry but forgetful. Arch Neurol. 2003;60(5):771–3.
131. Salvatore S, Serati M, Cardozo L, Uccella S, Bolis P. Cognitive dysfunction with tolterodine use. Am J Obstet Gynecol. 2007;197(2):e8.
132. Edwards KR, O'Connor JT. Risk of delirium with concomitant use of tolterodine and acetylcholinesterase inhibitors. J Am Geriatr Soc. 2002;50(6):1165–6.
133. Sand PK, Johnson Ii TM, Rovner ES, Ellsworth PI, Oefelein MG, Staskin DR. Trospium chloride once-daily extended release is efficacious and tolerated in elderly subjects (aged >/= 75 years) with overactive bladder syndrome. BJU Int. 2011;107(4):612–20.

134. Sand PK, Rovner ES, Watanabe JH, Oefelein MG. Once-daily trospium chloride 60 mg extended release in subjects with overactive bladder syndrome who use multiple concomitant medications: post hoc analysis of pooled data from two randomized, placebo-controlled trials. Drugs Aging. 2011;28(2):151–60.
135. Staskin D, Kay G, Tannenbaum C, Goldman HB, Bhashi K, Ling J, Oefelein MG. Trospium chloride has no effect on memory testing and is assay undetectable in the central nervous system of older patients with overactive bladder. Int J Clin Pract. 2010;64(9):1294–300.
136. Staskin D, Kay G, Tannenbaum C, Goldman HB, Bhashi K, Ling J, Oefelein MG. Trospium chloride is undetectable in older human central nervous system. J Am Geriatr Soc. 2010;58(8):1618–9.
137. Panel. AGSBCUE. American Geriatrics Society 2015 updated beers criteria for potentially inappropriate medication use in older adults. J Am Geriatr Soc. 2015;63(11):2227–46.

Chapter 17
Individualizing Drug Therapy

Ricardo Palmerola and Victor Nitti

Pharmacotherapy for overactive bladder (OAB) has been a mainstay of treatment for many years. Currently available oral, transdermal, and intravesical agents offer patients a significant reduction in urinary frequency, urgency episodes and urgency urinary incontinence episodes [1]. There are a number of pharmacologic agents and a mounting preponderance of evidence which suggest that overall, anticholinergic medications perform equally in their clinical efficacy [1, 2]. Furthermore, mirabegron has also been noted to have comparable clinical efficacy to anticholinergic medications for idiopathic OAB [3]. Oral, transdermal, and intravesical medication options have been shown to be superior to placebo in their effectiveness; thus the question becomes which medication is best suited for an individual patient. By exploiting a drug's particular characteristics, today's clinician can better tailor drug therapy using the vast menu of medical options. In the following chapter, the major oral drug classes for OAB will be reviewed with attention to pharmacological nuances that standout to clinicians. Next, considerations for individualizing therapy will be discussed for the major drug classes.

R. Palmerola (✉) · V. Nitti
Female Pelvic Medicine and Reconstructive Surgery Program, NYU Langone, Department of Urology, New York University, New York, NY, USA

L. Cox, E. S. Rovner (eds.), *Contemporary Pharmacotherapy of Overactive Bladder*, https://doi.org/10.1007/978-3-319-97265-7_17

Part I: Common Oral Pharmacotherapies' Review

Oral Pharmacotherapies

Antimuscarinic Agents

As per the American Urological Association (AUA)/Society of Urodynamics, Female Pelvic Medicine and Urogenital Reconstruction (SUFU) Guideline on OAB, first-line therapy for OAB consists of behavioral therapies (diet and fluid modifications, pelvic floor exercises, etc.). Medical therapy can be instituted along with first-line treatment or utilized alone as a second-line treatment [1]. Anticholinergics have been very effective in treating OAB symptoms by blocking the muscarinic receptors controlling uninhibited detrusor contractions, which are largely thought to play a role in OAB (see Chap. 6) [4]. As discussed in Chap. 6, muscarinic receptors (M1-5) are widespread through the body, while the M2/M3 receptors present in the urinary tract are frequently targeted for drug development [4]. The ubiquitous nature of the muscarinic receptors makes drug dosing challenging, particularly in patient populations where side effects may become problematic in successful management. Unfortunately, this drug class' therapeutic potential has been limited by drug tolerability, compliance to therapy, and persistence on therapy [5–8]. It has been demonstrated that up to 80% of patients will discontinue therapy within the first year and an even more staggering 50% will abandon therapy altogether [8, 9]. Nonetheless, antimuscarinics play a critical role in the management of OAB, and familiarity with the major drugs in this class should be in every treating clinician's armamentarium. Additionally, clinicians prescribing antimuscarinics should be familiar with dosing individual medications and titrating doses as dictated by clinical efficacy and tolerability. In general, beginning with a low dose of a medication and increasing the dose to meet the needs to the patient with consideration toward side effects and tolerability are recommended. Clinical trials for several antimuscarinics (solifenacin, oxybutynin ER, darifenacin, fesoterodine) have shown that nearly half of patients will request dose escalation if given the option and those that request higher doses of therapy tend to have more severe symptoms [10–14]. The following discussion will review some of the agents commonly used in clinical practice for idiopathic OAB.

Oxybutynin Chloride Oxybutynin has been a therapeutic option for almost five decades and has stood the test of time with regard to efficacy [15]. Along with other anticholinergics, its safety profile, particularly in the elderly, has been called into question [16–18]. Nonetheless, the drug will continue to be relevant as a therapeutic option as it is widely available for the majority of patients treated. Oxybutynin is available in an immediate-release (IR), extended-release (ER), transdermal gel, and transdermal patch. Oxybutynin exerts its effect on the detrusor smooth muscle by competitively antagonizing acetylcholine at post-ganglionic M1–M3 receptors and to a lesser degree, it also exerts a local anesthetic action on the bladder [15, 19, 20].

Pertinent Pharmacology Oxybutynin chloride is a small lipophilic drug that is metabolized by cytochrome P450A4 (CYP3A4) in the liver as well as the intestinal wall. The first-pass metabolite is N-desethyloxybutynin (DEO) which becomes clinically relevant as this compound is thought to produce unpleasant side effects like dry mouth [15]. Following ingestion of oral formulations of oxybutynin, approximately 6% is available as the parent compound, whereas DEO plasma levels are approximately 5–12 times greater [15, 21]. Furthermore, oxybutynin formulations that avoid first-pass metabolism have a significantly higher ratio of the desired parent compound vs. DEO [15]. Transdermal formulations that bypass hepatic metabolism benefit from a higher bioavailability of the desired compound oxybutynin and lower serum concentrations of the metabolite DEO which is largely responsible for anticholinergic side effects [22]. Ultimately these formulations translate into greater tolerability for the patient with the comparable efficacy with regard to reducing incontinent episodes [23]. For example, in the phase II study comparing immediate-release oxybutynin with transdermal oxybutynin, less than half of patients experienced dry mouth, and both treatment arms had a comparable decrease in incontinent episodes [23, 24].

Aside from the first-pass effect, several other properties need to be kept in mind when prescribing oxybutynin. First, patients using oxybutynin IR should be warned that ingestion with food causes a delay in absorption and an increase in bioavailability by 25% [15]. This may be helpful to the clinician when titrating the medication as one can potentially optimize medical therapy in select patients who need higher doses of oxybutynin (neurogenic bladder). On the other hand, elderly patients or those who have experienced unwanted side effects should be warned of this potential or be started on a lower dose (i.e., 2.5 mg bid for elderly) if the patient normally takes medications with meals. Other formulations of oxybutynin (extended-release, transdermal) have shown steady absorption regardless of food ingestion [20]. The pharmacokinetics of oxybutynin vary with the type of formulation. Briefly, oxybutynin IR is absorbed most rapidly (1 h) and achieves steady state at 72 h (as does oxybutynin ER), whereas steady state is achieved in 4 days and 1 week for the transdermal patch and gel, respectively [15]. The half-life is longest for the transdermal formulations, making them appealing for patients who may have difficulty committing to daily dosing [22]. Furthermore, transdermal formulations avoid peaks and troughs of serum concentrations that are associated with oral formulations [25]. For some patients, the quicker onset and shorter duration of action may be preferable, but for most patients the more consistent serum drug levels associated with extended-release formulations are preferred due to the lower side effects associated with avoiding high serum peak levels of oxybutynin and DEO.

Special consideration must be taken when prescribing oxybutynin as it metabolized by the liver enzyme CYP3A4. Drugs that induce this enzyme reduce the serum concentration of oxybutynin in contrast to drugs that inhibit the enzyme increase the serum concentration (Table 17.1). As illustrated in the table, caution should be taken when prescribing oral oxybutynin to patients with metastatic prostate cancer (enzalutamide), breast cancer (tamoxifen), leukemia (imatinib), fungal infections

Table 17.1 Common CYP4503A4 inhibitors and inducers

Inhibitors increase [serum][a]	Inducers decrease [serum][a]
Amiodarone	Carbamazepine
Cyclosporine	Dexamethasone
Diltiazem	Enzalutamide
Erythromycin	Phenytoin
Clarithromycin	Prednisone
Fluconazole	Rifampin
Ketoconazole	Phenobarbital
Itraconazole	Topiramate
Indinavir/ritonavir	Pioglitazone
Tamoxifen	Capsaicin
Verapamil	Modafinil
Imatinib	St. John's wort
Grapefruit	
Valerian root	

[a]Effect on anticholinergic drug [serum]

(azole antifungals), and certain immunosuppressed patients (cyclosporine). Transdermal formulations bypass metabolism by CYP3A4 enzymes in the liver, thus making them an option for patients at risk for potential drug-drug interactions.

Side Effects Review Dry mouth and constipation tend to be the most frequently encountered side effects that have a major impact on dose limitation for oral formulations. Dry mouth, in particular, has been reported in up to 60–70% of patients and is a major cause of drug discontinuation. However headache, dry eyes, blurred vision, and somnolence do occur in up to 10–20% of patients [20, 21]. One must use this medication judiciously in patients at high risk for incomplete bladder emptying (elderly, frail, detrusor underactivity, etc.); however, the risk of urinary retention remains low in most ambulatory patients. Certain patient populations that are at potentially higher risk of adverse effects should be offered other therapies. For example, patients with various gastrointestinal disorders should be counseled on potential adverse effects. Patients with inflammatory bowel disease must be warned of the risk of toxic megacolon as oxybutynin may affect gastric motility. Additionally, diabetic patients with gastroparesis should also use caution as to the risk of gastric retention. Patients with a history of constipation, or those who consume a low-fiber diet, should also be warned of a potential to exacerbate their symptoms.

As discussed, transdermal formulations avoid the first-pass effect and dissemination of the metabolite DEO, translating into a lower risk of undesirable side effects (namely, xerostomia). The risk of dry mouth is not completely eliminated but is greatly reduced to approximately 7% [26]. Transdermal application does come with unique side effects including application site erythema, rash, and pruritus. Although these reactions appear to be minor, they can occur between 3% and 32% of patients which lead to drug discontinuation [27, 28].

Dosing Please refer to Tables 17.2 and 17.3 and Chap. 6 for specific dosing protocols. Oxybutynin dosing varies across formulations and can be tailored to the needs of the patient. Oral oxybutynin for adults and children can be administered for immediate-release (IR), extended-release (ER), or liquid formulation (elixir). Oxybutynin IR can be dosed at 2.5 mg or 5 mg doses two or three times daily. For elderly patients, we recommend beginning therapy with 2.5 mg tablets two times daily and monitoring adverse effects closely. The 5 mg tablets may be cut in half by a caretaker, if acquiring 2.5 mg tablets becomes difficult. For most adults with idiopathic OAB, we begin therapy with 5 mg tablets three times daily. In our practice we prefer using extended-release formulations as we have found patients prefer a once-daily formulation and side effects seem to be better tolerated. For most adults on an extended-release formulation, we begin therapy at 5 mg daily and increase the dose up to a maximum of 20 mg per day. Dose increments of 5 mg can occur with at least 1 week intervals to assess for tolerability.

Liquid formulations can be useful when administering oxybutynin to children or adult patients who cannot tolerate oral pills. It is important to note that liquid oxybutynin or oxybutynin syrup is an immediate-release formulation and the dosing should be based according to this property. Oxybutynin liquid is dosed in milliliters (mL) where 1 mL is equivalent to 1 mg of oxybutynin. For adults the usual dose is 5 mL (5 mg) two to three times daily. Children over 5 years of age with neurogenic

Table 17.2 Dosing anticholinergic medications in patients with renal impairment and hepatic dysfunction

	Tolterodine ER	Tolterodine IR	Fesoterodine	Trospium	Darifenacin	Solifenacin
Level of renal impairment[a]						
Mild/moderate	Standard dosing	Standard dosing	Standard dosing	Standard dosing	Standard dosing	Standard dosing
Severe	2 mg daily	1 mg bid	4 mg daily	20 mg daily (extended-release not recommended)	Standard dosing	5 mg daily
Level of hepatic impairment[b]						
Mild/moderate	2 mg daily	1 mg bid	Standard dosing	N/A[c]	7.5 mg daily (moderate)	5 mg daily (moderate)
Severe	N/A[c]	N/A[c]	N/A[c]	N/A[c]	Contraindicated	Contraindicated

ER extended-release, *IR* immediate-release
[a]Mild renal impairment: creatinine clearance = 60–89 mL/min
Moderate renal impairment: creatinine clearance = 30–59 mL/min
Severe renal impairment: creatinine clearance <30 mL/min
[b]Mild/moderate hepatic impairment: Child-Pugh classifications A and B, respectively
Severe hepatic impairment: Child-Pugh classification C
[c]Data not available and thus dosing parameters are not defined

Table 17.3 Dosing protocols of antimuscarinic agents for overactive bladder

	Oxybutynin (IR/ER)	Oxybutynin (patch/gel)	Solifenacin	Fesoterodine	Tolterodine (IR/ER)	Darifenacin (IR/ER)	Trospium (IR/ER)
Lipophilicity[a]	+++	+++	+++	+	+	++	0
Molecular weight (Da) and charge	340 Neutral	357/340 Neutral	480.6 Positive	527.7 Positive	475.6 Positive	507.5 Positive	428 Positive
Hepatic enzyme	CYP3A4	CYP3A4	CYP3A4	CYP3A4 CYP2D6	CYP3A4 CYP2D6	CYP3A4 CYP2D6	None[b]
Active metabolites	Desethyl-oxybutynin	Desethyl-oxybutynin	None	5-HMT[c]	5-HMT	None	None
Half-life (hours)	2/13	7/62	45–68[d]	7–9	2–3/6[e]	3/13–19	20/35
Affect with food	Increased/–	–/–	None	None	Increased/–	None	Decreased
Binding affinity (K_i in nM)							
M_1	1.0	1.0	26	2.3	2.7	7.3	0.75
M_2	6.7	6.7	170	2.0	4.2	46.0	0.65
M_3	0.67	0.67	12	2.5	4.4	0.79	0.5
M_4	2.0	2.0	110	2.8	6.6	46.0	1.0
M_5	11.0	11.0	31	2.9	2.5	9.6	2.3

ER extended-release, *IR* immediate-release

[a]Not lipophilic 0, mild lipophilicity +, moderate lipophilicity ++, lipophilic +++

[b]Predominantly secreted in renal tubules

[c]5-Hydroxy-methyl-tolterodine

[d]Half-life can be up to 25% higher in patients 65–80 years of age

[e]Half-life can be higher for CYP2D6 poor metabolizer (10 h for tolterodine IR, 11 h for tolterodine ER)

bladder can be dosed up 15 mL daily; however, younger children should be dosed according to their weight. We typically use 0.2 mg/kg/dose every 8 h for children under 5 years of age.

Transdermal formulations are dosed according to their delivery system. Oxybutynin transdermal patches (Oxytrol®, Allergan, Irvine, CA, USA) contain 36 mg of oxybutynin in a 39cm^2 system and deliver 3.9 mg/day. The patch should be changed every 3–4 days by removing the old patch and reapplying the new patch in a different site. The patch must be placed on dry, intact skin, and we recommend patients avoid strenuous activity or bathing immediately after placement. Transdermal gel (Gelnique 3%®, Allergan; Gelnique®, Allergan) can be applied directly to the dry, intact skin and should also be covered with clothing to avoid transmission to close contacts. One heat-sealed sachet of Gelnique® should be applied daily, or three pumps of Gelnique 3%® can be applied daily. Although transdermal formulations are safe and effective in adults, their safety has not been well established in pediatric patients, and caution should be advised prior to prescribing.

Solifenacin Solifenacin (Vesicare®) is a competitive muscarinic antagonist that acts predominantly on the M_3 receptor. Solifenacin acts primarily in the bladder and has a lower affinity for the muscarinic receptors of the salivary glands. In vitro studies have shown that solifenacin is approximately 40-fold less potent than oxybutynin in inhibiting salivary secretions and in animal models there was a 3.5–6.5 functional selectivity for bladder smooth muscle over salivary tissue [29] . This offers some theoretical advantages, but unfortunately the side effect of dry mouth still limits its use in some patients.

Pertinent Pharmacology Solifenacin is a lipophilic compound that undergoes passive diffusion in all three segments of the small intestine. Absorption is not significantly affected by food intake and thus can be administered in the fasting or fed state without affecting serum drug levels [30]. Solifenacin's bioavailability is approximately 88% with less than 15% variability between subjects when administered orally. Solifenacin reaches Cmax (maximum plasma levels) within 3–8 h following administration and is widely distributed throughout the body reaching a volume of distribution of 600 liters [29, 30]. Steady state can be achieved in most patients after 10 days of consistent dosing; thus patients should be counseled appropriately upon treatment initiation. Although animal studies have demonstrated changes in EEG patterns following 4–52 weeks of treatment, similar studies have not been reproduced in humans [29]. Fortunately, solifenacin is ionized in neutral pH and is strongly bound to serum proteins (predominantly α_1-acid glycoprotein) making the drugs' blood-brain barrier (BBB) permeability less likely. The drug itself has less affinity for M_1 receptors present in the central nervous system, further limiting its effects in cognition [31].

Solifenacin undergoes hepatic metabolism primarily by CYP3A4 into four metabolites. Except for 4R-hydroxy solifenacin, the other metabolites are inert and do not have pharmacological activity. 4R-hydroxy solifenacin does have similar receptor-binding properties to the parent compound (M_3 receptor affinity) but is present as such low concentrations that it is not considered to have a significant effect on efficacy or side effects. Excretion of solifenacin and its metabolites occurs predominantly through the kidneys (approximately 23% in feces) with approximately 10% being excreted unchanged in the urine. The elimination half-life following chronic use is 45–68 h; however, in patients 65–80 years of age, the expected half-life is approximately 20–25% higher [30].

Drug Interactions Drug interactions can occur if solifenacin is administered with CYP3A4 inhibitors or inducers (see Table 17.1). The drug should be used with caution when used concomitantly with CYP inhibitors, and the dose should not exceed 5 mg daily in patients on such drugs.

Side Effects Solifenacin's side effect profile is similar to that of the other antimuscarinics used for the indication of OAB with the most common side effects being dry mouth, constipation, and blurry vision. Dry mouth seems to be dose related, occurring in less than 10% of patients with 5 mg dose and 17–28% of patients with the 10 mg dose [30, 32]. Constipation rates were similar irrespective of daily dose administered [33]. Solifenacin's rate of dry mouth is among the lowest in its class and thus should be considered for patients with preexisting symptoms of dry mouth (i.e., Sjogren syndrome) or in those that may have difficulty tolerating other medications in the antimuscarinic class when an antimuscarinic is truly desired.

QT interval prolongation has been reported with solifenacin, particularly at doses of 30 mg (three times higher than the highest recommended dose). Although this warning is rarely clinically relevant, one must consider this as a potential risk in patients who receive CYP inhibitors, patients with renal or hepatic impairment, or patients with cardiac risk factors.

Dosing Solifenacin is available in 5 mg and 10 mg tablets in the United States. Treatment can begin with a 5 mg daily dose and increased to 10 mg if necessary.

Tolterodine Tolterodine is a competitive muscarinic antagonist that is available as an immediate-release or as an extended-release formulation. Tolterodine purportedly has a stronger affinity for muscarinic receptors in the bladder over those in the salivary glands, and it is one of the first medications designed specifically for the treatment of OAB.

Pertinent Pharmacology Once administered, tolterodine is absorbed in the small intestine, and Cmax is attained within 2 h of administration. Extended-release tolterodine reaches Cmax between 2 and 6 h after administration [34]. It must be noted that food ingestion does affect the absorption of immediate-release tolterodine and increases the bioavailability by approximately 53%. Both extended- and immediate-release formulations are metabolized by the liver and mediated by CYP2D6, which produces the biologically active metabolite 5-hydroxymethyl metabolite (5-HMT) [35]. It must be noted that there is genetic polymorphism of CYP2D6, and this results in patients who are poor metabolizers and those that are extensive metabolizers. Approximately 7% of Caucasians are poor metabolizers and rely on a separate pathway mediated by CYP3A. The result in poor metabolizers will have a higher serum concentration of tolterodine in comparison with the 5-hydroxymethyl metabolite. Excretion is primarily in the urine, with a small portion in the feces with less than 1% being the intact parent compound. The half-life of IR formulations is 2–3 h and 10 h for poor metabolizers; ER has a half-life of 6 h and 11 h for poor metabolizers [34].

Side Effects Tolterodine produces adverse effects in approximately 20–30% of patients including dry mouth, constipation, and blurry vision [34, 36]. There have been reports of peripheral edema; however, specific incidence rates are unavailable. Tolterodine (among other antimuscarinics) have the potential to result in QT prolongation through effects on potassium channels in the heart [37]. It has also been noted to increase the QT interval at higher than the recommended doses; however, this should be considered as poor metabolizers which can reach higher serum plasma levels with normally prescribed doses. Tolterodine has the potential to produce CNS side effects; however, there are reports that show that there is minimal penetration of the blood-brain barrier, thus lowering its potential for CNS side effects [38].

Dosing Tolterodine IR is available in 1 or 2 mg tablets administered twice daily. Tolterodine ER is available in 2 mg and 4 mg tablets administered once daily. Although the drug undergoes its most extensive metabolism with CYP2D6, clinicians should exercise caution when prescribing with strong inhibitors of CYP3A4 in patients who are considered poor metabolizers.

Fesoterodine Fesoterodine is an extended-release medication used for the treatment of OAB. The parent compound is de-esterified rapidly in the serum to the active metabolite 5-HMT (the same active metabolite as tolterodine) which has activity as a competitive muscarinic receptor antagonist. The bioavailability of 5-HMT is approximately 52%, and Cmax (maximum plasma levels) is achieved after 5 h. Food intake does not affect bioavailability or plasma concentrations. Fesoterodine is converted to 5-HMT by non-specific esterases and then undergoes hepatic metabolism [39]. Approximately 15% of the administered dose is recovered in the urine as 5-HMT, which may contribute to local effects on the urothelium. The CYP2D6 and CYP3A4 enzymes are additional routes for elimination, and the metabolites that result from their actions are inert. The half-life of the medication spans 7–9 h after oral administration [40].

Side Effects Dry mouth occurs in approximately 19–22% of patients taking 4 mg and 34–36% for 8 mg doses [41]. Fesoterodine can cause an increase in heart rate as a result of its blockade of muscarinic receptors in the sinoatrial or atrioventricular nodes (M_2). Increases in heart rate are dose related with a mean increase in 3 bpm for the 4 mg dose and 4 bpm for the 8 mg dose [42]. Rates of constipation are low (5%), and thus this may be a suitable option for patients at risk of developing constipation or those with preexisting gastric motility disorders [13, 43].

Dosing Fesoterodine is available in 4 mg and 8 mg doses in the United States. For most adult patients and elderly, 4 mg can be administered daily. After assessing an individual patient's response, this dose can be increased to 8 mg.

Trospium Trospium is a quaternary amine with parasympatholytic properties by acting as a competitive antagonist of acetylcholine at the M_1, M_2,, and M_3 receptors. Trospium has a high affinity for muscarinic M1–M3 receptors and ultimately leads to smooth muscle relaxation at low serum concentrations. Ultimately, trospium binding to muscarinic receptors leads to decreased tone in smooth muscle, particularly in the bladder and gastrointestinal system. Most importantly, being a quaternary amine makes it a hydrophilic molecule that does not readily cross the blood-brain barrier [44]. Trospium is the only anticholinergic for OAB that does not cross the BBB.

Pertinent Pharmacology After ingestion, less than 10% becomes bioavailable, and peak plasma concentrations are reached approximately 6 h after ingestion. The medication should be taken on an empty stomach or 1 h prior to meals as its absorption can be decreased when taken concomitantly with food, and such administration may decrease plasma concentrations by over 50% [45]. The drug's metabolism has not been completely described, but in contrast to other OAB medications, cytochrome P450 is not thought to play a role in the elimination of the drug [44]. The half-life for the immediate-release formulation is approximately 20 h and 35 h for extended release [46].

Side Effects Due to several of this drug's pharmacologic properties, its side effect profile is unique. For example, approximately 60% of the drug is excreted in the urine unchanged from the parent compound [47]. Theoretically this could lead to local therapeutic effects and less systemic side effects than are observed with other anticholinergics; however, this has not been borne out in clinical trials. The most commonly reported side effect is dry mouth, which occurs in 4–20% of patients, and whereas constipation is encountered in approximately 10% of patients [44, 48].

Dosing Trospium can be administered as a 20 mg tablet twice daily or a single 60 mg extended-release tablet. As discussed, trospium should be taken orally, at least 1 h prior to meals. Dosing should be modified to 20 mg daily with patients with severe renal impairment (creatinine clearance<30 mL/min), and caution should be utilized in patients with hepatic impairment.

Darifenacin Darifenacin is a positively charged tertiary amine that is a competitive receptor antagonist with a very high affinity for M3 receptors (M3 > M1/M5> > M2/M4). In theory, the drug's affinity for M3 receptors should translate into better efficacy in reduction of OAB symptoms while minimally exacerbating side effects [49]. However this has not proven to be true in clinical practice as its efficacy in treating OAB is comparable to the other drugs in its class and constipation is a frequent concern due to its M3 selectivity.

Pertinent Pharmacology Extended-release darifenacin is absorbed throughout the small intestine and colon with peak plasma concentrations reached between 7 and 11.5 h. The drug reaches a steady state after 6 days, and the bioavailability is approximately 15% for the 7.5 mg dose and 19% for the 15 mg dose. Extended-release darifenacin bypasses first-pass metabolism and as a result has a twofold higher bioavailability. Darifenacin is distributed widely with a volume of distribution of 163 liters and largely bound to plasma proteins.

Darifenacin undergoes extensive hepatic metabolism; thus caution should be used in patients with multiple comorbidities. Hepatic metabolism is mediated by the enzymes CYP2D6 and CYP3A4. As discussed earlier there may be genetic variation in the community with regard to CYP2D6; however, poor metabolizers of CYP2D6 do not experience significant differences in plasma levels as the substrate is channeled to the CYP3A4 pathway. Darifenacin has a long half-life when steady state is achieved, which can range from 13 to 19 h. Most of the parent compound is metabolized into inert metabolites, and approximately 60% is excreted in the urine [50, 51].

Side Effects Due to darifenacin's high affinity for the M3 receptor, adverse effects including dry mouth and constipation are comparable to other antimuscarinics; however, this did not lead to excessive discontinuation of the drug in multicenter trials [52, 53]. Darifenacin is a large, charged molecule, and thus central nervous system (CNS) side effects (cognitive impairment, somnolence, and dizziness) are infrequently troublesome which makes it a particularly useful drug in the elderly. Furthermore, darifenacin is a substrate for the p-glycoprotein drug efflux transporter present in the CNS, thus limiting its ability to affect cognition.

Dosing Extended-release darifenacin is available in 7.5 mg and 15 mg tablets and can be taken with food. One can begin therapy at 7.5 mg and increase to 15 mg daily as dictated by the patient's clinical response and tolerability. Elderly patients should be started on 7.5 mg and monitored closely as serum levels have been found to be higher than younger patients beginning therapy. Patients with severe hepatic impairment should not be offered darifenacin, and caution should be exercised in those with moderate hepatic dysfunction (doses should not exceed 7.5 mg daily). Darifenacin can be used safely in patients with renal impairment as a result of chronic kidney disease, and dose modification is not required. Patients who take medications which are strong CYP2D6 inhibitors (cimetidine, terbinafine, paroxetine) and strong CYP3A4 inhibitors (fluconazole, erythromycin, grapefruit) should be monitored closely after starting at a dose of 7.5 mg.

β3-Agonists

The first β3-agonist approved for OAB was mirabegron, and it remains the only commercially available formulation worldwide. Like antimuscarinics, it is currently recommended as a second-line therapy for OAB or can be initiated simultaneously with behavioral therapy [1]. In contrast to antimuscarinic medications which inhibit stimulatory input to the bladder, mirabegron acts on an alternative pathway producing detrusor muscle relaxation during the storage phase by acting as an agonist on the most abundant β-receptor in the urinary bladder (β3-receptor) [54]. As a result, mirabegron does not produce the typical anticholinergic-related adverse effects common to most OAB pharmaceuticals (dry mouth, constipation, etc.) and contributes to better tolerability.

Pertinent Pharmacology The oral bioavailability of mirabegron is dose dependent and reaches up to 54% after ingestion. Peak serum concentration is attained after 3–5 h, and approximately 70% of the drug is plasma protein bound (albumin and α-1 glycoprotein). Mirabegron has a wide volume of distribution (1670 liters) and undergoes metabolism in the liver. Several liver enzymes are involved in the drug's metabolism including uridine diphospho-glucuronosyltransferase, alcohol dehydrogenase, butylcholinesterase, and to a minor extent CYP3A4/CYP2D6. It does act as a minor to moderate CYP2D6 inhibitor; thus medications should be reviewed prior to administration [55]. Approximately ten metabolically inert metabolites are produced during the drug's metabolism, and the elimination half-life is 50–65 h. The drug is most likely secreted in the renal tubules, and this leads to a significant increase in the Cmax in patients with mild to severe renal impairment [56]. Cmax is also affected by hepatic impairment, and patients with mild and moderate disease can have plasma levels rise by approximately 19% and 65%, respectively [56].

Side Effects One of the advantages of treatment with mirabegron is that the clinician can circumvent the bothersome adverse effects associated with anticholinergic medications. Rates of dry mouth, constipation, and headache were comparable to placebo groups in phase III studies [57]. Cardiovascular side effects can potentially occur with mirabegron and include hypertension and tachycardia. Hypertension has been reported to be associated with treatment (and is listed as a side effect in many countries); however, this was not observed to be a dose-related phenomenon in phase III studies, and its incidence was comparable to placebo [57]. Urinary side effects can occur, with urinary tract infection being the most common. Although urinary retention is a potential risk, it should be noted that the drug acts by decreasing the frequency of involuntary detrusor contractions with little effect over detrusor contractility during the voiding phase [58, 59]. Overall, the drug is well tolerated with a low potential for serious adverse events or drug interactions [54].

Dosing Mirabegron is available in both 25 mg and 50 mg doses in the United States and Canada. The recommended starting dose is 25 mg daily, and in most healthy patients, the dose can be increased to 50 mg daily. Based on tolerability and side effects reported in clinical trials, we feel comfortable starting healthy patients on 50 mg daily; however, caution must be exercised when beginning therapy at this dose. Food does not affect the bioavailability of the medication, and all efforts should be made to take the medication at a consistent dosing interval. There are few medications that interact with mirabegron; however, caution is advised for CYP2D6 substrates like metoprolol. Patients with mild to moderate renal disease may be prescribed 25 or 50 mg daily, meanwhile patients with severe renal impairment should not exceed 25 mg daily. Although most patients taking mirabegron do not experience worsening hypertension, patients with renal impairment should be monitored closely as they are higher risk of uncontrolled hypertension secondary to their disease state. Patients with moderate hepatic impairment should not exceed 25 mg daily, while patients with mild hepatic disease do not need dose adjustment.

Part II: Individualizing Therapy

In order to achieve maximum efficacy of OAB pharmacotherapy, compliance with medications must be assured by understanding the pitfalls of medical therapy in the context of the patient being treated. Similar to other chronic syndromes, OAB medication persistence rates are poor. There are multiple reasons for discontinuation, and they are similar to other medications, including poor patient education and communication [7, 60, 61]. Thus, prior to beginning medical treatment for OAB, one must consider several factors to optimize pharmacotherapy. First, patient expectations and goals should be assessed so that the clinician can educate the patient on realistic outcomes. Patient education is paramount prior to beginning therapy to help patients understand how therapy can be tailored to their needs and most importantly so that they understand options are available if oral pharmacotherapy is not sufficient to control their symptoms. Initial therapy offered should be customized to the patient's goals with oral pharmacotherapy, with emphasis on their expectations and comfort level with potential side effects. Despite the clinical efficacy of many oral pharmacotherapies, patient persistence on therapy for OAB is one of the lowest when considering all chronic conditions [9]. For example, in one recent study after 1 year of therapy, 65–85% patients discontinued anticholinergic agents, and up to 62% discontinued mirabegron [62]. Although it is easy to conclude that medication side effects, inconvenience of administration, and/or cost may be limiting persistence rates, if it was simply a result of these factors, it would be difficult to explain the patients who remain on pharmacotherapies when they perceive an improvement while simultaneously being affected by side effects. The reality is that a large proportion of patients discontinue prescribed OAB medications as a result of unmet treatment expectations [7]. One can also assume that many patients who discontinue oral therapy abandon OAB therapies altogether based on the equally disappointing numbers of patients that progress to third-line therapies (onabotulinumtoxinA, neuromodulation) [63]. Therefore, the most critical aspect of managing pharmacotherapy for OAB is not only setting proper expectations but also knowing how to individualize therapy to optimize patient satisfaction and assure compliance. Knowing when to "pull the trigger" and move on to another therapy (be it drug or other) requires a firm understanding of the patient's goals and symptom severity. Therefore, attempts at enhancing their ability to enjoy overall satisfaction with treatment outcomes may lead to better persistence rates. This underscores the importance of selecting the proper agents and doses to maximize the therapeutic efficacy and minimize side effects. Some patients desire maximum efficacy and are willing to tolerate a certain degree of side effects to achieve that, while other may be satisfied with less improvement in OAB symptoms if side effects can be minimized or avoided. Thus, a sound assessment of the patient's most bothersome symptoms must be factored into the therapeutic plan in order to balance expected drug efficacy with tolerability. Regular follow-up should also be instituted when initiating therapy or when modifying a drug's doses. This becomes important when managing side effects, evaluating treatment outcomes, and deciding whether to implement third-line agents [64]. Without adequate follow-up, the opportunity to intervene and dose titrate (up or down), change medication, consider combination therapy, and introduce third-line therapy to a dissatisfied patient may be missed. Patient comorbidities should always be assessed, as treatment plans should always aim at improving quality of life while not adding unnecessary harm. Finally, cost of therapy should also be considered when counseling patients on treatments, and attempts to provide a reasonable alternative should be implemented when medications are cost prohibitive.

Although current options for initial pharmacotherapy may include both anticholinergic medications and β3-agonists, for the purposes of this discussion, the anticholinergic class will be discussed first. As discussed anticholinergic medications have been the mainstay of medical therapy for years and treatment with these medications having resulted in improvements in mean daily urgency episodes, number of incontinence episodes, and number of micturitions per day. Furthermore, therapy with anticholinergic medications can improve quality of life for patients with OAB, and significant improvements can be seen in most quality-of-life domains studied [65]. Despite the improvements in symptom control, persistence rates remain low as described above. The most commonly quoted reasons for discontinuation include bothersome side effects and insufficient symptom control; however, other factors such as cost must be considered in today's healthcare environment [66]. Studies to compare the relative efficacy of anticholinergic medications have been performed and concluded that there is no significant difference in efficacy between these drugs [1]. However, there are differences between the anticholinergic medications in terms of drug tolerability which may translate into longer persistence rates [2]. Thus, when initiating therapy one must consider how to maximize the efficacy and compliance for a particular drug, minimize side effects, and determine an adequate cutoff point to either change oral medications or move on to third-line OAB treatments (onabotulinumtoxinA, neuromodulation).

The AUA/SUFU OAB Guideline stresses several general considerations when considering which antimuscarinic medication to begin. First, extended-release formulations should be prescribed whenever possible in order to decrease risk of dry mouth as a side effect. For example, 40% of patients taking oxybutynin ER will experience dry mouth in comparison with 69% in those prescribed the immediate-release agent [1]. Extended-release formulations are also preferable as many extended-release anticholinergics can be dosed once daily. Furthermore, extended-release formulations are not affected by food intake and can potentially improve compliance especially for patients taking other medications. This not only becomes important for practical reasons, but extended-release formulations lead to a predictable pharmacokinetic response which is not affected by external variables (patient administers medications sporadically, concomitant food intake, etc.). Second, for patients who experience dry mouth as a result of oxybutynin, transdermal formulations may be considered as the serum levels of the active metabolite N-desethyloxybutynin are significantly lower [15]. It should be noted that at the time of this publication, access to transdermal oxybutynin has been limited, and certain pharmacies may not carry the medication. Furthermore, the cost to the patient has become comparable to nongeneric antimuscarinics further limiting its use [22].

Several factors must be considered prior to beginning anticholinergic therapy including the patient's medical comorbidities, the current medications, and the properties of the drugs being considered. In general, anticholinergic medications for OAB are well-tolerated and safe to use in most patients. However, there are certain considerations that must be taken prior to prescribing the medication. One medical condition that must be evaluated is narrow-angle glaucoma [1]. Patients should be discouraged from anticholinergic therapy if the patient has not been treated, for this condition as administration of an anticholinergic can induce acute glaucoma which is considered a medical emergency [67]. In most circumstances, narrow-angle glaucoma is very symptomatic, and patients are treated expeditiously. Most community-dwelling patients being treated for glaucoma have the open-angle variety. However, if the history is unclear, one must consult with the patient's ophthalmologist prior to starting treatment. Additionally, two conditions that may be exacerbated by anticholinergic therapy include gastroparesis and urinary retention. Patients with gastroparesis or those at high risk (poorly controlled diabetes mellitus) should also be screened, and appropriate consultation is recommended with a gastroenterologist prior to beginning therapy. Similarly, anticholinergic medications should be used judiciously with patients at high risk of urinary retention. Special consideration should be taken for patients with a history of inflammatory bowel disease including ulcerative colitis and Crohn's disease as several extended-release formulations depend on colonic absorption (oxybutynin ER). Elderly and frail patients frequently present with symptoms of OAB and frequently have several comorbidities that interfere with dosing therapeutic agents. Although there are studies to suggest safety in patients older than 65 years old, particularly with fesoterodine, one must consider the effects on cognitive function and potential side effects (see below) [68, 69].

Serious life-threatening toxicity is rarely encountered in clinical practice as supratherapeutic doses are quite difficult to attain with recommended doses and higher dosing than recommended, often results in intolerable anticholinergic side effects. However, patients with renal and hepatic impairment can be vulnerable to supratherapeutic serum levels that may reach inappropriately high levels if dosing is unsuitable (see Table 17.2). Similarly, patients with multiple medical comorbidities may be taking several medications with the potential to cause drug-drug interactions. Many of the medications in this class are metabolized by cytochrome P450 enzymes, specifically CYP3A4 and CYP2D6. Depending on the medication co-administered with the anticholinergic, this may cause an increase or a decrease in serum levels (see Table 17.1). This could lead to potentially high or low serum levels, which may affect therapeutic plasma levels or exacerbate side effects, respectively. Although rare in normal dosing protocols, cardiac toxicity including QT prolongation and increased heart rate may become apparent with unsafe serum levels of a medication.

Patients at high risk for central nervous system (CNS) side effects should be warned of the potential side effects including cognitive impairment, dizziness, and somnolence [41]. Since the publication of the Beers Criteria and its subsequent revisions, the use of medications with anticholinergic effects in the elderly has been criticized due to their contribution to total anticholinergic burden. Although there are studies indicating a detrimental effect of anticholinergic medications on cognitive function, several studies investigating anticholinergics for the indication of OAB demonstrate less concerning perceivable cognitive effects [68–70]. High-risk individuals considered in clinical practice should not solely be limited to the frail and elderly. Younger patients operating heavy machinery, pilots, drivers, physicians, etc. should also be counseled on these risks and medications tailored to suit the demands of their lifestyle. Furthermore, the clinician should recognize and reconcile any medications the patient is already taking with anticholinergic properties in order to reduce the anticholinergic burden (Table 17.4). This becomes particularly important in patients with Alzheimer's disease or other neurological diseases who are being treated with acetylcholinesterase inhibitors. If one is concerned with CNS side effects, selecting the appropriate medication based on pharmacologic properties becomes paramount. One must recall that all muscarinic receptor subtypes (M_1–M_5) are present in the brain and selecting the best medication to prevent CNS side effects is not guided by simply choosing the most "uroselective" (M_3) [71]. Surely, medications that antagonize M1 receptors in the brain can potentially lead to cognitive impairment; however, there are other considerations that must be addressed

Table 17.4 Common anticholinergic medications

Antihistamines
Diphenhydramine, meclizine, hydroxyzine, promethazine, dimenhydrinate
Parkinson's disease medications
Benztropine, trihexyphenidyl, orphenadine, proyclidine
Muscle relaxants
Cyclobenzaprine, methocarbamol
Tricyclic antidepressants
Amitriptyline, imipramine, nortriptyline
Antipsychotics/antidepressants
Aripiprazole, clozapine, olanzapine, chlorpromazine, haloperidol, risperidone, paroxetine, bupropion, trazadone
Antispasmotics
Hyoscyamine, dicyclomine, scopolamine, clidinium-chlordiazepoxide

[72]. In general, starting at the lowest dose possible and titrating based on urinary symptom control and tolerability are important as serum concentration determines how much of the medication cross the blood-brain barrier (BBB) by passive diffusion. Next, selecting an agent based on the physiochemical properties of the parent compound and its active metabolites becomes important. Medications that have a low molecular weight, lipophilic, and neutral at physiologic pH tend to cross the BBB more readily than their counterparts (see Table 17.3). Suitable options for those at risk of CNS side effects, particularly patients >65 years old, these may include trospium, solifenacin, and darifenacin. Additionally, trospium and darifenacin are substrates for a permeability glycoprotein in the blood-brain barrier that facilitates active transport out of the CNS [73, 74]. These medications are particularly useful when treating elderly patients as they are at risk of cognitive impairment but may also have other patient-specific factors that must considered. For example, nocturia affects approximately 71% of nursing home residents and a significant number of community-dwelling elderly patients, and solifenacin and trospium have been shown to specifically decrease the number of nocturia episodes [32, 48, 75], though neither of these medications has nocturia as an indication. Polypharmacy is also a common issue in this population, and trospium may be a suitable option for elderly patients who are on concomitant medications that may be metabolized by the CYP enzyme system. Furthermore, all three medications are readily available in extended-release formulations, which contribute to their ease in administration and favorable side effect profile. Fesoterodine is another medication that can be considered in the elderly and those patients concerned about cognitive impairment as it has a low propensity to cross into the blood-brain barrier due [76]. Its clinical safety has been reported in patients greater than 65 years old with significant medical comorbidities and a comparable adverse effect profile to younger patients [69]. Ultimately the clinician and patient must weigh the risk of beginning pharmacotherapy against the benefit pharmacotherapy may impart. Surely the benefit of anticholinergic medications has been well documented in clinical trials; however, improvement in quality of life must be considered against potential complications in this population. For example, one must consider that an appreciable decrease in urinary frequency, urgency episodes, or incontinence can reduce the risk of falls or the burden of diaper changes in an already physically limited population. Furthermore, the consequences of untreated OAB including incontinence-related dermatitis, depression, and sleep disturbance must be imparted upon patients when beginning therapy [77]. Prior to beginning therapy in this population, one must assess the patient's individual goals and tailor drug dosage to simultaneously provide relief while avoiding complications. In cases where the patient's medical condition, symptoms, or goals conflict with starting anticholinergic therapy, one must consider alternatives. For these patients, alternative pharmacotherapies including mirabegron and onabotulinumtoxinA are suggested.

Proactive management of potential side effects of antimuscarinics should be practiced in order to improve drug tolerability. For those patients with increased risk (or preexisting) of dry mouth or constipation, clinicians should educate patients on methods to prevent and treat these potentially dose-limiting side effects [1]. Maintaining good oral hygiene is important for patients at risk as well as sugar-free chewing gum, mucin sprays, and betaine [78]. Patients at risk of constipation should be counseled on the importance of dietary changes that increase fiber content. Consideration should also be given to introducing psyllium-based fiber supplements as well as polyethylene glycol supplementation. Finally, patients should be counseled that inadequate fluid intake might exacerbate both symptoms, although this may be challenging as patients tend to fluid restrict in order to control their symptoms.

For patients with idiopathic OAB, mirabegron can be initiated as a monotherapy to anticholinergic naïve patients, as an alternative to patients that have failed anticholinergic medications, or in combination with anticholinergics [1, 55]. Its use in combination medical therapy is not strictly limited to OAB. For example mirabegron has been used safely for the treatment of bothersome lower urinary tract symptoms in men with bladder outlet obstruction (combination medical therapy is discussed in detail in Chap. 8). Mirabegron works through an alternative pathway utilizing the β3-adrenergic receptor, which is found in the human bladder and sparingly throughout the body (as opposed to the ubiquitously distributed muscarinic receptors). As a result of its selectivity, mirabegron use is not associated with the adverse effects commonly experienced in patients using anticholinergic medications and has been shown to have the most favorable tolerability profile of OAB medications [3]. Mirabegron's efficacy on improving OAB symptoms is apparent across several trials; however, its improvements in patient-reported outcomes indicate its potential for long-term persistence [79]. Studies have also found that persistence rates have also been higher at 6 months when compared to antimuscarinic medications, particularly at the extremes of age [80, 81]. Although it seems reasonable to assume that persistence rates are higher as a result of improved tolerability, a study by Chapple et al. found that up to 62% of patients discontinued mirabegron within 12 months [62]. Mirabegron has proven to be a cost-effective treatment in the United States, United Kingdom, and Canada; therefore overall cost to the population must be considered as well [82–84].

In addition to its use as a monotherapy in adults with idiopathic OAB, it is beneficial in certain patient populations that may have relative contraindications or a propensity to develop adverse reactions with anticholinergic medications. For example, this medication is particularly useful in the elderly population who may have preexisting dry mouth as a result of other medications (diuretics, antipsychotics, etc.) and constipation which are frequently encountered in this population [85]. Furthermore, patients with preexisting psychiatric and neurologic disorders who may already be on several medications with antimuscarinic properties should be considered for treatment with mirabegron as tolerability and resultant compliance may be improved.

Combination Therapy

As discussed in previous sections, both anticholinergic and β3-agonists are superior to placebo in the treatment of lower urinary tract symptoms due to overactive bladder and lead to significant improvements in quality of life. Despite their effectiveness in treatment, oral medications may be ineffective in meeting the patient's goals in symptom relief. In order to maximize efficacy of treatment plans, the use of combination therapy may be instituted with the initiation of pharmacotherapy. Combination therapy with medication and behavioral therapy may be initiated early in the treatment course; however, they have been shown to be effective in improving treatment outcomes in patients dissatisfied with oral medication [86]. Interventions including bladder training, pelvic floor exercises, and fluid management have all been shown to be effective without introducing side effects [1]. Furthermore, initiating behavioral therapy may help engage the patient in their treatment plan, which may have a positive effect on medication compliance and satisfaction with therapy.

Combination medical therapy (detailed in Chap. 8) can also be considered for patients with unsatisfactory improvement of symptoms with either antimuscarinic medications or β3-agonists. It is also useful for patients who have experienced adequate relief at higher anticholinergic doses at the expense of increasingly bothersome side effects [87]. For example, by introducing a second agent and reducing the dose of the anticholinergic, a patient's symptoms may be adequately controlled. As described in Chap. 8, combination medical therapy has proven to be effective for several indications. When specifically addressing idiopathic OAB, the combination of an antimuscarinic and mirabegron has proven to be effective in patients in reducing urinary frequency, and urinary urgency. The use of an anticholinergic and mirabegron introduced a marginal increase in risk of side effects, and most patients tolerate the medications well [88]. The benefits in improving urinary symptoms produced a perceivable difference in OAB symptoms and improvement in OAB-q scores [89]. In order to maximize this form of medical therapy, one must consider whether the benefit of two oral therapies outweighs progressing to third-line therapies. Several considerations must be addressed including medication compliance, cost, and polypharmacy when one is deciding to add another medication. Alternatively, treatment with onabotulinumtoxinA is associated with a higher likelihood of achieving a > 50% decrease in urge urinary incontinence when compared to all the frequently prescribed oral OAB medications [90]. Ultimately, one must decide whether combination medical therapy would effectively treat the patient's symptoms while remaining congruent with the patient's goals and expectations.

Conclusion

OAB is a symptom-driven disorder that can cause substantial distress to a person's well-being and has a major impact on quality of life. The condition is not life threatening, and the therapies recommended should be individualized by weighing the treatment benefits against the risks of treatment. Therapies available have been proven to be effective; however, patients should be educated on the realistic expectations of treatment success based on their presenting symptoms. Furthermore, clear communication regarding potential side effects and future therapeutic options should be discussed. Appropriate follow-up to monitor symptoms and tolerability ensures that the patient's treatment plan is further tailored as their clinical condition evolves. For patients whose symptoms are refractory to oral pharmacotherapies, experience dose-limiting side effects, or have medical comorbidities that preclude oral therapy, serious consideration should be given to third-line therapies including onabotulinumtoxinA and neuromodulation.

References

1. Gormley EA, Lightner DJ, Faraday M, Vasavada SP. Diagnosis and treatment of overactive bladder (non-neurogenic) in adults: AUA/SUFU guideline amendment. J Urol. 2015;193(5):1572–80.
2. Chapple CR, Khullar V, Gabriel Z, Muston D, Bitoun CE, Weinstein D. The effects of antimuscarinic treatments in overactive bladder: an update of a systematic review and meta-analysis. Eur Urol. 2008;54(3):543–62.
3. Maman K, Aballea S, Nazir J, Desroziers K, Neine ME, Siddiqui E, et al. Comparative efficacy and safety of medical treatments for the management of overactive bladder: a systematic literature review and mixed treatment comparison. Eur Urol. 2014;65(4):755–65.
4. Abrams P, Andersson KE, Buccafusco JJ, Chapple C, de Groat WC, Fryer AD, et al. Muscarinic receptors: their distribution and function in body systems, and the implications for treating overactive bladder. Br J Pharmacol. 2006;148(5):565–78.
5. Basra RK, Wagg A, Chapple C, Cardozo L, Castro-Diaz D, Pons ME, et al. A review of adherence to drug therapy in patients with overactive bladder. BJU Int. 2008;102(7):774–9.
6. Wagg A, Compion G, Fahey A, Siddiqui E. Persistence with prescribed antimuscarinic therapy for overactive bladder: a UK experience. BJU Int. 2012;110(11):1767–74.
7. Benner JS, Nichol MB, Rovner ES, Jumadilova Z, Alvir J, Hussein M, et al. Patient-reported reasons for discontinuing overactive bladder medication. BJU Int. 2010;105(9):1276–82.
8. Chancellor MB, Migliaccio-Walle K, Bramley TJ, Chaudhari SL, Corbell C, Globe D. Long-term patterns of use and treatment failure with anticholinergic agents for overactive bladder. Clin Ther. 2013;35(11):1744–51.
9. Yeaw J, Benner JS, Walt JG, Sian S, Smith DB. Comparing adherence and persistence across 6 chronic medication classes. J Manag Care Pharm. 2009;15(9):728–40.
10. Chapple CR, Rosenberg MT, Brenes FJ. Listening to the patient: a flexible approach to the use of antimuscarinic agents in overactive bladder syndrome. BJU Int. 2009;104(7):960–7.
11. Cardozo L, Hessdorfer E, Milani R, Arano P, Dewilde L, Slack M, et al. Solifenacin in the treatment of urgency and other symptoms of overactive bladder: results from a randomized, double-blind, placebo-controlled, rising-dose trial. BJU Int. 2008;102(9):1120–7.
12. Staskin D, Khullar V, Michel MC, Morrow JD, Sun F, Guan Z, et al. Effects of voluntary dose escalation in a placebo-controlled, flexible-dose trial of fesoterodine in subjects with overactive bladder. Neurourol Urodyn. 2011;30(8):1480–5.
13. Wyndaele JJ, Goldfischer ER, Morrow JD, Gong J, Tseng LJ, Guan Z, et al. Effects of flexible-dose fesoterodine on overactive bladder symptoms and treatment satisfaction: an open-label study. Int J Clin Pract. 2009;63(4):560–7.
14. Cardozo L, Amarenco G, Pushkar D, Mikulas J, Drogendijk T, Wright M, et al. Severity of overactive bladder symptoms and response to dose escalation in a randomized, double-blind trial of solifenacin (SUNRISE). BJU Int. 2013;111(5):804–10.
15. Kennelly MJ. A comparative review of oxybutynin chloride formulations: pharmacokinetics and therapeutic efficacy in overactive bladder. Rev Urol. 2010;12(1):12–9.

16. Katz IR, Sands LP, Bilker W, DiFilippo S, Boyce A, D'Angelo K. Identification of medications that cause cognitive impairment in older people: the case of oxybutynin chloride. J Am Geriatr Soc. 1998;46(1):8–13.
17. Kay G, Crook T, Rekeda L, Lima R, Ebinger U, Arguinzoniz M, et al. Differential effects of the antimuscarinic agents darifenacin and oxybutynin ER on memory in older subjects. Eur Urol. 2006;50(2):317–26.
18. Klausner AP, Steers WD. Antimuscarinics for the treatment of overactive bladder: a review of central nervous system effects. Curr Urol Rep. 2007;8(6):441–7.
19. Noronha-Blob L, Kachur JF. Enantiomers of oxybutynin: in vitro pharmacological characterization at M1, M2 and M3 muscarinic receptors and in vivo effects on urinary bladder contraction, mydriasis and salivary secretion in Guinea pigs. J Pharmacol Exp Ther. 1991;256(2):562–7.
20. Ditropan XL® (oxybutynin chloride) (package insert). Raritan: Ortho-McNeil-Janssen Pharmaceuticals; 2009.
21. Ditropan® (oxybutynin chloride) (package insert). Raritan: Ortho-McNeil Pharmaceuticals; Feb 2008.
22. Cohn JA, Brown ET, Reynolds WS, Kaufman MR, Milam DF, Dmochowski RR. An update on the use of transdermal oxybutynin in the management of overactive bladder disorder. Ther Adv Urol. 2016;8(2):83–90.
23. Davila GW, Starkman JS, Dmochowski RR. Transdermal oxybutynin for overactive bladder. Urol Clin North Am. 2006;33(4):455–63, viii.
24. Davila GW, Daugherty CA, Sanders SW, Transdermal Oxybutynin Study G. A short-term, multicenter, randomized double-blind dose titration study of the efficacy and anticholinergic side effects of transdermal compared to immediate release oral oxybutynin treatment of patients with urge urinary incontinence. J Urol. 2001;166(1):140–5.
25. Nitti VW, Sanders S, Staskin DR, Dmochowski RR, Sand PK, MacDiarmid S, et al. Transdermal delivery of drugs for urologic applications: basic principles and applications. Urology. 2006;67(4):657–64.
26. Dmochowski RR, Nitti V, Staskin D, Luber K, Appell R, Davila GW. Transdermal oxybutynin in the treatment of adults with overactive bladder: combined results of two randomized clinical trials. World J Urol. 2005;23(4):263–70.
27. Sand P, Zinner N, Newman D, Lucente V, Dmochowski R, Kelleher C, et al. Oxybutynin transdermal system improves the quality of life in adults with overactive bladder: a multicentre, community-based, randomized study. BJU Int. 2007;99(4):836–44.
28. Yamaguchi O, Uchida E, Higo N, Minami H, Kobayashi S, Sato H, et al. Efficacy and safety of once-daily oxybutynin patch versus placebo and propiverine in Japanese patients with overactive bladder: a randomized double-blind trial. Int J Urol. 2014;21(6):586–93.
29. Doroshyenko O, Fuhr U. Clinical pharmacokinetics and pharmacodynamics of solifenacin. Clin Pharmacokinet. 2009;48(5):281–302.
30. VESIcare® (solifenacin succinate) tablets. (packet insert). Northbrook: Astellas Pharma US; Feb 2016.
31. Abrams P, Andersson KE. Muscarinic receptor antagonists for overactive bladder. BJU Int. 2007;100(5):987–1006.
32. Cardozo L, Lisec M, Millard R, van Vierssen Trip O, Kuzmin I, Drogendijk TE, et al. Randomized, double-blind placebo controlled trial of the once daily antimuscarinic agent solifenacin succinate in patients with overactive bladder. J Urol. 2004;172(5 Pt 1):1919–24.
33. Haab F, Cardozo L, Chapple C, Ridder AM, Solifenacin Study G. Long-term open-label solifenacin treatment associated with persistence with therapy in patients with overactive bladder syndrome. Eur Urol. 2005;47(3):376–84.
34. Detrol® (tolterodine tartrate) (package insert). Kalamazoo: Pharmacia & Upjohn; 2004.
35. Nilvebrant L, Gillberg PG, Sparf B. Antimuscarinic potency and bladder selectivity of PNU-200577, a major metabolite of tolterodine. Pharmacol Toxicol. 1997;81(4):169–72.

36. Appell RA, Sand P, Dmochowski R, Anderson R, Zinner N, Lama D, et al. Prospective randomized controlled trial of extended-release oxybutynin chloride and tolterodine tartrate in the treatment of overactive bladder: results of the OBJECT study. Mayo Clin Proc. 2001;76(4):358–63.
37. Roden DM. Drug-induced prolongation of the QT interval. N Engl J Med. 2004;350(10):1013–22.
38. Clemett D, Jarvis B. Tolterodine: a review of its use in the treatment of overactive bladder. Drugs Aging. 2001;18(4):277–304.
39. Malhotra B, Guan Z, Wood N, Gandelman K. Pharmacokinetic profile of fesoterodine. Int J Clin Pharmacol Ther. 2008;46(11):556–63.
40. Toviaz® (fesoterodine fumarate) (package insert). New York: Pfizer Inc.; 2014.
41. Leone Roberti Maggiore U, Salvatore S, Alessandri F, Remorgida V, Origoni M, Candiani M, et al. Pharmacokinetics and toxicity of antimuscarinic drugs for overactive bladder treatment in females. Expert Opin Drug Metab Toxicol. 2012;8(11):1387–408.
42. Nitti VW, Dmochowski R, Sand PK, Forst HT, Haag-Molkenteller C, Massow U, et al. Efficacy, safety and tolerability of fesoterodine for overactive bladder syndrome. The J Urol. 2007;178(6):2488–94.
43. Herschorn S, Swift S, Guan Z, Carlsson M, Morrow JD, Brodsky M, et al. Comparison of fesoterodine and tolterodine extended release for the treatment of overactive bladder: a head-to-head placebo-controlled trial. BJU Int. 2010;105(1):58–66.
44. Rovner ES. Trospium chloride in the management of overactive bladder. Drugs. 2004;64(21):2433–46.
45. Tadken T, Weiss M, Modess C, Wegner D, Roustom T, Neumeister C, et al. Trospium chloride is absorbed from two intestinal "absorption windows" with different permeability in healthy subjects. Int J Pharm. 2016;515(1–2):367–73.
46. Sanctura® (trospium chloride) 20mg tablets (package insert). Irvine: Allergan; 2004.
47. Kim Y, Yoshimura N, Masuda H, De Miguel F, Chancellor MB. Intravesical instillation of human urine after oral administration of trospium, tolterodine and oxybutynin in a rat model of detrusor overactivity. BJU Int. 2006;97(2):400–3.
48. Zinner N, Gittelman M, Harris R, Susset J, Kanelos A, Auerbach S, et al. Trospium chloride improves overactive bladder symptoms: a multicenter phase III trial. J Urol. 2004;171(6 Pt 1):2311–5. quiz 435
49. Andersson KE. Potential benefits of muscarinic M3 receptor selectivity. Eur Urol Suppl. 2002;1(4):23.
50. Skerjanec A. The clinical pharmacokinetics of darifenacin. Clin Pharmacokinet. 2006;45(4):325–50.
51. Zinner N. Darifenacin: a muscarinic M3-selective receptor antagonist for the treatment of overactive bladder. Expert Opin Pharmacother. 2007;8(4):511–23.
52. Zinner N, Tuttle J, Marks L. Efficacy and tolerability of darifenacin, a muscarinic M3 selective receptor antagonist (M3 SRA), compared with oxybutynin in the treatment of patients with overactive bladder. World J Urol. 2005;23(4):248–52.
53. Chapple C, Steers W, Norton P, Millard R, Kralidis G, Glavind K, et al. A pooled analysis of three phase III studies to investigate the efficacy, tolerability and safety of darifenacin, a muscarinic M3 selective receptor antagonist, in the treatment of overactive bladder. BJU Int. 2005;95(7):993–1001.
54. Chapple CR, Cardozo L, Nitti VW, Siddiqui E, Michel MC. Mirabegron in overactive bladder: a review of efficacy, safety, and tolerability. Neurourol Urodyn. 2014;33(1):17–30.
55. Leone Roberti Maggiore U, Cardozo L, Ferrero S, Sileo F, Cola A, Del Deo F, et al. Mirabegron in the treatment of overactive bladder. Expert Opin Pharmacother. 2014;15(6):873–87.
56. Dickinson J, Lewand M, Sawamoto T, Krauwinkel W, Schaddelee M, Keirns J, et al. Effect of renal or hepatic impairment on the pharmacokinetics of mirabegron. Clin Drug Investig. 2013;33(1):11–23.
57. Nitti VW, Auerbach S, Martin N, Calhoun A, Lee M, Herschorn S. Results of a randomized phase III trial of mirabegron in patients with overactive bladder. J Urol. 2013;189(4):1388–95.

58. Gillespie JI, Palea S, Guilloteau V, Guerard M, Lluel P, Korstanje C. Modulation of non-voiding activity by the muscarinergic antagonist tolterodine and the beta(3)-adrenoceptor agonist mirabegron in conscious rats with partial outflow obstruction. BJU Int. 2012;110(2 Pt 2):E132–42.
59. Caremel R, Loutochin O, Corcos J. What do we know and not know about mirabegron, a novel beta3 agonist, in the treatment of overactive bladder? Int Urogynecol J. 2014;25(2):165–70.
60. Brubaker L, Fanning K, Goldberg EL, Benner JS, Trocio JN, Bavendam T, et al. Predictors of discontinuing overactive bladder medications. BJU Int. 2010;105(9):1283–90.
61. Veenboer PW, Bosch JL. Long-term adherence to antimuscarinic therapy in everyday practice: a systematic review. J Urol. 2014;191(4):1003–8.
62. Chapple CR, Nazir J, Hakimi Z, Bowditch S, Fatoye F, Guelfucci F, et al. Persistence and adherence with mirabegron versus antimuscarinic agents in patients with overactive bladder: a retrospective observational study in UK clinical practice. Eur Urol. 2017;72(3):389–99.
63. Moskowitz D, Adelstein SA, Lucioni A, Lee UJ, Kobashi KC. Use of third line therapy for overactive bladder in a practice with multiple subspecialty providers: are we doing enough? J Urol. 2018;199(3):779–84.
64. Marschall-Kehrel D, Roberts RG, Brubaker L. Patient-reported outcomes in overactive bladder: the influence of perception of condition and expectation for treatment benefit. Urology. 2006;68(2 Suppl):29–37.
65. Khullar V, Chapple C, Gabriel Z, Dooley JA. The effects of antimuscarinics on health-related quality of life in overactive bladder: a systematic review and meta-analysis. Urology. 2006;68(2 Suppl):38–48.
66. Schabert VF, Bavendam T, Goldberg EL, Trocio JN, Brubaker L. Challenges for managing overactive bladder and guidance for patient support. Am J Manag Care. 2009;15(4 Suppl):S118–22.
67. Weinreb RN, Aung T, Medeiros FA. The pathophysiology and treatment of glaucoma: a review. JAMA. 2014;311(18):1901–11.
68. Wagg A, Arumi D, Herschorn S, Angulo Cuesta J, Haab F, Ntanios F, et al. A pooled analysis of the efficacy of fesoterodine for the treatment of overactive bladder, and the relationship between safety, co-morbidity and polypharmacy in patients aged 65 years or older. Age Ageing. 2017;46(4):620–6.
69. Dubeau CE, Kraus SR, Griebling TL, Newman DK, Wyman JF, Johnson TM 2nd, et al. Effect of fesoterodine in vulnerable elderly subjects with urgency incontinence: a double-blind, placebo controlled trial. J Urol. 2014;191(2):395–404.
70. Lackner TE, Wyman JF, McCarthy TC, Monigold M, Davey C. Randomized, placebo-controlled trial of the cognitive effect, safety, and tolerability of oral extended-release oxybutynin in cognitively impaired nursing home residents with urge urinary incontinence. J Am Geriatr Soc. 2008;56(5):862–70.
71. Volpicelli LA, Levey AI. Muscarinic acetylcholine receptor subtypes in cerebral cortex and hippocampus. Prog Brain Res. 2004;145:59–66.
72. Anagnostaras SG, Murphy GG, Hamilton SE, Mitchell SL, Rahnama NP, Nathanson NM, et al. Selective cognitive dysfunction in acetylcholine M1 muscarinic receptor mutant mice. Nat Neurosci. 2003;6(1):51–8.
73. Chancellor MB, Staskin DR, Kay GG, Sandage BW, Oefelein MG, Tsao JW. Blood-brain barrier permeation and efflux exclusion of anticholinergics used in the treatment of overactive bladder. Drugs Aging. 2012;29(4):259–73.
74. Wagg A, Nitti VW, Kelleher C, Castro-Diaz D, Siddiqui E, Berner T. Oral pharmacotherapy for overactive bladder in older patients: mirabegron as a potential alternative to antimuscarinics. Curr Med Res Opin. 2016;32(4):621–38.
75. Tani M, Hirayama A, Fujimoto K, Torimoto K, Akiyama T, Hirao Y. Increase in 24-hour urine production/weight causes nocturnal polyuria due to impaired function of antidiuretic hormone in elderly men. Int J Urol. 2008;15(2):151–4. discussion 5
76. Kerdraon J, Robain G, Jeandel C, Mongiat Artus P, Game X, Fatton B, et al. Impact on cognitive function of anticholinergic drugs used for the treatment of overactive bladder in the elderly. Prog Urol. 2014;24(11):672–81.

77. McGhan WF. Cost effectiveness and quality of life considerations in the treatment of patients with overactive bladder. Am J Manag Care. 2001;7(2 Suppl):S62–75.
78. Millsop JW, Wang EA, Fazel N. Etiology, evaluation, and management of xerostomia. Clin Dermatol. 2017;35(5):468–76.
79. Wagg A, Nitti V, Kelleher C, Auberbach S, Blauwet MB, Siddiqui E. Effects of the beta-3-adrenoceptor agonist, mirabegron, on quality of life in older patients with overactive bladder: a post-hoc analysis of pooled data from 3 randomised phase 3 trials (abstract). J Urol. 2014;191(4 Suppl):e339.
80. Wagg A, Franks B, Ramos B, Berner T. Persistence and adherence with the new beta-3 receptor agonist, mirabegron, versus antimuscarinics in overactive bladder: early experience in Canada. Can Urol Assoc J. 2015;9(9–10):343–50.
81. Nitti VW, Rovner ES, Franks B, Muma GN, Berner T, Fan A, Ng DB. Persistence with mirabegron versus tolterodine in patients with overactive bladder. Am J Pharm Benefits. 2016;8(2):e25–33.
82. Wielage RC, Perk S, Campbell NL, Klein TM, Posta LM, Yuran T, et al. Mirabegron for the treatment of overactive bladder: cost-effectiveness from US commercial health-plan and medicare advantage perspectives. J Med Econ. 2016;19(12):1135–43.
83. Herschorn S, Nazir J, Ramos B, Hakimi Z. Cost-effectiveness of mirabegron compared to tolterodine ER 4 mg for overactive bladder in Canada. Can Urol Assoc J. 2017;11(3–4):123–30.
84. Nazir J, Maman K, Neine ME, Briquet B, Odeyemi IA, Hakimi Z, et al. Cost-effectiveness of mirabegron compared with antimuscarinic agents for the treatment of adults with overactive bladder in the United Kingdom. Value Health. 2015;18(6):783–90.
85. Schaefer DC, Cheskin LJ. Constipation in the elderly. Am Fam Physician. 1998;58(4):907–14.
86. Klutke CG, Burgio KL, Wyman JF, Guan Z, Sun F, Berriman S, et al. Combined effects of behavioral intervention and tolterodine in patients dissatisfied with overactive bladder medication. J Urol. 2009;181(6):2599–607.
87. Visco AG, Fraser MO, Newgreen D, Oelke M, Cardozo L. What is the role of combination drug therapy in the treatment of overactive bladder? ICI-RS 2014. Neurourol Urodyn. 2016;35(2):288–92.
88. Herschorn S, Chapple CR, Abrams P, Arlandis S, Mitcheson D, Lee KS, et al. Efficacy and safety of combinations of mirabegron and solifenacin compared with monotherapy and placebo in patients with overactive bladder (SYNERGY study). BJU Int. 2017;120(4):562–75.
89. Robinson D, Kelleher C, Staskin D, Mueller ER, Falconer C, Wang J, et al. Patient-reported outcomes from SYNERGY, a randomized, double-blind, multicenter study evaluating combinations of mirabegron and solifenacin compared with monotherapy and placebo in OAB patients. Neurourol Urodyn. 2018;37(1):394–406.
90. Drake MJ, Nitti VW, Ginsberg DA, Brucker BM, Hepp Z, McCool R, et al. Comparative assessment of the efficacy of onabotulinumtoxinA and oral therapies (anticholinergics and mirabegron) for overactive bladder: a systematic review and network meta-analysis. BJU Int. 2017;120(5):611–22.

Index

L. Cox, E. S. Rovner (eds.), *Contemporary Pharmacotherapy of Overactive Bladder*, https://doi.org/10.1007/978-3-319-97265-7

Q

R

S

T

Printed by Printforce, the Netherlands